Old and Sick in America

STUDIES IN SOCIAL MEDICINE

Allan M. Brandt, Larry R. Churchill, and Jonathan Oberlander, *editors*

This series publishes books at the intersection of medicine, health, and society that further our understanding of how medicine and society shape one another historically, politically, and ethically. The series is grounded in the convictions that medicine is a social science, that medicine is humanistic and cultural as well as biological, and that it should be studied as a social, political, ethical, and economic force.

MURIEL R. GILLICK, M.D.

Old and Sick in America
The Journey through the Health Care System

The University of North Carolina Press Chapel Hill

© 2017 The University of North Carolina Press
All rights reserved.
Set in Arno Pro by Westchester Publishing Services
Manufactured in the United States of America

The University of North Carolina Press has been a member of the
Green Press Initiative since 2003.

Library of Congress Cataloging-in-Publication Data
Names: Gillick, Muriel R., 1951– author.
Title: Old and sick in America : the journey through the health care system /
    Muriel R. Gillick, M.D.
Other titles: Studies in social medicine.
Description: Chapel Hill : University of North Carolina Press, [2017] |
    Series: Studies in social medicine | Includes bibliographical references
    and index.
Identifiers: LCCN 2017029456 | ISBN 9781469635231 (cloth : alk. paper) |
    ISBN 9781469635248 (pbk : alk. paper) | ISBN 9781469635255 (ebook)
Subjects: LCSH: Older people—Medical care—United States. | Older
    People—Health and hygiene—United States. | Medicare. | Older
    People—Long-term care—United States. | Medical care, Cost of—United States.
Classification: LCC RA413.7.A4 G55 2017 | DDC 362.1084/6—dc23
    LC record available at https://lccn.loc.gov/2017029456

Cover illustrations: "Walker" icon by Koen Voogd and "Heart"
icon by Alice Noir, from thenounproject.com.

In memory of my father, Hans Wolfgang Garfunkel, 1924–2016

Contents

Prelude

For over seventy-five years, Americans have been arguing over whether medical care is a right or a privilege. We began arguing during the 1930s, when the first private insurance companies began to appear and when prepaid health care was born. We argued after World War II, when President Truman tried to introduce national health insurance. And seven years after the passage of the Affordable Care Act, which provided a path for every citizen to get health insurance, we are still arguing. But it's only the young and the middle-aged whose rights and needs are being debated. For those over age sixty-five, the right to health insurance coverage is a done deal and it has been since the passage of Medicare in 1965. Seeing a physician, going to the hospital, getting rehabilitative care and, along the way, undergoing tests and taking medicines, are all part of the fabric of modern life for older Americans. So much so that we tend to assume that the way things are in health care—the organization of medical care—is the way things have to be. Physicians are rushed and the office is difficult to get to? That's just the way it is. Hospitals make the oldest and frailest of patients disoriented and discharge them so quickly they have to go to rehab before returning home? That's the way the system works. Medications are expensive and produce side effects? That's the price you have to pay for a cure. Procedures are risky and perhaps unnecessary? That's the chance you must take if you want the marvels medicine has to offer.

What happens to people as they journey through the health care system is actually not nearly so inevitable and immutable. It's a product of our uniquely American version of medical care. How people react to sickness and to its treatment reflects their personalities, their culture, and the organization of medical care. The patient's experience today is different from what it was fifty years ago and from what it is in other parts of the developed world. But it's not just the patient's reaction that has changed; what happens, what is done or not done, the tests they have, the drugs they take, in the most general sense, *how they are treated*, has changed. The question is, what determines the shape of medicine today and how did it get this way?

In the course of my last thirty years as a practicing physician, I've repeatedly asked why things are the way they are. How do large machines—computerized tomography (CT) scanners and magnetic resonance imaging

(MRI) equipment and radiotherapy machines—end up in hospitals? Why is most medical training in the hospital even though most medical care is delivered in the office? And most fundamentally, what aspects of the health care system shape the patient's experience? What forces mold and influence that experience, where by "experience" I mean something more than just the patient's degree of satisfaction with care, although that's part of what shapes experience. I'm interested in not only what happens to patients but also the ways that the structure and practice of medicine affect the patient's well-being, level of functioning, and recovery from acute illness.

I first realized that what doctors and patients take for granted could look very different—and perhaps be dramatically better for patients—when I was in medical school. I was on a "clinical rotation," a two-month, intensive experience on the cardiology service of a major teaching hospital in Boston. A group of us, two medical residents, two interns, and me, were on "rounds," going from the bed of one patient to another, checking on their progress, reviewing their lab test results, ordering more tests and more medications. Suddenly, the public address system crackled and came to life, announcing a "code blue": a cardiac arrest.

The pager worn by the medical resident with whom I was working went off, along with a chorus of other ring tones. We—the resident who was head of the "code team," two medical interns, a technician wheeling an electrocardiogram (EKG) machine, and I—all ran to the room of the patient whose heart had stopped and who was no longer breathing. The resident in charge spoke briefly with the patient's nurse and then summarized what he'd learned: "Ninety-year-old white female, admitted with congestive heart failure, found in bed unresponsive." He took up a position next to the EKG machine, which began spitting out an extended strip of paper with the patient's heart rhythm. There wasn't much to see—the rhythm was "flat line," showing no electrical activity at all.

One of the residents leaned over the patient and, one hand on top of the other, began methodically compressing the chest while a second resident squeezed oxygen into the patient's lungs through an "ambu bag," a rubber bag connecting an oxygen tank to a mask over the patient's face. The resident barked out orders: ten milligrams of this medication, ten milligrams of that, everyone stand back, get ready to shock, resume chest compressions. For half an hour, the drama went on. And then, when the EKG still showed a flat line, the resident "called the code" and everyone backed off. He looked up at the clock and solemnly intoned the time of death, which was duly recorded by the nurse who had been keeping track of every medication administered and every heart rhythm reported.

The physicians in training filed out of the small single room where the attempted resuscitation had taken place. They were joined by several other young physicians in training who were not part of the code team. "What did you get to do?" one of the interns asked, a hint of jealousy in his voice. "I put in a central line," his fellow house officer told him—a catheter inserted into a large vein in the neck that leads directly to the heart. "I almost got to put in a temporary pacemaker," a second resident said, "but they called the code." He sounded disappointed.

I glanced at the patient, unclothed and lifeless on the bed. The nurses were removing the intravenous lines, the EKG electrodes, and the urinary catheter from her small, shriveled body. All that remained was her watch and a wedding ring. Her face was frozen in a frown. I noticed a vase of pink and yellow flowers on the windowsill: somebody had been thinking of her. A nephew? A granddaughter? A friend? Did the person who sent the flowers know she was gone? The room was suddenly very, very quiet.

Why, I wondered, had the house staff even tried to resuscitate someone who was ninety years old and had a failing heart? Had anyone spoken to her family? Had she known how seriously ill she was? Had the possibility of death even been raised? Who was going to contact her family now? Did she even have a family? I never found out.

Other people—physicians, lawyers, and the budding profession of medical ethicists—were also asking how and by whom important medical decisions were made. Over the ensuing decade, medical care was transformed to include far more communication between doctors and patients. Patients were increasingly expected to become engaged in their care, and their doctors were supposed to offer them the possibility of participating in medical decision making and in monitoring and treating disease. Evidently, merely asking why things are the way they are can lead to a change in the practice of medicine. It is the first step on the road to reforming the health care system, and so the importance of understanding the forces behind the patient's experience is the first theme of this book.

Asking what mysterious forces shape the reality that both patients and doctors tend to take for granted has become something of a habit for me. As a physician, I know I need to conform to professional standards. I have to act in the ways that everyone expected: I have to order the recommended tests, prescribe the customary medications, and make the usual referrals. But whenever a new technology becomes available—CT scans were just appearing when I was an intern, and MRI and positron emission tomography (PET) scans had yet to be developed—I always wonder where it came from, and how it made its way into medical practice. The same for medications: when I was starting out, we often used the drug reserpine in the treatment of high blood pressure; today, reserpine is dismissed as causing cancer (it produced tumors in mice when administered in doses many times greater than the usual therapeutic dose), and far more expensive medicines such as angiotensin converting enzyme (ACE) inhibitors are used instead. Even the institutions in which patients receive care have changed dramatically: when I was in training in the late seventies and early eighties, patients stayed in the hospital until they were well enough to go home. If they were unable to return home, perhaps because they had had a stroke and did not have anyone to care for them at home, they would enter a nursing home. Today, by contrast, patients stay only a short time in the hospital and then recover either at home or in a post-acute care facility, a short-term, less intensive site of inpatient care.

Sometimes the answer to the question of why medical practice changed is rooted in science; it is what has come to be called "evidence-based." Medical scientists conduct a study that shows that a new medication or test or procedure works better than its predecessor, and soon everyone is using the new product. Sometimes the answer to why comes from outside medicine altogether—consumerism in the surrounding society trickles down into medicine, resulting in better-informed patients who demand a role in their care. Suddenly, "patient-engagement" and "self-management" of disease are all the rage. And sometimes the answer to why the patient experience is the way it is proves to be more complex.

Just how complex became evident when my friend Joanna told me about her eighty-three-year-old uncle who lived alone in a condominium in Florida. Uncle Ned, my friend explained, had always been a bit of a loner—he was a widower who had no children and had worked as a chemical engineer in a job that didn't call for a great deal of human interaction. He had a strong stubborn streak that had only become more pronounced with age. My friend and her sister, neither of whom lived in Florida, were his only surviving relatives. They were concerned because Uncle Ned was not eating well, which was particularly problematic since he was a diabetic taking insulin and at risk of developing dangerously low or excessively high blood sugars. Moreover, both he and his condominium were—Joanna struggled to find a diplomatic way of expressing her concern—untidy.

My friend felt her uncle would do better in an assisted living facility that would provide housekeeping, meals, and opportunities for socializing. Short of that, she hoped he would accept a housekeeper. She also felt he needed a medical evaluation as she strongly suspected his cognition was not what it had once been. Uncle Ned said there was no way he was moving into "one of those places for old people." He made it quite clear that he believed he did not need any help at home. But he did agree to see his primary care physician, ostensibly to see how well he was controlling his diabetes. When he went to the doctor, she performed only a cursory examination of his mental status and ordered blood tests and a CT scan of his brain. When those were all negative, the doctor said she would not be able to prescribe any medications for Ned—or do anything else to help him—unless he got a PET scan that she claimed could definitively diagnose Alzheimer's disease.

That's when my antennae went up. A PET scan to diagnose Alzheimer's disease? There is no test to definitively diagnose Alzheimer's disease short of a brain biopsy (or autopsy). A careful history and physical exam, however, can correctly diagnose the disorder in 90 percent of cases. But a PET scan is an expensive radiologic exam that I was reasonably certain was of no proven value in diagnosing Alzheimer's. Did Ned's primary care physician really insist on a PET scan?

Apparently she did. She went so far as to say she would not even arrange for a visiting nurse to check Ned's blood sugars at home or a home health aide to help him bathe until she had the results of the PET scan. Intrigued, I decided to look into the situation.

The facts about PET scans and dementia were reasonably straightforward. The American Academy of Neurology, a leading professional society, does not recommend routine use of PET scans in establishing the diagnosis of Alzheimer's disease. Medicare, after initially refusing to reimburse for any PET scans done in the course of a work up of dementia, relented slightly and agreed to pay for PET scans in the one circumstance in which they had been shown to be useful—when explicitly performed to distinguish an unusual form of dementia called frontotemporal dementia (seldom found in people over age seventy-five) from Alzheimer's.

The facts about Florida and x-rays were also fairly straightforward. Florida is the Medicare radiology capital of the United States. In the era when Ned was sent for his scan, Florida was number two in the country in spending on "imaging," as radiologic tests of all sorts are called, for patients with chronic disease in the last two years of life. And while federal anti-kickback laws prevent doctors from referring patients for tests in a practice that they own, physicians have come up with all kinds of lucrative self-referral arrangements to get around the restrictions. These involve leasing deals or time-share arrangements, which Florida uses in abundance. Sometimes physicians and hospitals simply flout the law and hope they will get away with it. The Baptist Hospital of South Florida, for example, began paying community physicians to refer patients to an MRI facility that the hospital owned—and ended up forking over $7.8 million to the U.S. Department of Justice as a settlement for its illegal behavior.[1] Why was there a PET scanner in the small Florida community where Uncle Ned lived? And how did his primary care physician know about it and believe it would be useful to diagnose Alzheimer's disease? After all, if the equipment had not been available nearby, getting a scan would not have been an option. And if the doctor hadn't ordered the test, Ned certainly wouldn't have gotten it.

Apparently, Florida is fertile territory for all things medical. Florida has one of the highest percentages of elderly patients of any state. And the culture in Florida is conducive to the use of more and more health care resources: the social life of many older people revolves around their doctors' appointments, their tests, and their medicines.[2] The net effect is that Medicare spends more per capita on Floridians in their last two years of life than the national average: in 2011–12, Medicare spent an average of $78,998 per patient in Florida, topped by $84,489 in New Jersey, but overshadowing North Dakota, where expenditures were a mere $47,183 per person.[3]

It's not surprising that a radiology facility would want to set up shop in Florida, given the high level of interest in medical technology. But once established, it would need to attract customers. That means persuading doctors and patients that PET scans offer something special, which is exactly what Florida imaging centers tried to do through advertising. One facility boasted about its PET scan capacity on its website, claiming (falsely) that "PET can diagnose Alzheimer's disease years before symptoms begin," and asserting (misleadingly) that "Medicare approves the use of PET scans in the diagnosis of Alzheimer's disease."[4]

Physicians are not just influenced in their behavior by local hospitals, whether through television spots, newspaper ads, billboards, or direct appeals; they are also influenced by the device manufacturers themselves. An Institute of Medicine report on conflict of industry in medicine found that 94 percent of physicians had some kind of relationship with industry, and physicians in solo practice or very small group practices were far more likely to have such interactions than other doctors—and far less likely to adhere to clinical practice guidelines, the evidence-based advice issued by professional societies. This kind of pernicious influence can take the form of industry-sponsored "educational programs" that are sometimes thinly veiled propaganda sessions or one-on-one "detailing" in which an industry representative personally makes the case for a device or drug.[5]

I cannot be sure why a primary care physician in Florida insisted on a PET scan for my friend's Uncle Ned, but I'm reasonably certain there was no medical justification for the test. And I can make a pretty good guess as to what happened. PET scanners in the early 2000s were a technology in search of a disease—ultimately, they would be widely used in determining the extent of many types of cancer and monitoring the progress of treatment—and their use in the diagnosis of Alzheimer's was a promising possibility. About 500,000 people develop dementia each year; if all of them had a PET scan as part of their evaluation, that decision alone could keep the machines whirring. Imaging centers everywhere decided to invest in PET scanners, particularly facilities that were aided and abetted by the availability of Medicare reimbursement in states like Florida with large concentrations of older individuals. Medicare's decision to reimburse for the scan under select circumstances was in turn influenced by political pressure, but that's another story.[6] As soon as the imaging facilities brought in the new technology, they sent out brochures to area physicians, they gave lectures at hospitals, and they may even have sent representatives to visit physicians' offices to introduce their test. At the same time, they raised awareness of their new capability by targeting prospective patients and their families with advertising. Their promotions emphasized that the scan was approved for diagnosing dementia, with the small print explaining that Medicare would pay for the test provided the physician mentioned the phrase "frontotemporal dementia." When Ned's doctor was faced with a patient who clearly had something very wrong with his thinking and his judgment, she knew just what to do—she would order a PET scan.

The key to understanding Uncle Ned's experience isn't quite so simple as the case of the ninety-year-old woman undergoing attempted CPR. Why Uncle Ned's doctor ordered a PET scan when there was no clinical evidence that this was necessary or even useful, and why Ned couldn't even access home services unless he obtained the test, wasn't just due to a few "bad apples," doctors who are incompetent or corrupt. It can't be explained by greedy capitalists who wanted to make a lot of money by peddling their machine. In fact, the inventors of the PET scanner no doubt believed strongly in the value of their creation, though they needed to find the ideal applications for their machine. It's not just a consequence of our health insurance system, in which patients often regard tests as free because they don't have to pay for them out of their own pockets. Ned's experience with the health care system was shaped by the interplay of several powerful actors on the health care stage: physicians, device manufacturers, health insurance companies, and popular culture. This is the second major theme of this book: lurking behind the scenes whenever an older patient undergoes medical care are many forces that interact with each other, reinforcing one another, creating elaborate feedback loops, and together comprising a complex system. As with any such complex system, the components seek to maintain their prevailing relationships; they will adapt to any perturbation in ways that attempt to preserve the status quo.

One part of the ecosystem that I'd never paid very much attention to was the Medicare program. But then I began writing an article about the influence of Medicare on the experience of death and dying, and I quickly realized that the Medicare program—both as it was initially created in 1965 and as it evolved over the years—affects just about every aspect of end of life care.[7] The most obvious way that Medicare affects the way people die, and what everyone first thinks of, is through its hospice benefit. Enacted in 1982, seventeen years after the passage of the initial Medicare legislation, hospice was introduced as a special variant of Medicare. People who develop an illness that, in the normal course of events, could be expected to be lethal within a matter of six months or less, are eligible to enroll—if they want to. What they get is a very different model of care, focused on keeping them home and comfortable until they die. But there is a quid pro quo. In exchange for enhanced home care services, patients are asked to forgo any curative treatment of their disease and to restrict hospital care.

Hospice has grown to the point where over 40 percent of Medicare enrollees who die have received hospice services. But because Medicare hospice is limited to people with a very poor prognosis, and because hospice requires giving up various treatment options in exchange for intensive home care, patients typically end up getting hospice care for little more than two weeks. More than a third of patients get hospice care for a week or less.[8] The rules and regulations governing Medicare hospice clearly influence *how* we die. But it turns out that Medicare affects far more than just the last six months of life.

Medicare also influences *when we die*, that is, how long we live. After the introduction of Medicare, mortality rates among older people began a steep decline. The most dramatic fall was in the death rate for heart disease, and since heart disease is the leading cause of death in older people, the net effect is that life expectancy at age sixty-five increased shortly after the passage of Medicare and has continued to increase since then.[9]

It's impossible to prove that it was Medicare that produced this salubrious effect and, in fact, death rates fell in the 1960s throughout the developed world, both in countries that had recently expanded insurance coverage to elders and in those that had not. But some analyses suggest that the American Medicare program *did* affect age-adjusted death rates in the ten years after it was introduced.[10] It is also striking that the United States currently performs poorly in all international rankings of the quality of health care *except* in the quality of care for people over age sixty-five, making a compelling case that providing universal insurance coverage for older people has had an impact.[11] Medicare matters. It seems very likely that, at the very least, Medicare *promoted* changes that led to longer lives for older people.

Medicare also influences *how we die*: the procedures we have and the medications we take. Once again, the way it does this is indirect. But by reimbursing generously for technology-intensive, hospital-based care, and poorly for labor-intensive, home-based care, the program tends to favor an aggressive approach to care near the end of life. Among elderly Medicare enrollees who died in 2008, nearly one-third underwent a surgical procedure in the last year of life—including 18 percent who had surgery in what would prove to be their last month of life and 8 percent in their last week.[12]

By mandating that Medicare drug plans cover essentially all chemotherapy drugs, Medicare assures that older patients have access to even the most marginally beneficial medications. This financial incentive, combined with the reluctance of many oncologists to discuss prognosis with their patients, results in patients receiving chemotherapy in the last two weeks of life, although this is generally regarded as a marker of poor quality care.[13]

If Medicare has such diverse effects on what happens to patients as they approach the end of life, perhaps Medicare could also affect people like my friend's Uncle Ned—even though a variety of different forces appeared to impact his situation. We know that many complex adaptive systems, as big complicated systems such as health care are often called, turn out to have just such levers; perhaps what happens to patients as they journey through the health care system can similarly be understood in this way.[14] Demonstrating that Medicare plays an outsized role in shaping medical care for older individuals in the United States is the third theme of this book.

Old and Sick in America: The Journey through the Health Care System is about what happens to older people when they become patients, it is about the hidden forces that mold their experience, and about the way those forces together form an ecosystem. And it offers some suggestions about how that ecosystem can be modified to create better care for patients: improved outcomes, greater satisfaction, and more attention to those needs of the older patient that truly matter because they determine quality of life.

I begin where most patients begin their health care journey, with a visit to the doctor. For the majority of older individuals, this means seeing a primary care physician, usually an internist or a family practitioner, in an office setting, so Part I is concerned with office care. Chapter 1 focuses on the specific experience of a particular patient—my father-in-law, Saul. What it was like for him, sometimes a positive experience, sometimes not so positive, highlights some of the crucial aspects of being a patient as it is in the office that the doctor-patient relationship grows and develops. Recognizing that one person's experience may not be representative—though I have chosen the vignette to embody what I take to be the most important features of ambulatory care—chapter 2 asks whether other practice arrangements make a difference. Ownership, reimbursement, and organization vary, with arrangements ranging from solo practice at one extreme to large, multispecialty group practices at the other, from physician-owned to hospital-owned, and from exclusive, cash-only concierge practices to models in which all forms of insurance are accepted. Chapter 3 examines how various powerful actors within the health care system—physicians, hospitals, device manufacturers, the pharmaceutical industry, and Medicare—shape what happens to patients in the office. Chapter 4 contrasts the small, intimate, low tech practice of outpatient medicine fifty years ago with the multiphysician, rule-driven, computerized practice of today and asks what factors are responsible for the change. I look for the answer in three distinct domains: scientific advances in medicine, social trends, and legislative developments.

The next encounter with the health care system for many older patients, and the subject of Part II of *Old and Sick in America*, is with the hospital. The modern hospital offers an unprecedented array of diagnostic procedures and treatments, from biopsies to surgery—to attempted cardiopulmonary resuscitation (CPR), as I observed early on in my medical training. Chapter 5 begins with a sample patient's experience, the story of Barbara Ellis, who was admitted to an academic teaching hospital for treatment of congestive heart failure. Her acute medical problem was successfully treated, but not until after she had developed multiple complications. Chapter 6 broadens our view of the prototypical hospitalization by putting Barbara's experience in perspective. I compare the world of the teaching hospital to that of the small community hospital, the for-profit hospital to the not-for-profit hospital, the free-standing hospital to the hospital that is part of an entire health system. Chapter 7 shows how the medical profession, the hospital CEO, drug and device manufacturers, and Medicare influence what happens to patients in the hospital. Chapter 8 contrasts the modest-sized, nonprofit hospital of the early 1960s with the streamlined, high tech, business-oriented hospital of today and asks what produced the change. Once again, I identify scientific advances, social trends, and health policy as all playing a role.

Part III takes us to the next stop on the health care journey, the skilled nursing facility (SNF). Each year, 20 percent of all Medicare fee-for-service beneficiaries (and probably an equal number of Medicare Advantage patients) are transferred to a SNF (pronounced 'sniff') for "post-acute" or "rehabilitative" care upon discharge from the hospital. Chapter 9 tells the story of Taylor Bryan, one of the 1.7 million Medicare patients each year who spend time in a SNF. Admitted for recuperation and rehabilitation after a long hospital stay for heart disease and its complications, Taylor suffered a setback on the road to recovery and was readmitted to the hospital. Chapter 10 moves beyond Taylor's experience in a free-standing, not-for-profit nursing facility to explore how for-profit nursing homes, chains, and teaching nursing homes affect patient care. Following the now familiar pattern, chapter 11 examines the role of nursing home administrators, hospitals, drug and device companies, the medical profession, and government in shaping the SNF experience. Chapter 12 contrasts the nursing home of the early 1960s, which was a residential facility housing those who could not care for themselves, with the medical institution focused on post-acute care that it has become today. I review the advances in medicine, the social trends, and the legislation that are responsible for the changes.

The book's finale opens with another patient story, this time tracing a single patient over a five-year period as she shuttled back and forth between all three major sites of health care—the office, the hospital, and the SNF—ending up in an assisted living facility where she ultimately enrolled in hospice. Rosa Gottlieb's story illustrates how the many forces that act on the institutions of health care also interact with each other and together shape what happens to patients. I then contrast the experience of the four patients described in *Old and Sick in America* with ideal geriatric care, and conclude by discussing how we can get from the current reality to where we should be, in light of the forces that conspire to maintain the status quo.

Old and Sick in America depicts the patient's experience of the health care system through a series of vignettes. The cases presented are based on real patients in whose care I was in some way involved, suitably modified to protect confidentiality. The cases were chosen to be representative: their diagnoses include congestive heart failure, coronary artery disease, stroke, and cancer (the leading causes of death), as well as high blood pressure, elevated cholesterol, dementia, falls, incontinence, and infection (the most widely reported outpatient medical problems). I also selected patients with varying personal characteristics and different family constellations, some men and some women, although capturing the diversity of ethnicities and socioeconomic class in American society with a sample of four was not possible so I made no attempt to do so. It should be apparent that patients' needs are tremendously variable, even among a group of primarily middle-class individuals with well-educated adult children. If members of this superficially homogenous collection differ in what they need from the health care system, how much more will the entire older population vary in its needs?

It is my hope that *Old and Sick in America* will open the door to understanding health care as older patients experience it, and that it will also point the way to reforming a great but imperfect system. It is also a very personal story. In addition to the data and the references and the examples I have amassed for this book—and I've put additional statistics in the notes for readers who want even greater detail—I have felt free to share my view of what's good and bad about American health care and how it could be improved. In over thirty years as a practicing geriatrician and palliative care physician, I have developed my own perspective about the health care system. It is that perspective that colors my depiction of what it is like to age and to ail in the United States today, and how we can revamp our deeply flawed approach to caring for older patients. In the end, I hope we will be able to provide outstanding medical care to *all* geriatric patients, including those who are the most vulnerable and sickest of them all.

Abbreviations in the Text

ACA	Affordable Care Act (full name—the Patient Protection and Affordable Care Act)
ACE unit	Acute Care for the Elderly
ACO	Accountable Care Organization
AHRQ	Agency for Healthcare Research and Quality
AIM	Advanced Illness Management
AMDA	American Medical Directors Association (former name of the Society for Post-Acute and Long-Term Care Medicine)
BBA	Balanced Budget Act
BIDMC	Beth Israel Deaconess Medical Center (Boston)
BWH	Brigham and Women's Hospital (Boston)
CAHPS	Consumer Assessment of Healthcare Providers and Systems (survey)
CHF	congestive heart failure
CMS	Centers for Medicare and Medicaid Services
CNA	Certified Nursing Assistant
CPR	cardiopulmonary resuscitation
CT	computerized tomography
DNR	do not resuscitate
DRG	diagnosis-related group
EKG	electrocardiogram
EMR	electronic medical record
FDA	Food and Drug Administration
GPO	Group Purchasing Organization
GRACE	Geriatric Resources for Assessment and Care of Elders
HCA	Hospital Corporation of America
HDL	Health Diagnostic Laboratory

HEDIS	Healthcare Effectiveness Data and Information Set
HIPAA	Health Insurance Portability and Accountability Act
ICU	Intensive Care Unit
IMRT	Intensive Modulated Radiation Therapy
MAC	Medicare Administrative Contractor
MedPAC	Medicare Payment Advisory Commission
MGH	Massachusetts General Hospital (Boston)
MRI	magnetic resonance imaging
NIH	National Institutes of Health
NP	nurse practitioner
OBRA	Omnibus Budget Reconciliation Act
OIG	Office of the Inspector General
P&T	Pharmacy and Therapeutics
PA	physician assistant
PAMC	Palo Alto Medical Center
PAMF	Palo Alto Medical Foundation
PET	positron emission tomography
RUG	Resource Utilization Group
RVU	Relative Value Unit
SHEP	Systolic Hypertension in the Elderly Program
SNF	skilled nursing facility
VA	Veterans Administration

Old and Sick in America

Part I
The Office

CHAPTER ONE

Going to the Doctor

Every so often during my years as a primary care geriatrician, a new patient landed in my practice who hadn't seen a doctor for forty or fifty years. Sometimes, the last direct personal encounter with a physician had been during childbirth. I faced patients like that with a shiver of dread because they usually turned out to have something terrible wrong with them, like the woman who had been healthy all her life, who exercised regularly and ate a good diet, and who came to see me because she'd woken up one day feeling as though she'd been hit by a Mack truck. She might as well have been hit by a truck: she proved to have widely metastatic cancer and would be dead within six weeks. Or there was the 82-year-old woman who had never been sick a day in her life and, according to her, still wasn't. She was dragged into the office over her vociferous protests by her son and daughter because she went out into the snow wearing sandals and left the teapot burning on the stove long after all the water had evaporated. She had Alzheimer's disease which had progressed to the point where she could no longer safely live alone. Her judgment, markedly impaired by her dementia, didn't allow her to grasp her situation. She refused to accept the various creative compromises her family and I devised to provide support for her while allowing her to maintain a measure of autonomy. I thought that if only I had known her for years and been able to establish a relationship with her, I could have chipped away at her denial. She might have trusted me and let me gradually arrange increases in the amount of supervision she had, allowing her to stay at home. Instead, she lost her zest for life after her daughter, at her wit's end, placed her in a nursing home.

These health care virgins were the exceptions that proved the rule—almost all older people have a long history of interactions with the health care system, and most of those interactions take place in the doctor's office. Even the outliers, like my patient who had stayed away from the medical profession for decades, sought help in the outpatient setting when they finally developed problems that either they or their families could no longer ignore. The doctor's office, for the vast majority of patients, is where the journey through the health care maze begins. And the tour guide, the person most likely to accompany them through sickness and through health, is their personal physician.

At last count, Americans made over one billion office visits a year, slightly more than a quarter of those visits involving people over the age of sixty-five, although they account for only 12 percent of the population.[1] And older people don't just go to the physician once a year for a checkup: they make an average of seven visits to the doctor over the course of a year. Not only do they have many appointments, but they typically see more than one doctor. Fewer than half of their visits are to a primary care physician, with the remainder involving either a medical subspecialist—such as a cardiologist, hematologist, nephrologist or rheumatologist—or a surgeon.[2]

The office practice of medicine is a crucial component of medical care not just because of the sheer volume of visits, but also because it is the gateway to the rest of the health care system. It is in the office that most blood tests, x-rays, and other procedures are ordered. It is in the office that primary care physicians discover or elicit medical problems that lead to a subspecialty referral. It is in the outpatient setting that much of community-based, long-term care, such as visiting nurse services and physical therapy, is initiated. Typically, it's the outpatient physician who directs patients to the hospital, and from there to the skilled nursing facility. And it's in the office that the doctor-patient relationship is most often established and developed—the relationship that is at the heart of the patient's experience of the health care system.

Over the years, I've seen patients in the hospital, in the skilled nursing facility, and in my consultative outpatient practice. Some of these patients arrived at my doorstep from solo or small group practices. Some got their care in a multispecialty group practice. But while the office practice of medicine looks very different depending on whether the practice is large or small, urban or rural, hospital-affiliated or free-standing, I've been struck by how many of its basic features are the same. This homogeneity reflects the interests of physicians, hospitals, government regulators, health insurers, and the drug and device industries that shape the essential characteristics of contemporary ambulatory care. These same interests determine what happens to the patient when he or she has an appointment. I came to appreciate just what "going to the doctor" means for older individuals not just through my own patients, but also thanks to my father-in-law.

Saul's Story

The man usually dies first, but that's not how life unfolded for my in-laws. After forty-four years of marriage, Ada succumbed to colon cancer. She died at home, with hospice services. And then Saul's world fell apart.

Ada had been the family's chief executive, as I'd learned when I first met my future in-laws. She and Saul had complemented each other perfectly. She was sociable, vivacious, and gregarious; he was one of the shyest men on the planet. She organized the couple's social life, which mainly involved visiting her sisters and brothers and their families; he worked in their pharmacy six and a half days a week. She arranged things, from hiring an interior decorator when they first moved to a new apartment after they retired, to college visits when their son (my future husband) was a high school junior; and Saul handled the finances. She made the decisions, whether about getting a new car, which they did every ten years, or going on vacation, which they did with just about the same frequency; he was the family breadwinner. His life was his family and his drugstore.

For a year after Ada died, Saul stayed on in the Philadelphia high rise apartment complex where the couple had lived since Saul sold his struggling pharmacy. He managed, but barely, despite a housekeeper who came in weekly, then twice a week, and then daily. My husband began traveling to Philadelphia every couple of months to check on his father. He began worrying about his father after his first car accident, in which mercifully only the car was hurt. He worried more when he discovered his father wasn't able to balance his checkbook and sometimes paid the same bill several times. Ultimately, he concluded that the status quo was no longer viable, and he persuaded his father first to give up driving and then to move into an assisted living facility in Boston, near us. Seventy years after arriving in the United States, a refugee from the Russian civil war and Ukrainian pogroms, Saul left Philadelphia.

Compared to the other disruptions associated with moving, starting over with a new physician was relatively minor. But Saul had gone to the same doctor for fifteen years. And before that, he hadn't gone to a doctor at all. Only when he'd had emergency surgery for an abscess and was found to have very elevated blood pressure—which he'd probably had for some time, judging by the abnormalities on his electrocardiogram that indicated permanent heart damage—did he start seeing a primary care physician regularly.

I didn't think that finding a new doctor would be difficult. Surely, only remote rural communities suffered chronic severe doctor shortages. And Saul had particularly good health insurance—in addition to Medicare Part A (hospital coverage) and Part B (physician and lab test coverage), he had supplementary coverage, the so-called "gap insurance" for co-pays and deductibles. Not only that, he didn't have many medical problems apart from his high blood pressure, chronic constipation, and a little trouble with his memory:

he'd be an easy patient. My assumption that it would be easy to find a new doctor couldn't have been more wrong.

Access to Primary Care

After the passage of Medicare, resulting in health insurance coverage for virtually everyone over age sixty-five, access to primary care was in principle not an issue for older people in the United States.[3] The reality has been a bit different. Some of the vaunted universal access is illusory if the patient lives in what is euphemistically called an "underserved area," a region with an insufficient number of physicians to meet the demand. And some of that access is eroding as more and more physicians decide they will not accept *any* Medicare patients. Disappointed by the levels of reimbursement available from government insurers, particularly but not exclusively Medicaid (the combined federal-state program for the poor), 15 percent of self-employed physicians in a recent survey indicated they are not taking patients with either Medicare or Medicaid, and another 25 percent indicated they are undecided about what their policy will be in the coming year.[4]

A growing number of primary care physicians are shunning conventional practice models in favor of a "concierge practice." In this arrangement, they either bill patients a "retainer"—usually many thousands of dollars a year, while not accepting payments from Medicare—or they charge a "membership fee" for various "extra" services on top of what they can bill Medicare for. These extras include round-the-clock physician telephone availability, same-day appointments, and longer, more leisurely visits. This structure allows physicians to have smaller patient panels—often considerably smaller.[5] But these practices are not an option for poor patients, and they have the potential to further decrease access to primary care by creating a two-tier medical system.[6] Currently, concierge practices are relatively rare but the number of such practices has been growing dramatically, with more and more practicing physicians saying that they are considering a transition to this model.[7]

On top of the defections to concierge medicine, the older patient has to contend with a shrinking pool of primary care doctors. By some estimates, the United States already had a shortage of primary care doctors in 2010, and by 2020 that deficit is projected to grow five-fold. In part, this is related to the lower salaries that generalists (internists, family physicians, and pediatricians) command compared to specialists: the average starting salary for a family physician is less than half that for a urologist.[8] In addition, primary care doctors are retiring, cutting back their hours, or leaving the practice of medicine altogether.[9] And they're not being replaced by young new physicians at anything near a sufficient rate: a survey of doctors in internal medicine residency programs between 2009 and 2011 found that only one-fifth of them planned to become generalists; the remainder expected to specialize in a field such as cardiology, nephrology, or oncology.[10] Recent surveys hint at a reversal of this trend, with growing numbers of medical school graduates opting for family medicine or primary care internal medicine residencies, but how many will remain committed to primary care rather than moving into administration, or leaving the field altogether, remains to be seen.[11]

First Steps

Saul had a great deal of adjusting to do after he moved to the Boston area. He still missed his wife terribly. He had to get used to waking up in a strange apartment and he had to learn to find his way around his new neighborhood. With more important things on his mind than medical care, he took a laissez-faire approach to finding a new physician. He did ask his fellow residents at the assisted living facility for suggestions, and one chatty woman at the dinner table recommended her own doctor, but that physician's practice was full. Saul mentioned to the director of the assisted living facility that he was looking for a doctor and she provided a list of local physicians, but half of them had moved away and the other half weren't taking new patients. After he'd lived in the Boston area for several months and still hadn't found a doctor, I decided to intervene. As a physician who had lived and worked in the area for over twenty years, I felt confident that my connections would suffice. I was mistaken. Many phone calls and false leads later, a friend of a friend led me to Dr. Walker Wilson, an internist with a practice affiliated with a nearby community hospital. I didn't know him personally, but I was told he was a good doctor.

Once I'd found a doctor for Saul, I figured the access problem had been solved. I'd forgotten, or maybe I never appreciated, how many steps remained before Saul would actually meet Dr. Walker Wilson—and how hard it would be for him to climb those steps. Even calling to make an appointment was a challenge. Saul wasn't used to dealing with an "interactive voice response" program, which is what he encountered when he called to set up an appointment. It took him a while to realize he was speaking to a machine—he had grown up in an era when a real person always answered the phone. He became so flustered that he couldn't remember whether he needed to press one (for prescription renewals), two (for an appointment), three (for a referral), or four (to speak to a human being). He finally managed to push the right button, only to be kept on hold for what seemed like eternity, and then, just when he thought surely he would be put through, the line was disconnected. But Saul was both patient and persistent, so after several tries over the course of a few days, he succeeded in making an appointment with Dr. Wilson.

Scheduling an appointment did not guarantee that Saul would end up at the right place at the right time. First he had to get to the doctor's office. The office was in a low-rise building conveniently located down the street from a small community hospital. At least the arrangement was convenient for the doctors working in the building who could go back and forth between the hospital—where some of them saw patients or taught medical students—and their offices. For patients, it wasn't quite so convenient. The building wasn't near a bus or subway stop. And if Saul were still driving, which he wasn't, he would have had to park in a narrow, winding garage with multiple levels that was a nightmare to navigate, and where the distance between the upper levels and the office itself was considerably longer than he could have managed.

Saul took the "Ride" from his assisted living residence to the doctor's office building; he had given up driving and didn't want to bother my husband and me. The van driver dropped him off in front of the building, leaving him to make his way to Dr. Wilson's office. That strategy would have been fine except that the building was filled with doctors' offices, all of which, Saul discovered when he went to the wrong suite by mistake, looked more or less identical. They had the same ochre rugs, the same check-in window that looked like it belonged in a bank, and the same warren of examining rooms and offices lining the corridors radiating from a central waiting room. Nothing like the atmosphere in his previous doctor's office, which resembled the living room of an old Victorian mansion.

When Saul finally walked in and the receptionist told him that yes, he was in the right place, he could have hugged her—if he hadn't been so reserved and if a glass panel hadn't separated him from the area where the support staff sat in front of their computers. She didn't smile at him, and she didn't ask whether he was new to the area and welcome him when he said that he was. She just requested his insurance card and handed him a sheaf of forms to fill out that involved answering questions about his past medical history (which he had already provided on his pre-visit questionnaire), providing the name and telephone number of his next of kin (which he couldn't remember), and authorizing the doctor to examine him after supplying him with detailed information about his rights under HIPAA (sometimes referred to as the "Health Information Privacy Act"). He next encountered a "practice assistant" who looked to be about eighteen, and who called him into the office by addressing him as "Saul" rather than as "Mr. Gillick," after which she weighed him and took his blood pressure, pulse, and temperature. The assistant, he would later discover, changed with each visit; sometimes it was a nurse and sometimes a nurse's aide, or sometimes just a high school graduate with a few hours of on-the-job training.

If Saul had been given a customer satisfaction questionnaire then, Dr. Wilson's practice would not have fared very well. And that was before he'd even seen the doctor.

The Patient Satisfaction Industry

The hospitality industry has become the principal model for the outpatient practice of medicine. And the way hotels evaluate their services is increasingly the standard way that physician practices assess theirs. Patients are customers—and customers are always right, according to the service industry. Patient satisfaction does matter: it is correlated with better self-management of chronic disease, with higher rates of adherence to recommended treatment and, for physicians, to lower malpractice risk and less staff turnover. The association between patient satisfaction and clinical effectiveness holds across a range of different diseases, from cancer to heart disease, and in a variety of patient populations and practice types.[12] But while satisfaction is just one component of the patient's experience, it has increasingly come to be its sole measure. And that, in large part, is thanks to a pioneering medical anthropologist named Irwin Press and his statistician partner, Rod Ganey.

Professor Press began with the assumption that understanding the patient's social, personal, and cultural needs could improve the quality of medical care—and reduce malpractice suits. In the mid-1980s, he set out to design surveys, with Ganey's help, that measured the degree of patient satisfaction with their physicians. Were they respectful? Did they answer questions clearly? Were they available by phone or in person in a timely fashion? His genius was to devise different surveys for the hospital, for the office, and for health plans (the insurers), and to feed back the results to the relevant health care organization to allow them to modify their practice—producing happier patients who wouldn't leave the practice, who would recommend it to others, and who wouldn't sue. They might also be more likely to do what their doctor recommended and—the new buzzword—be *engaged* in their health care.

Press Ganey Associates, Inc. soon became a wildly successful organization. It used "scientifically rigorous" tools to determine what questions to ask and how to ask them, and it sold its products to thousands of physician practices, hospital systems, and health plans. In May 2015 Press Ganey went public, and as of early 2016, it had just under a thousand employees and a market capitalization of $1.58 billion. Its chief executive officer is paid over a million dollars and its chief medical officer almost as much.[13] As the company says in its web profile, suitably dressed up in corporate lingo, it now provides "patient experience measurement, performance analytics, and strategic advisory policies for healthcare organizations across the continuum of care."[14]

Other organizations concerned with improving the quality of medical care have also been persuaded that patient involvement in their care was key, and that surveys were an invaluable tool for assessing patients' concerns.[15] The Agency for Healthcare Research and Quality (AHRQ), a government agency devoted to promoting the quality, appropriateness, and effectiveness of care, decided to fund its own initiative to survey patients. The result was the Consumer Assessment of Healthcare Providers and Systems survey, or CAHPS, which initially focused on the quality of private health plans but more recently on patients' satisfaction with their physicians.

The questionnaires capture only those parts of the patient's experience that involve access, communication, customer service, and coordination of care, where access means the ability to get an appointment promptly, communication deals with the clinician's ability to explain medical issues to patients and to answer their questions, customer service refers to having helpful, competent, and respectful staff, and coordination of care deals with whether the results from one doctor are available to another doctor involved in the patient's care. But there are other aspects of "the patient's experience" beyond the *service*. There is the whole question of what happens to patients: what medical problems do doctors pay attention to and what problems do they ignore? What kinds of medication do they prescribe—cheap and effective drugs or expensive and questionable drugs? What sorts of procedures do doctors order—simple, painless tests or high-tech, risky ones? How is medical care delivered—by an individual? By a team? Where is it delivered—in an inaccessible office? Around the corner from the patient's home? In the patient's home? And then there's the patient's *interpretation* of what happens: does the treatment make the patient feel like a machine that just needs an oil job to be restored to perfect functioning? Does the approach to care reinforce the belief that chronic, ultimately fatal medical conditions are curable? Does it promote the view that ill health is due to bad behavior—to inadequate exercise, a poor diet, or lack of virtue—or that it is due to chance? Or maybe to genes or environmental toxins?

Whatever their limitations, patient satisfaction surveys seem to be here to stay. Government regulators are enthusiastic about them, and so are private accreditation organizations and administrators concerned with marketing. Satisfaction surveys even made their way into the Affordable Care Act: as of 2017, all practices with more than two physicians will be required to administer patient surveys and submit the results to Medicare; the level of their reimbursement will hinge, in part, on their performance on these questionnaires.

In the Office

Saul moved from the waiting room to the examining room—and continued waiting. After about fifteen minutes, a young woman walked in and introduced herself as Dr. Wilson's nurse practitioner, Nancy Sheridan. Saul didn't know what a nurse practitioner was, but this young woman acted much like a doctor. She even sported a white coat, complete with a pen, flashlight, and tongue depressor tucked into her front pocket, and wore a stethoscope like a necklace. Ms. Sheridan was organized and efficient, but at the same time cheerful and reassuring. She asked Saul questions about any current symptoms and about his past medical history, then entered all the information into his medical record. She even asked whether he had any trouble getting dressed or going to the bathroom, and she wanted to know how his spirits were after the move from Philadelphia. When she was finished asking questions, she performed a physical examination, proceeding methodically from head to toe: she checked his vision and made him take off his socks so she could inspect his feet.

Ms. Sheridan was a perfectly nice lady, Saul told my husband and me afterwards, but she wasn't a doctor. The doctor had put in a brief appearance at the end of the visit. His main concern, Saul reported, was with what he called "health maintenance," a phrase which sounded to Saul like something a car mechanic might discuss. He wanted to be sure Saul's blood sugar was normal, even though Saul didn't have a problem with his sugars; he'd had an elevated reading once when he'd been hospitalized for a minor surgical procedure and, ever since then, "diabetes" had consistently appeared on his problem list. Dr. Wilson also wanted to check whether Saul had any blood in his stool, though at age eighty-five, Saul wasn't too worried about colon cancer. He figured that he wouldn't agree to surgery even if he turned out to have a malignancy. He knew all about colon cancer because it's what had killed his wife, Ada, but now he was older than she had been when she underwent surgery. And look where an operation had gotten her.

After spending perhaps five minutes with him, Dr. Wilson sent Saul for a blood test, a urine test, and a chest x-ray. He also told him to schedule an appointment with a cardiologist—only because he had had an abnormal electrocardiogram during the fateful hospitalization a few years earlier that had marked him for life as a diabetic—and an appointment with a podiatrist to cut his toenails, and an appointment with an ophthalmologist to check his eyes, since all diabetics were supposed to have regular eye exams (even though he wasn't actually a diabetic). And, of course, Saul was to set up a follow-up appointment with Dr. Wilson to take place after he had had the tests and subspecialty exams.

Saul didn't look forward to all those additional appointments. He later commented to my husband—not a complaint, just an observation—that Dr. Wilson seemed to be in a tremendous hurry. He frequently glanced down at his watch, conveying the distinct impression that he was eager to be done with Saul so he could move on to someone or something more interesting. When he wasn't checking the time, he was staring at his computer screen, entering data directly into the electronic medical record. It was true, Saul admitted, that he moved slowly. He got undressed slowly. He stumbled in telling his medical history. But he'd done his best. He wasn't like some of his wife's friends who had a long list of complaints—joints that ached, hearts that palpitated, lungs that wheezed.

Saul didn't like to say anything critical, especially not about a physician, but he wondered why his doctor hadn't bothered to explain to him why he needed all those tests and referrals.

Mid-Levels

Physicians are increasingly turning to "mid-level practitioners" to help them in the office, as well as in the hospital and the skilled nursing facility. We rely on these nurse practitioners (NPs) and physician assistants (PAs) because we find ourselves rushed. That's not surprising, since primary care doctors are typically expected to see between twenty and thirty patients a day. As a result, the majority of appointments are short, commonly lasting somewhere between thirteen and sixteen minutes.[16]

Primary care doctors see mid-levels as a welcome safety valve to help deal with mountains of paperwork: authorizations for services to submit to the Visiting Nurse Association, pre-approvals for pricey prescription drugs to send to pharmacies, and requests for durable medical equipment—wheelchairs or bedside commodes—to give to health insurers. Already in 2008, American physicians spent about one-sixth of the work day on administration. That amount of time has been rising steadily, with the "practice profitability index," or the percent of physicians who spend a day or more every week on paperwork, reaching 70 percent in 2014.[17] Since professional satisfaction is inversely proportional to the time spent on paperwork (with physicians working in hospital-run practices suffering the most), physicians find the opportunity to off-load some of those responsibilities extremely attractive.[18]

All those forms and, more generally, the activities spent in coordinating care and arranging services such as home-delivered meals or adult day care programs, are a reflection of the reality that older patients today suffer from chronic diseases. They have high blood pressure, elevated cholesterol, ischemic heart disease, arthritis, and diabetes, just to list the most common diagnoses. Most of them don't have only one chronic condition, they have multiple conditions. And the older they get, the more diseases they have. By the time they reach eighty-five, the majority will have four or more different chronic diseases.[19]

The enthusiasm for mid-levels has resulted in 56 percent of primary care physicians practicing together with a mid-level practitioner. In larger group practices, the percentage of physicians employing NPs or PAs reaches 80 percent.[20] These new members of the practice do far more than alleviate the stress or boredom that plague physicians. They also directly affect what happens to patients, and what they bring to the practice has a great deal to do with their education and training.

On the surface, the training for PAs and for NPs looks very similar: both groups go through two-year programs that culminate in a master's degree and certification to practice, and both programs involve a mixture of lecture classes devoted to topics such as physiology and pharmacology and "rotations" or "practicums" focused on experiential learning. But there are differences, and those differences affect the patients that mid-levels care for.

A physician assistant, as the training program at Northeastern University in Boston explains, is "a health care provider who practices medicine under physician supervision." To become a PA, you have to have a BA and have fulfilled prerequisites in biology and chemistry, and you should have a few years of health care-related experience. In an accredited PA program, you spend a year taking courses, both in core subjects such as anatomy, physiology, and pharmacology, and in applied subjects such as physical diagnosis, orthopedics, and obstetrics and gynecology. The second year of the program involves clinical rotations, similar to what medical students go through in the last two years of their training, but typically compressed into five weeks each. Usually, students can expect a standard sequence that includes ambulatory medicine, emergency medicine, inpatient medicine, pediatrics, and surgery. At the end of the program, which at Northeastern University in 2015 cost just under

$40,000 per year, students sit for the PA National Certifying Examination, which is required for licensure in all states. Once they pass the exam, they can go out and get a job that includes doing physical exams, ordering diagnostic tests, making diagnoses in consultation with their supervising physician, prescribing medications, and advising and educating patients on prevention and disease management.[21] Fully one-quarter of PAs work for surgeons, and the majority are employed in hospitals rather than the outpatient setting, reflecting the profession's historical origins in the 1960s when former military corpsmen were commonplace in the student body.

Nurse practitioner students have considerable practical knowledge when they start their programs. They generally already have a bachelor's degree in nursing. When they enroll in a master's in nursing program, they must select a particular track. The University of Massachusetts NP program in Boston, for instance, offers a family nurse practitioner concentration and two types of adult-gerontological nurse practitioner concentrations, one tailored to the ambulatory setting and one to the acute care setting. Each path involves two semesters of classroom work and two semesters of supervised clinical practice. Training is holistic and focuses on the patient as part of a family or community. Tuition at private universities is comparable for PA and NP courses of study.

As a result of their interdisciplinary training, their skills in coordinating care, and their interest in working with patients as part of a family or community, mid-levels can bring a missing element to primary care office practice: they can serve as the glue that allows older patients with multiple chronic conditions to get the kind of coordinated care they need. But, to achieve this end, they have to be utilized in this way by the physicians who employ them and patients and families need to understand their role. All too often, nurse practitioners and physicians are deployed interchangeably, or advanced practice clinicians evaluate acute problems—walk-in patients or urgent care visits—while physicians address chronic conditions at regularly scheduled visits, an arrangement that fails to take advantage of the physician's diagnostic skills and the NP's expertise in coordination and functional assessment.

Seeing the Subspecialist

After Saul's first visit to Dr. Wilson, he was anxious about getting to the doctor's office for a follow-up visit. He was even more concerned about how he would find his way to the various subspecialists he was supposed to see, all of whom had offices elsewhere. He quietly wondered whether those other doctors would talk down to him or use language he didn't understand to an even greater extent than Dr. Wilson did.[22] He had experience with surgeons from when he'd had an operation in Philadelphia for a twisted bowel, and his recollection was that they did a good job of describing the operation they wanted to perform, but were not so good at exploring his concerns about the surgery.[23]

The trip to the podiatrist was helpful since Saul could no longer cut his own toenails and they were badly in need of attention. The visit to the eye doctor was also useful because Saul left it with a prescription for new reading glasses. But the visit to the cardiologist was another matter.

Dr. Smith was young, female, and brusque. Saul couldn't believe she was old enough to be a doctor, let alone a heart doctor, though in fact she was in her mid-thirties, having spent four years in medical school, three years in residency, and another three years specializing in cardiology. Saul had never had a woman doctor before: his image of the quintessential physician was of an older man—at least sixty and more likely over sixty-five—who was overbearing, intimidating, and had a beard. He'd never found that kind of doctor particularly endearing, but it's what he expected—even though only a minority of physicians in office practice today are over sixty-five, and a substantial number of both family doctors and internists are women.[24] Dr. Smith didn't look the part, but she was as efficient and inscrutable as Saul's archetype.

Dr. Smith ordered the same lab tests that Dr. Wilson had obtained just a few weeks earlier. She sent him down the hall for an echocardiogram to determine how well his heart was pumping and to evaluate the status of his heart valves, and told him tersely that the test was "fine" when he returned to her office. The results never made it back to Dr. Wilson.

The medical assistant in the office measured Saul's blood pressure which, as happened every time he went to the doctor, was high. Saul had high blood pressure but he also had "white coat hypertension," a condition in which his pressure rose when he was anxious, and he was always anxious at the doctor's office. The cardiologist nonetheless felt obligated to adjust his blood pressure medicines, although neither she nor Saul knew what drugs had already been tried and in what doses. And when Dr. Smith gave Saul yet another prescription for blood pressure pills, she didn't tell his primary care doctor what new pill she had selected. She didn't think she needed to since she had entered all the relevant information in Saul's electronic medical record. But Dr. Wilson used a different, incompatible electronic medical record, so he never learned of the change.

Subspecialists and the Geriatric Patient

The trouble with specialists is that they are principally interested in a single organ system or a specific disease. The very essence of specialization in medicine is an intense focus on one body part—the heart or the lungs or the kidneys, or on a particular type of disorder—infections or cancer. But what's unique about older patients is that optimizing the operation of the individual parts is often not as important as maximizing the functioning of the whole person. Excellent blood sugar control is the sine qua non of good diabetes care—but not if it results in dangerously low blood sugars, sugars so low that the patient gets confused or falls down. Maintaining systolic blood pressure below 140 is similarly the goal of organ-focused medical care—but if the medication that brings the blood pressure into the desirable range also causes a marked drop in pressure when the patient goes from sitting to standing, enough of a drop to make him dizzy and faint, then that medicine is too strong.

What matters most to older patients is their daily activities, and their ability to walk and talk and hear and think. That kind of functioning requires the integration of lots of different body parts. Walking, for example, involves the muscles of the legs and the circulation to those muscles, it requires balance and awareness of the environment (ideally good vision and intact hearing), and it entails judgment. Attending to each of the component parts without looking at their integration into the whole person or, worse yet, focusing exclusively on one piece without regard for how its treatment will affect all the others, isn't good enough for the geriatric patient.

A laser-like focus on a single organ or disease is problematic for another reason: the physician needs to be fully aware of all the other medical problems the patient has in order to assess whether standard care is likely to work. New medical treatment—and medication is the paradigmatic example—is typically tested in people who have nothing wrong with them except the problem for which they're being treated. That's a great strategy for figuring out whether the treatment ever works, or works better than an alternative medication. But it doesn't answer the question of whether the treatment will work in a patient with five other serious, chronic medical conditions. Sometimes the conventional treatment would make perfectly good sense—if only the patient lived long enough to reap its benefits. I remember seeing a patient once who had both severe coronary heart disease and metastatic cancer. Her cardiologist wanted to do the right thing for her and, according to the usual algorithms, she should have recommended bypass surgery to treat the narrowing in her coronary arteries. That approach would have made perfectly good sense if the patient could expect to live for a few more years, but her advanced cancer was likely to kill her before her coronary disease did. It took a good deal of reassurance to persuade the cardiologist that she wasn't a bad doctor because she didn't advise surgery.

In principle, subspecialists know about *all* their patient's diagnoses, but they don't always appreciate the implications of those conditions. I remember seeing a homebound patient with advanced Parkinson's disease whose neurologist had prescribed a medication he was supposed to take every two hours. That regimen, the neurologist argued, was superior to taking a long-acting medication once or twice a day. There was just one problem with this scenario. The patient had mild dementia and couldn't remember to take pills more than once a day. For him to take medication six times a day, he would have needed almost constant supervision. That, in turn, would have meant going into a nursing home or paying for an aide, but he didn't have the money for an aide and had no desire to move to a nursing facility. He was quite happy to substitute a very good medical regimen for an excellent medical regimen in exchange for the satisfaction he derived from staying in his own home.

Subspecialty medicine is part of what makes American medicine great—patients are offered the latest and most sophisticated treatments. But, for the oldest and the frailest patients, the latest and greatest may not be so great. What matters more is having a team of physicians who work collaboratively. Ideally, the primary care doctor is the manager, the person who can explain to the cardiologist just how advanced the patient's cancer actually is and can estimate his life expectancy. In the best of all worlds, the primary care doctor would review the recommendations of specialists and decide, together with the patient, which ones to implement. But the tendency of many subspecialists is to assume they know best about "their" diseases and make unilateral decisions, without involving or, in some cases, informing the primary care doctor. Or the subspecialists simply work in a different health care system from the primary care physician—one is hospital-based, the other is at a different hospital or works in an independent practice—and they seldom communicate.

Fewer than half of the office visits made by patients over the age of sixty-five are to primary care doctors.[25] The remaining visits are either to medical subspecialists such as cardiologists, nephrologists, rheumatologists, neurologists, and oncologists, or to surgeons, including orthopedists, general surgeons, and surgical subspecialists. Saul had sufficient difficulty coping with one new doctor—he didn't need any additional physicians in his life.

Ongoing Primary Care

For the next year, Saul stuck with Dr. Wilson. At least Dr. Wilson spoke English and didn't have a foreign accent, a problem Saul's companions at the assisted living facility complained about bitterly because they had so much trouble understanding their doctors. But Dr. Wilson rarely talked to Saul. When my husband or I accompanied Saul to the office, Dr. Wilson addressed himself to us. Whenever he spoke to Saul directly, he mumbled, he spoke quickly, and he didn't speak loudly enough for Saul to hear him. He seemed to regard Saul as a healthy eighty-five-year-old who was doing very well. I found that perspective puzzling.

What I saw when I looked at Saul was a man whose life had been a paradox: on the one hand, he had been fiercely independent and determined to make a living running his own pharmacy; on the other hand, he had relied heavily on his wife for his social life, for filling what little leisure time he had, and even for some of his business decisions. Now that he was without his life partner, he was flailing. In addition, he was failing: his thinking and his judgment were increasingly impaired, as was his walking. He sometimes referred to my husband as his father; he jaywalked across the busy street outside the assisted living complex, believing he could dart past the oncoming cars. I felt he should use a cane; Saul didn't believe in assistive devices and his doctor was agnostic on the subject. On one occasion, Saul thought he was in his own apartment when he was actually in the assisted living common room and he began taking his clothes off to get ready for bed. Knowledge of the episode was transmitted to the director of the assisted living facility, who reacted promptly and dramatically, demanding that his "behavioral problems" be addressed immediately or they would evict him. Fortunately, at about the same time, Saul found a lady friend among the other residents, a strong-willed older woman who was physically frail but mentally intact. She watched him like a hawk and intervened swiftly to halt any attempts on his part to disrobe in public.

Saul's incontinence proved a greater challenge. He began wearing adult diapers, but they were sometimes insufficiently absorbent. Nursing homes make it a practice to offer "scheduled toileting" (or they are supposed to) in order to decrease the frequency of incontinence by escorting residents to the bathroom on a regular basis, but assisted living facilities are not set up to do anything of the kind. As a result, Saul sometimes had wet spots on his pants. Worse, he occasionally left a puddle on the dining room chair. Worse still, he sometimes smelled. My husband attempted to help by keeping him supplied with adult diapers, trying different brands in hopes of finding a leak-proof variety, and purchasing new underwear every few weeks; Saul had developed a tendency to discard his underwear after he'd had an accident. My husband wondered why Dr. Wilson didn't do anything about the problem. He didn't do anything about it because he didn't realize it existed—he never asked.

When Saul could no longer remain in the assisted living facility because his dementia and his incontinence had progressed to the point that attention from his lady friend and supplemental private help were no longer sufficient for his needs, he moved to a nursing home. Dr. Wilson did not take care of nursing home patients—he would have had to see them on-site, initially every thirty days, and then every sixty days once they were medically stable, and his practice was not set up to accommodate what were essentially home visits. As soon as Saul moved to the skilled nursing facility, we had to find him a new primary care doctor, one of the very small number of physicians who were willing to include long-term care patients on their roster of cases. For Saul, that meant getting to know someone new at a point in his life when he was having increasing difficulty remembering names and faces. It meant getting medical care from someone who had never known him when he was able to carry on a lengthy conversation and ask intelligent questions about his condition. Saul would depend for his medical care on a doctor who obtained information about the signs and symptoms of disease from the facility nurses and who relied on family members for knowledge of Saul's goals of care. The absence of any semblance of a patient-doctor relationship was just one more loss in the mounting series of losses that constituted Saul's life.

Geriatrics and Primary Care

What little time Saul spent with his doctor when he lived in assisted living was typically devoted to the doctor's agenda. His physician didn't talk about incontinence or dementia or depression or, indeed, any of Saul's major concerns because he, like most internists, hadn't had much geriatric training. What he never learned about because internal medicine didn't traditionally address them were geriatric syndromes. These are disorders that span multiple organ systems: incontinence, for instance, is not necessarily exclusively a bladder problem. More commonly, it is a disturbance that arises from the bladder and the prostate and the brain. It may be triggered by medications, drugs given for problems such as insomnia or nasal congestion that have nothing to do with the urinary tract. And it is often made worse, as in Saul's case, by something as seemingly unrelated as a slow gait. By the time Saul's brain sensed that he needed to empty his bladder, it was often too late; he couldn't get to the bathroom in time. Other geriatric syndromes such as dementia, depression, and falls also typically arise from problems involving more than one organ system.

The medical specialty of geriatrics is relatively new: before 1978, there were no formally trained geriatricians. Without geriatric specialists, there was no one to develop a model geriatric clinical program, nobody to educate medical students, and no one to do research in the physiology, pathophysiology, or care of older people.[26] Geriatrics still isn't regarded by the American College of Graduate Medical Education as a specialty analogous to cardiology or nephrology. Instead, physicians can be awarded a "Certificate of Added Qualifications" in Geriatrics after doing a one-year clinical fellowship and passing a certification examination.

Diagnosing and treating geriatric syndromes differs from the conventional medical or surgical approach to symptoms. In addition to taking a medical history (asking when the problem began, and what makes it better and what makes it worse) and performing a physical examination (listening to the lungs, palpating the abdomen, checking the reflexes), geriatrics requires a different kind of assessment. Geriatricians are concerned with function, with how well a person gets up out of a chair and walks across the room; we ask whether a patient can feed and dress himself and whether he can perform other activities essential to living independently such as cooking, shopping, telephoning, driving, or taking public transportation. Geriatricians rely both on patients and on their families and caregivers for the answers to our questions, as well as on direct observation. Geriatrics is fundamentally interdisciplinary: it requires the input of physical therapists, nurses, and social workers, and, in some instances, of pharmacists, psychiatrists, or occupational therapists.

Very few physicians are geriatric specialists. In 2005 the United States had only 7,128 board-certified geriatricians. The field is not growing fast enough to meet the demand: by 2030, the projections are that the United States will need 36,000 geriatricians but will be lucky if it has 7,500. Fellowship slots, the positions in post-residency programs that train doctors to become geriatricians, have been unfilled in recent years.[27] The lack of geriatric specialists wouldn't matter so much if generalists—internists and family doctors—were extensively trained in geriatrics, but they are not. A survey of residents in these two fields at the time they completed their programs found that half felt unprepared to care for geriatric patients.[28]

Practicing physicians agree that most doctors don't have the requisite knowledge or skills to provide first-rate care to older patients; they also say that they don't think their colleagues knew how to manage the common geriatric syndromes. And the trouble starts before residency: medical schools also don't teach much about the aging process. Too many other subjects vie for time, from the basic sciences like anatomy, biochemistry, and physiology, to established clinical domains such as cardiology and dermatology. The lack of available faculty to teach geriatrics just makes the situation worse.

The Office: Final Grade

Saul was a dutiful patient. He took whatever pills his doctors prescribed—he cycled through a long list of antihypertensive medications before his primary care doctor hit on one that worked without side effects; he peed in a cup and proffered his arm for a blood sample. He never had a harsh word for Dr. Wilson. After all, the doctor was a cut above average. He was at least interested in having older patients. He had hired a nurse practitioner who cared about the problems unique to older people. He neglected to inquire about precisely those issues that affected patients like Saul far more than their cholesterol level or tight control of diabetes, but he did manage to keep Saul out of the hospital during the two years he served as his primary care physician. He, or more often than not, his nurse practitioner, prescribed the antibiotics that nipped his bronchitis in the bud before it blossomed into a more severe infection, vaccinated him against pneumonia, and adjusted his blood pressure medications while keeping his blood chemistries in balance.

Saul did not much care for going to the doctor. The entire experience made him feel incompetent: he had trouble finding the office, he had difficulty answering questions and filling out forms, and he felt rushed. Saul came to rely on my husband and me for transportation to his doctor's visits, but he didn't like that either. He regarded relying on us for something as basic as a ride to be a worrisome sign of dependency, and if there was one thing he dreaded about old age, it was dependency.

Like the vast majority of older patients, if you asked Saul whether he was satisfied with his primary care doctor, he would have said yes.[29] He was one of the lucky ones for whom high out-of-pocket costs did not prevent him from seeing his doctor, from getting recommended tests, or from taking prescribed medications. He was able to see his primary care physician reasonably promptly when he got sick, unlike many patients who cannot and end up going to the local hospital's emergency department.[30] But Saul had no idea that there was so much else his physician could have done for him. He didn't know about advance care planning—discussing preferences for future care in the event he would be unable to participate in making decisions at the time he became acutely ill. He didn't know about comprehensive geriatric assessment—a systematic evaluation that would have focused on his ability to do the daily activities he needed to remain independent, rather than on organ systems and diseases. He had no idea that primary care medicine could be integrated into specialty care, so that physicians could regularly communicate with each other.

Saul experienced one type of office practice. His physician was one of three who owned their own practice and were affiliated with the local community hospital. Perhaps other models of office practice would have led to a different patient experience.

CHAPTER TWO

The Lay of the Land

The prophets of doom say that the era of small, independent medical practices that operate in a fee-for-service model is over.[1] As with other similarly dire forecasts, most famously of Mark Twain's impending death when he was alive and well, this claim may well be exaggerated. What is true is that solo practice is fading from view: thirty years ago, roughly 40 percent of American doctors were in solo practice; by 2012, only 18 percent were solo practitioners, although the majority of doctors still practice in groups of fewer than ten physicians.[2] What is also true is that there are now many models of office practice other than one- or two-person private practices that charge for each service they provide. And those models vary enormously in size, ownership, reimbursement, and structure.

The most obvious difference among medical practices is their *size*, but size can be misleading. Small groups are often nestled within larger ones and large ones are often subdivided into semi-autonomous units. When I started out in primary care after completing my residency in internal medicine and a fellowship in geriatrics, I worked at a neighborhood health center that felt like a small group practice—we were about five internists, a comparable number of pediatricians, and a psychiatrist. But the entire center was owned by Massachusetts General Hospital (MGH), a mammoth tertiary referral center that operated a number of health centers like ours. My primary care patients got their hospital care at MGH—but there were so many internal medicine interns and residents, and the attending staff was so large, that I seldom saw a familiar face when I went to the hospital to check on them. Later, I practiced in a large, teaching nursing home where medical care was provided by what was a medium-sized group practice—we had about a dozen primary care doctors on the staff along with a number of consultants in orthopedics, neurology, and ophthalmology who saw patients several hours a week. We were affiliated with a major Boston teaching hospital, which meant our patients were hospitalized at that institution, and we each spent a few weeks every year teaching and seeing patients at the hospital. But working in our closed nursing home environment (unlike most nursing homes, we did not allow outside doctors to see patients in the facility) with the same nursing staff day after day and year after year, caring for patients who lived in the facility where we worked, was actually far more insular, far more intimate than anything I had previously experienced. After ten years spent practicing in that environment, I joined a very large, multispecialty group practice with over 600 physicians (including both primary care internists and pediatricians, medical subspecialists, psychiatrists, and surgeons), where I served as a palliative care consultant rather than a primary care doctor. That was by far the largest practice I'd ever been a member of, but my day-to-day interactions centered on the small, interdisciplinary team with which I worked: the nurse practitioner, social worker, psychiatric nurse, and chaplain who comprised the palliative care team. Size alone doesn't shape the nature of office practice for the physician—and more than likely does not for the patient either.

From the patient's perspective, a small group may not feel substantially different from a solo practice. Most of the time, the patient sees his or her own doctor; sometimes, when that physician is on vacation, someone else will substitute. In neither case will other services be available on-site—at most, the practice will employ a technician to draw blood and do EKGs, but for physical therapy or social work or x-rays, the patient will have to go elsewhere. Coordination with specialists is likely to be spotty except in those cases where the primary care doctor has a strong personal relationship with the physicians to whom he refers patients, and neither solo practices (which only rarely use an electronic medical record) nor small groups (which often have electronic records but may not use the same system as other area groups) have a convenient way to communicate with other practitioners. And small groups, like individual practitioners, are unlikely to offer comprehensive geriatric assessment, home visits, transitional care in the skilled nursing facility, or any other geriatric-specific service.

Reimbursement, the way physicians are paid for their services, is at least as important as the size of the practice in determining what happens to patients when they go to the doctor, though patients may be completely unaware of how their doctors are paid. Reimbursement may subtly influence the physician's proclivity to order tests and willingness to coordinate care. Fee-for-service medicine, the style most doctors have practiced for the last fifty years, is notorious for encouraging doctors to do more, to see patients often, and to order numerous tests and procedures because the more they do, the more money they earn, regardless of how much, if at all, the interventions benefit patients. A capitated payment system, by contrast, in which a practice receives a fixed amount of money per patient per year and is at risk for all the expenses the patient incurs—lab tests, subspecialty visits, and in many cases hospital and even skilled nursing facility care—encourages prudence; some would say underutilization. Newer variants such as Accountable Care Organizations are essentially capitated, at-risk models with various safeguards built in to prevent doctors from doing too little; the savings the practice gains through efficiency are contingent on meeting a variety of quality standards. Large practices that accept patients who have Medicare Advantage—a capitated form of Medicare—can afford to pay for case management services that coordinate care for complex patients with chronic diseases, a strategy that can both improve outcomes and simplify life for patients.

Concierge practices are a type of office practice in which physicians opt for still another form of reimbursement: they charge a fee to the patient that either replaces or supplements Medicare, in exchange for additional, personalized attention. This arrangement clearly affects how patients are cared for. First and foremost, it affects the individual's wallet—retainer fees vary tremendously, but typically range between $1,500 and $5,400 per year.[3] It allows for longer visits, shorter wait times to get an appointment, and easier telephone access to the doctor. For older people with multiple chronic conditions and problems in their daily activities, the kind of individual attention available from a concierge practice can be a lifesaver. As one geriatrician who gave up practicing medicine in a large multispecialty group practice to form a solo concierge practice says, this is the way medicine ought to be practiced. "This is a beautiful life," she says of her experience providing highly personalized care to older or disabled individuals in their homes. Instead of a panel of 2,000 patients, she has 50 patients and she's not looking for more. She charges between $4,000 and $6,000 per person per year, depending on how far she has to drive to reach the patient. And she comments anecdotally that her patients seldom go to an emergency room: she makes emergency home visits and can usually stave off hospitalization. She's happy and her patients are happy.[4]

Ownership affects the style of practice, as do size and reimbursement. Physicians used to own their practices. They still do, to some extent—as of 2012, just over half of all practicing physicians owned part or all of their practices. Among internists and family practitioners, ownership rates are even lower.[5] Ownership matters for physician autonomy; for patients, it can determine the shape of care delivery. And increasingly the owner, in part or entirely, is a hospital.

The American Hospital Association estimates that 20 percent of physicians are employed by a hospital—but as many as 45 percent have some kind of contractual financial relationship with a hospital.[6] What happens in these arrangements is that the hospital takes over the business side of the practice: the billing, paying taxes, renting space, arranging for malpractice insurance.

The hospital typically contracts with outside vendors for all the supplies and services the practice needs in order to function, including the all-important purchase of an electronic medical record system. By virtue of the size of its institutional parent—and often the hospital is itself part of a still larger health care system—the practice may benefit from economies of scale. But it also typically has to conform to the hospital's standards for how to practice medicine, perhaps eliminating visits by primary care physicians to their hospitalized patients and abolishing home visits. The hospital may require the members of the group to adhere to certain practice guidelines or to use the hospital medication formulary, which translates into changes in medical care for patients.

Finally, there's the *organization* of the practice, which sometimes overlaps with the way services are reimbursed as well as with ownership. The number of options for how to structure a practice continues to multiply. There are the simple ones: form a practice that is made up exclusively of internists—or orthopedists, or radiologists, or pediatricians (50 percent of practices follow the single-specialty model); or set up a multispecialty group practice, allowing patients the convenience of one-stop shopping. But joining together with one or more other doctors is not the only way that physicians have found to reorganize their office practices. They can form an independent practice association, an organization in which physicians retain their independent corporate status but integrate financially or even clinically, and contract with payers and vendors as a group. They can decide to outsource the management of their individual practices to a for-profit practice management company. They can retain nominal independence but agree to be acquired by a health insurer.[7] Or, encouraged by the Affordable Care Act to provide coordinated, integrated care, they can join with hospitals, nursing homes, and other groups to form an Accountable Care Organization (ACO). In this arrangement, all the parties to the ACO collectively share the risk for the costs of care with the insurance company.

Among these myriad forms of organization, the multispecialty group practice has garnered the attention of both pundits and politicians because of its track record in providing efficient, high-value care. Practices such as Geisinger Health Systems in Pennsylvania and Intermountain Healthcare in Utah, both of which are not-for-profit health care systems with multispecialty practices at their core, stand out.[8] Such practices are growing in number and in patient volume, although they currently employ only about a quarter of all physicians.[9] And because the large multispecialty group practice is about as different from a small generalist practice as it's possible to get, this model is worth a closer look.

The Palo Alto Medical Foundation

Route 101 covers over 1,500 miles as it meanders from the state of Washington to southern California, hugging the rugged Pacific coast and traversing stately redwood forests. The fifty-mile stretch from San Francisco to San Jose is one of the busiest sections of what is already a very heavily traveled road. It is there that the road passes through Mountain View, home to the Googleplex, and through Palo Alto, site of the verdant and prosperous campus of Stanford University. A brief detour will take you to Cupertino, which houses Apple's main campus, to the Menlo Park headquarters of Facebook, and to other thriving Silicon Valley cities and towns. And visible from Interstate 101, just about midway between San Francisco and San Jose and looking for all the world like a luxury hotel, is the newest branch of the Palo Alto Medical Foundation (PAMF).

The Palo Alto Medical Foundation is a multispecialty group practice whose selling point is that it offers high-quality, integrated, comprehensive care. Its focus is on the population it serves—young families at some sites, older patients at others, and professionals in the booming tech industry at still others. That's exactly the approach to care that Dr. Russel Van Arsdale Lee wanted when he established what one day would become PAMF in 1930.

Lee was always a bit of an iconoclast. He supported national health insurance when it was just a gleam in President Harry Truman's eye, he endorsed birth control when it was widely seen as a threat to marriage and the family, and he supported group practice at a time when the American Medical Association regarded anything other than solo, fee-for-service medicine as un-American. Born the son of a Presbyterian minister in Spanish Fork, Utah, in 1895, he reportedly chose medicine over chemical engineering while an undergraduate at Stanford after discovering he was color blind, a decision that would have widespread ramifications for both him and the practice of medicine.[10] When he moved back to Palo Alto in 1924 to set up his own medical practice, he quickly gathered a group of partners who shared his interest in providing primary care to the community. He called the practice the Palo Alto Medical Center (PAMC).

Dr. Lee and his partners soon concluded that the best way to address community needs was to take care of medical problems throughout the age spectrum. That meant they needed a pediatrician as well as an obstetrician and an internist. It meant addressing the various kinds of problems that their patients were most likely to develop, conditions for which they would need surgical care and subspecialty medical care in areas such as cardiology and oncology. By 1946, PAMC had recruited twenty physicians, representing most of what were then the critical areas of medicine. As a direct outgrowth of its awareness that members of particular communities often had common needs, PAMC began providing medical care to all Stanford University students for a flat fee. And, in keeping with its mission to enhance care, PAMC established its own research foundation, with many faculty members holding joint appointments with Stanford University. Hoping to imbue the next generation of physicians with its patient- and community-centered philosophy, PAMC also became involved in medical education. What had begun as a strictly clinical practice had morphed into a multifaceted organization with clinical, research, and educational arms. This diversification was embodied in a new structure, and in 1981 the Palo Alto Medical Foundation (PAMF) was born, encompassing health care, education, and research divisions.[11]

The leadership of PAMF came to recognize that without integrating hospital care into their system they couldn't provide the full spectrum of care, so in 1993 PAMF added the missing piece by affiliating with Sutter Health. The merger allowed it to offer—and maintain control over—medical care throughout the continuum of care, from the office to the hospital.[12] Since that time, the organization has continued to grow, acquiring new medical group practices and integrating them into PAMF, forming a coordinated, unified whole that benefits from a shared mission, extensive resources, and economies of scale. As of 2013, the entire system includes nearly 1,200 physicians. All told, its patients make just over 2.5 million visits a year.[13]

The latest branch of PAMF is the San Carlos Medical Center, the gleaming facility visible from Route 101 in Silicon Valley. In keeping with the high-tech environment where it's located, the building itself is environmentally sophisticated; PAMF was at pains to ensure that the $230 million multispecialty campus was built from locally harvested or recycled materials, and conformed to prevailing green standards. It's also a quintessentially Californian facility, featuring a roof garden covered with drought-resistant plants and irrigated with a high-efficiency drip system.

The four-story San Carlos Medical Center started out by hiring seventy-five physicians and, within a year after opening, its staff had doubled in size. In addition to its primary care center, with its twenty internists and family physicians, the facility includes an ambulatory surgery center where patients can undergo colonoscopies or have a cataract removed. It also houses a diagnostic imaging center where patients can have a CT scan or an MRI, a laboratory where they can have blood and other specimens processed, and an urgent care center where they can be evaluated between seven A.M. and nine P.M. seven days a week. Coming soon but not yet under construction is a ninety-four-bed hospital, to be fully owned and operated by the Palo Alto Medical Foundation.[14]

What this means for patients is one-stop shopping. They still have to get to the Center—there is ample parking and even a shuttle from the nearest train station—but once they've made the trip, they can see their primary care doctor or a specialist, get a test or have a procedure. They can even have their toenails cut in Podiatry, improve their mobility in Physical Therapy, learn about a special diet in Nutrition, or have their hearing tested in Audiology. For most geriatric patients, this arrangement works well, but for the frailest and the sickest, getting good care remains a challenge.

Geriatric Care at PAMF

Despite the impressive array of services offered by the San Carlos Center, several essential services are missing from the list. Many of them are available elsewhere in the PAMF system, and perhaps someday they will come to San Carlos if its population of older patients grows, but at present there is no neurologist or psychiatrist on staff. And it is neurologists and psychiatrists, more than any other physicians apart from geriatricians, who are likely to address the problems of dementia, depression, and delirium that are so common in older patients.

There are thirteen physicians on staff at PAMF whose practice is almost exclusively geriatric; another three are board certified in geriatrics but see themselves principally as family physicians, internists, or palliative care doctors. The geriatric group was initially set up to follow PAMF patients into nursing homes, and much of its work continues to be based at the eleven nursing homes in the PAMF orbit. The practice has grown to encompass outpatient geriatric consultation as well, a service offered in principle to all PAMF patients, though it is only available at select locations. But it doesn't include primary care geriatrics, and the consultative model falls short of true interdisciplinary comprehensive geriatric assessment.

Comprehensive Geriatric Assessment

The idea of geriatric assessment is simple: if primary care physicians don't routinely address quintessentially geriatric problems such as falls, cognitive impairment, and incontinence, and if they aren't likely to start paying attention to these matters any time soon, then the next best alternative is to send patients for geriatric consultation. Sometimes consultation just involves an examination by a physician who has extra training in geriatrics beyond the basics that all internists and family practitioners acquire in their residency programs. Ideally, the consultation takes the form of a multifaceted evaluation, typically involving a team of professionals rather than just a physician.

I have been a member of several different geriatric interdisciplinary teams, each with a slightly different composition, but usually the core includes a geriatrician, a nurse, and a mental health professional. Roughly speaking, the physician pays attention to diseases, medications, and "geriatric syndromes," conglomerations of symptoms that don't fit neatly into a single organ system.[15] The nurse—often a nurse practitioner—pays attention to function, to activities such as walking, seeing, and hearing. And the mental health worker— often a social worker but sometimes a nurse with behavioral health expertise or even a psychiatrist—explores family dynamics and looks for depression and dementia.

My initial role, as the team geriatrician, is to see if a patient has a geriatric syndrome. Delirium, for instance, is a classic geriatric syndrome. It strikes its victims suddenly, causing disorientation and inattentiveness, and it has a nasty tendency to fluctuate over the course of the day, abruptly getting much worse just after it seemed to be improving. It's not, strictly speaking, a neurologic problem, although diseases of the brain such as meningitis or stroke can cause delirium. It's not just an adverse drug reaction, although many different medications, including anti-anxiety drugs and anti-diarrheal agents, can produce delirium. Delirium may have many different causes, but each of those triggers, whether an infection, a chemical imbalance in the blood, or even severe constipation, results in a very similar picture.

The nurse then turns to function, to what the patient can do. It's this focus on function that distinguishes geriatric assessment from other holistic approaches to health care. For older patients, how they get along every day— whether they can walk or see or hear, and whether they can shower or dress themselves or make dinner—is at least as important as what diseases they have. Arguably, it's more important, since patients can often live quite comfortably with nasty sounding diseases such as breast cancer or prostate cancer, conditions that may never cause them problems during their lifetime, but when they have problems with function, they run into trouble in the here and now. Nurses will typically evaluate the "activities of daily living" (core functions such as dressing and bathing and eating) and the "independent activities of daily living" (more sophisticated functions such as cooking and shopping and handling finances).

The third component of comprehensive geriatric assessment is the psychological and psychosocial dimension. The mental health professional evaluates the older person's cognitive function and mood and looks into the environmental factors that influence those domains. Older people rarely exist in isolation: usually they have family or community supports. Even when they live alone, their physical surroundings affect both physical and mental functioning.

The physician then synthesizes the findings of the individual interdisciplinary team members and sends a report, together with recommendations, to the primary care or other referring physician. It is then typically up to that physician to act on the team's suggestions. When this evaluation is targeted to high-risk patients, and when primary care doctors follow the team's advice, patients are less likely to lose function or to become depressed.[16] For older patients who are not merely at risk of functional decline and hospitalization, but who also have a serious, life-limiting disease, palliative care is another alternative.

Caring for Patients near the End of Life at PAMF

Outpatient palliative care is unusual: most palliative care services are found in hospitals. In California, only 8 percent of acute care hospitals had an outpatient program in 2011.[17] However, PAMF, which has ten physicians on staff who are board certified in hospice and palliative medicine (three of whom combine geriatrics and palliative care), is an impressive outlier. But the service offered by PAMF is limited to selected sites and the San Carlos Center is not one of them—though in principle, patients can travel to a remote site for specialized care.

What PAMF provides for all its patients if they are sick enough, and if they're interested, is the Advanced Illness Management program (AIM), a service developed by Sutter Health, which merged with PAMF in 1993. Targeted to people in the last twelve months of life with two or more chronic conditions, AIM in Northern California uses a multidisciplinary team to provide support. Its explicit goal is to promote hospice enrollment, rather than to help patients choose whatever course makes most sense for them, which is the usual approach taken by palliative care teams. The way the program works is that a nurse or social worker goes to the home and does an assessment, and after the initial meeting primarily offers telephone advice, with occasional in-person visits in the office or the hospital. In fact, AIM is more of a transitional care program than an ongoing management service.[18]

Palliative Care

Palliative care burst onto the American medical scene as a new discipline in the last twenty years. The idea of providing supportive care to patients nearing the end of life has been around a good deal longer than that—in the Middle Ages, hospices were created for the dying, and Dame Cecily Saunders, a British physician and social worker, created the first modern hospice with the foundation of St. Christopher's in London in 1967. But in the United States, hospice and palliative medicine only became a recognized specialty, certified by the American Board of Medical Specialties, in 2006. And while palliative medicine includes hospice care, it is much more than that. Hospice care, as enshrined in the Medicare program, is an approach to care that focuses exclusively on comfort and is restricted to patients who will likely live no more than another six months. Palliative care is for patients with an advanced illness—and for their families. It offers management of symptoms—most serious, progressive illnesses are associated with pain, shortness of breath, nausea, or some other unpleasant symptom. It provides advance care planning—the team sits down with patients and families to discuss their options in light of the realities of their condition and their personal goals. And palliative care gives psychosocial support to both patients and families. Having a disease that is almost certainly fatal is not easy for patients or those who love them. It frequently leads to depression, anxiety, or, when patients and families disagree about strategy, to interpersonal conflict. Palliative care, like comprehensive geriatric assessment, is inherently interdisciplinary, with different team members taking on various responsibilities and working together to make those last weeks, months, or sometimes years of life as rewarding and meaningful as possible.

Palliative care is for younger as well as older people. But fortunately, the vast majority of individuals with serious, advanced illness are elderly: the thirty-five-year-old dying of cancer may be the poster child for palliative care, but the eighty-five-year-old with severe heart failure or advanced Alzheimer's disease is the more frequent client.

The field of palliative care has made the greatest inroads in the hospital. Hospital administrators increasingly recognize the potential financial as well as human value of a consultative service that often saves patients from unnecessary, burdensome, and expensive procedures in their dying days.[19] But it has an equally important role to play in the outpatient setting—before patients are hospitalized and subjected to the glittering array of modern technological tools. Office-based palliative care seems to improve the quality and sometimes even the quantity of life when it's delivered alongside conventional treatment. In one startling example, patients with the most common form of advanced lung cancer—a uniformly fatal condition with a very poor prognosis—but who saw a palliative care team in addition to their oncologist did better than their counterparts who were cared for only by the oncologist, even though they received many of the same chemotherapy drugs. Fewer of them were depressed and, on average, they lived two and a half months longer, a significant difference in the lung cancer world, where half of all patients die within a year.[20]

The secret of palliative care's success is uncertain. Some have speculated it's the "added layer of support" that patients with advanced illness get from the palliative care team. Others point to more vigorous treatment of depression. My personal suspicion is that it's not that palliative care prolongs life, but rather that usual care shortens life by encouraging patients to opt for last-ditch therapies that actually hurt more than they help. In the context of a relationship with a palliative care clinician, patients are more apt to forgo this sort of Hail Mary treatment. They realize that declining a toxic, risky drug isn't giving up or giving in—it's just rationally recognizing that the potential harms of treatment outweigh the remote chance of benefit.

Integrating Care: The Medical Home

At PAMF, only a small minority of patients will end up with geriatric or palliative care services. Everyone, however, has access to a whole host of specialists. But for older patients with multiple chronic medical problems, having access to different services is not good enough; the various clinicians have to communicate with each other to assure good quality care and avoid redundancy. The physical therapist has to know just what the orthopedist thought the patient's problem was in order to prescribe the optimal exercises. The rheumatologist has to have the most up-to-date medication list to choose the right drug for treating the patient's arthritis. The surgeon has to have access to the cardiologist's assessment to figure out whether the patient is eligible for a surgical procedure that would require general anesthesia. The primary way that PAMF promotes communication among physicians is through its electronic medical record; PAMF staff members have been using EPIC, the largest supplier of electronic medical records to outpatient practices, since 1999. But complex older patients need more—they need coordination and integration of services, and that is best achieved through use of a "Medical Home."

The idea of a single place or "home" that centralizes and coordinates all aspects of a patient's medical care, and that is comfortable and accessible, has been around for over fifty years. First designed to provide interdisciplinary team care to children with special needs, the model didn't catch on for vulnerable adults until the early 2000s. But recently, a group of professional physician societies banded together to issue a set of guiding principles for medical homes.

The guidelines are rigorous and they are tough to achieve. To qualify as a medical home, a primary care practice must offer comprehensive care (preventive care, treatment of acute illness, and management of chronic diseases); it must be patient-centered (attentive to the patient's family, culture, values, and preferences); it has to coordinate care (facilitating transitions and communication across multiple sites including the hospital, the skilled nursing facility, and other doctors' offices); it has to be accessible (not just with elevators and ramps but also by offering enhanced in-person hours, around-the-clock telephone access to a team member, and regular email communication); and it must demonstrate a commitment to safety and quality (demonstrated by the use of evidence-based medicine and clinical decision-support tools).[21]

While PAMF endorses the medical home concept and its Palo Alto site won the coveted certification, it's not clear how well the model is working. When Group Health in Washington and Idaho, another multispecialty group practice, studied whether the medical home idea worked in their system, they came up with some surprising results. In response to the new initiative, Group Health shrank the panel size of its participating physicians substantially, while simultaneously increasing both the time allocated for visits and that for coordinating care. As a result, patients were happier and quality improved with no major change in costs.[22] But the doctors found it hard to adjust to the patient-centered medical home. The approach challenged their basic philosophy of care. It required a cultural shift away from a physician-centered model, one that is set up for the convenience of the physician, to a patient-centered system, one that is meant to be user-friendly. The physicians at Group Health liked having more face time with patients. They appreciated having thirty-minute appointments rather than the rushed twenty-minute visits they were used to. But they were less enthusiastic about all the email exchanges they were suddenly expected to carry on with patients, and the evening and weekend hours they were supposed to offer. And they were not used to working as part of a team, sharing patient care responsibilities with a nurse or heeding the advice of a pharmacist.[23]

Making the Medical Home Work

To make the medical home model work, a practice needs to incorporate a true interdisciplinary team into routine care. A handful of practices have figured out how to do that. At Wishard Health Services in Indianapolis, Indiana, recently renamed Eskenazi Health after receiving a multimillion-dollar donation, physicians partnered with the geriatrics program of the Indiana University School of Medicine to form one of the most innovative and elaborate programs in the country. The GRACE model (an acronym for a cumbersome name, Geriatric Resources for Assessment and Care of Elders), specifically targeted to a low-income elderly population, makes use of two interdisciplinary teams: a core team composed of a nurse practitioner and a social worker; and an extended, supporting team that includes a pharmacist, a mental health specialist, and others.

The program starts out with a home visit by the core team to perform a comprehensive geriatric assessment. The team members attend to quintessentially geriatric concerns such as vision, hearing, gait, balance, and cognition. In addition to evaluating the patient and getting to know the family, they assess the home, looking for poor lighting, cluttered rooms, and slippery floors that may be hazardous for a frail older patient. The team doesn't just perform an assessment; it also meets with the patient's primary care physician to actually design a plan of care, a plan that takes into account the patient's health status, medical needs, resources, and preferences. Implementation of the plan entails a follow-up home visit and typically utilizes community services such as adult day care, home health aides, or transportation. The details of the care plan are entered into a web-based care management tracking tool to which all team members have access. The program works: when just under 1,000 high-risk older adults were randomized to the GRACE program or usual care, those in the intervention arm showed greater improvement in both general and mental health. In addition, already by the second year of the program, their emergency department visits and hospitalization rates were lower than among patients getting standard medical care.[24]

Several other programs throughout the country offer promise in addition to GRACE, which is available only in Indiana.[25] Guided Care, originally designed and tested at Johns Hopkins University Medical School in Maryland, uses a nurse as the linchpin for numerous services, including comprehensive assessment, ongoing monitoring of chronic diseases, care coordination, transitional care, and coaching for self-management. The approach has spread to a number of communities. However, while patients who participate in the program report that it delivers a higher quality of care than conventional medical practices, the program does not appear to lead to lower emergency department visits or hospitalization rates.[26]

As of 2012, only 10 percent of medical practices in the United States had applied for accreditation and been certified as medical homes.[27] Even fewer medical practices offer longitudinal home care—more than just a single home visit followed by telephone management. But home-based primary care, with doctors who make house calls, is just what the frailest of the frail need.

Home Visits

Back in 1930, fully 40 percent of all physician visits took place in the home; by 1950, the rate was down to 10 percent, and by 1980 it had fallen to 1 percent. Recent increases in Medicare reimbursement for home visits have led to a rise in the number of such visits: in 2009, Medicare was billed for 2.3 million visits. But most doctors don't make any house calls at all, and those who do typically make between one and two house calls per year.[28] Most home visits occur within a special home care program, many of them part of the Veterans Administration (VA) medical system. Patients who are fortunate enough to be able to participate in such a program are the lucky ones.

The VA Connecticut Healthcare System set up such a "Home-Based Primary Care Program" for vets with disabilities, frailty, or dementia for whom travel to the local VA hospital's outpatient department had become too burdensome. Anna Reisman is one physician who was attracted to the home care model. She had been practicing office-based primary care, also in the VA health care system, until she was too fed up to continue. Her motivation wasn't that she didn't like primary care: she delighted in "fixing one man's dizziness" and helping someone else "give up a fifty-year smoking habit." It wasn't that she didn't like her patients; they were a diverse and complicated group, and both she and they shed lots of tears when she announced she was leaving the practice.

It wasn't even that she didn't like the system within which she practiced. The VA office system was pretty good, with its best-in-the-country electronic medical record and the many services it provided for patients, including reasonably priced prescription medications. She enjoyed working in a single-payer system (the VA is the only major segment of American health care that is truly government-run), so she didn't have to deal with multiple insurance companies and complicated billing procedures. Dr. Reisman simply reached a point where she felt the practice was becoming impossible, despite the VA offering a unique combination of "cutting edge medicine" and "small town practice." She had to write down a diagnosis and a special identifying code for every visit, which she found increasingly arcane and arduous as the number of codes proliferated. She felt oppressed by the amount of time she spent on the phone, writing follow-up letters, and responding to the endless electronic reminders to screen for depression, to administer a flu shot, or to refer a patient to a podiatrist. Her job was encroaching on her life: she was regularly late picking her children up from their after school program and, in the evenings, when she should have been having family time, she often sat down at her computer and spent a few hours finishing her chart notes and other business.

In the Home-Based Primary Care Program, by contrast, Dr. Reisman has the support she needs to take care of patients. She works with a multidisciplinary team that includes a nurse, a social worker, a physical therapist, and various other professionals such as a pharmacist. She can take all the time that she needs to see her patients at home.[29] And if she's anything like other geriatricians who practice home-based medicine, she will find that the number of trips her patients make to the emergency department and the number of hospitalizations they experience fall dramatically, while patient outcomes improve and satisfaction increases. In one study of over 700 high-risk elders enrolled in a home visit program matched to over 2,000 controls of similar age, cognitive status, degree of frailty, race, and gender who received conventional medical care, the two groups were comparable in terms of mortality but the home care patients had fewer hospitalizations and substantially lower Medicare costs—the program saved an average of nearly $8,500 per patient.[30]

The Wide World of Multispecialty Group Practices

The Palo Alto Medical Foundation is not the only large multispecialty group practice in the United States, nor was it the first. That distinction goes to the Mayo Clinic, established in the late 1880s in the small town of Rochester, Minnesota. According to legend, William Worrall Mayo and his two sons, Charlie and Will, would have been quite happy to continue their small town medical practice in Rochester if the area hadn't been struck by a tornado in 1889.

The tornado devastated the community, killing and injuring dozens. The Mayos did their best to treat the victims but could offer little more than first aid since the town had no hospital and no way to transport patients to the nearest hospital in a safe and timely way. Responding to the tragedy, the founder of the local Sisters of Saint Francis made a proposal to the older Dr. Mayo: she would raise the money to build a hospital in Rochester if Dr. Mayo agreed to run it once it was built. Mother Alfred was evidently a persuasive and persistent woman—she wore down Dr. Mayo's resistance and, that same year, the forty-five-bed St. Mary's Hospital opened its doors. Initially, it was primarily a surgical facility, reflecting both the town's needs and the Mayo family's area of expertise. But increasingly, Dr. Mayo senior came to believe that the only way to provide first-rate care to patients in an era of expanding medical knowledge was to offer multiple specialties under one roof. The Mayos brought on additional partners, and in 1914 opened a new building with offices, exam rooms, and laboratories to complement the inpatient facility.[31] The Mayo model would always be firmly linked to hospital care and would boast a strong surgical component, but it would also become synonymous with innovative, multispecialty care.

Other multispecialty groups grew up elsewhere the country, including the Lahey Clinic in Massachusetts, the Marshfield Clinic in Wisconsin, and the Geisinger Health System in Pennsylvania. Some of these practices were built on a radically different model from either PAMF or the Mayo Clinic. Kaiser Permanente, for example, was from its inception both a health insurance company and a provider of health services. Kaiser had its roots in the Mojave Desert of California, where Dr. Sidney Garfield offered medical care to workers building an aqueduct in the early 1930s. Unfortunately, the workers were ill-equipped to pay for much needed medical services and the practice was on the verge of going under when Dr. Garfield came up with a novel and, as it turned out, life-saving scheme. He proposed to an area insurance company that they set up a system that would guarantee workers medical care in exchange for a small fee to be deducted from each paycheck. The scheme was so successful that the industrialist Henry Kaiser asked Dr. Garfield to replicate the model for workers on the Grand Coulee Dam project in the state of Washington. He went on to offer the same service to shipyard workers during the Second World War. When, after the war, those same workers wanted to continue the plan even after they had stopped building ships and moved on to other jobs, Garfield agreed to open the plan to the public and Kaiser Permanente was born.[32]

Today's Kaiser is an umbrella organization for the Kaiser Foundation Health Plan (the insurance component), the Permanente Medical Groups (where patients pay a fixed monthly fee to receive all-inclusive medical care), and the Kaiser Foundation Hospitals (where enrollees receive medical care from Kaiser Permanente physicians). Like PAMF and the Mayo Clinic, Kaiser is a large, multispecialty group practice. Like them, it engages in research and educational activities designed to study and teach its model of care. But unlike the others, it is also a prepaid health plan. Kaiser Permanente as of 2014 has just over ten million members, with sites in eight states and the District of Columbia, though over one-fourth of its members belong to one of several California plans. It has close to 18,000 physicians and 50,000 nurses and operates 38 hospitals, generating total revenues of $56.4 billion.[33]

Despite the considerable growth of each of the pioneer multispecialty group practices, and even with the appearance of new exemplars of this mode of health care delivery such as the academically affiliated Harvard Community Health Plan in the Boston area in the 1960s, and the religiously affiliated DuPage Medical Group in the Chicago area in the 1990s, they constitute a minority of practices. As of 2014, approximately one-fourth of all physicians work in such groups.

Does Practice Site Matter for Geriatric Patients?

There is a great deal in between the solo practice or small, single-specialty group, and the large, multispecialty group practice. And yet, they all have much in common: they feature short visits in a building that patients often must drive to; the focus of the visits is on the functioning of the various organ systems; they use electronic medical records; and they start with measuring vital signs and taking a brief history, and end with an order for blood tests and x-rays along with a prescription for a medication.

For the frailest of the frail and the oldest of the old, none of these arrangements work very well. The ideal would be medical care at home provided by a team composed of a physician, nurse practitioner, social worker, and sometimes a physical therapist or nutritionist. Next best is a single health center that provides all the services the geriatric patient needs—and a good way of getting back and forth from that centralized location. Wherever care is delivered, it has to be coordinated and integrated, so if the patient does end up in the hospital or the SNF, the physician taking care of them, if it's someone other than the primary care doctor, has to communicate with the regular physician. In addition to coordination and interdisciplinary care, frail geriatric patients need a plan of care that is tailored to their particular conditions, physical, mental, and social, a plan that takes into account their preferences, their resources, and the supports available in their community. Only rarely does an outpatient practice conform to this model.

Most medical practices, regardless of size, ownership, reimbursement, and structure, deviate substantially from the geriatric ideal, although the multi-specialty group practice comes closest. But generally, the various types of office practice are remarkably similar in what they do offer. The reason they are more alike than different is that they are all influenced by the same forces—the hospital, Medicare, pharmaceutical companies, and device manufacturers, as well as physicians and patients themselves. To a great extent, it is these external agents that shape what doctors do when they meet with a patient in the office, what tests they order, what specialists they refer to, what drugs they prescribe, and even what subjects they do—or don't—discuss with their patients.

CHAPTER THREE

From the Outside In

For four years, medical school steeped me in evidence-based medicine. I learned about the merits of double-blind, controlled randomized trials—and the weaknesses of observational studies. I came to understand that to shine on rounds in the hospital wards, I needed to cite data and quote the "medical literature," as journal articles are known, though they are decidedly not literary. I was told that medicine was a science and that treatments should be subjected to rigorous testing to determine if they work. And then for three years of residency in internal medicine, when I was supposedly learning how to be a real doctor, my teachers continued to promulgate evidence-based medicine in lectures and at the bedside, even while much of the day-to-day learning was far more practical and of the "see one, do one, teach one" variety.

After eight years of education and training—following residency I spent a year doing a geriatrics fellowship—I was ready to enter the office practice of medicine. Armed with theoretical knowledge from medical school, applied knowledge from residency, and the ability to critically evaluate new information and, if it passed muster, integrate it into practice, I accepted my first job—as a primary care physician at Bunker Hill Health Center, a neighborhood clinic. I was pretty certain that I knew exactly what I was supposed to do in order to be a good doctor, not that I thought it would be easy or that I was confident I actually would be able to function well without the constant camaraderie of the hospital. Even in a group practice, where there are always colleagues down the hall, outpatient medicine is mainly a solitary pursuit. It's all about the interaction between the doctor and the patient, with no supervising senior physician to check up on what's happening in the privacy of the office. But I knew the drill. I subscribed to the *New England Journal of Medicine*, and eagerly looked forward to Thursdays when it arrived at my doorstep. I would scan the table of contents, then read the abstracts of the most interesting articles and decide which ones to read more carefully. I also subscribed to the *Annals of Internal Medicine*, which at the time came out monthly, and also, because I needed to keep up with my field of specialization, the *Journal of the American Geriatrics Society*. Every year I went to the national meeting of the American Geriatrics Society plus a few day-long courses or seminars on a topic of interest. Later, I would also have resources such as the spectacularly successful *UpToDate*, a continuously updated on-line textbook that helps doctors remain current.

My assumption was that, whatever I learned from all this reading, studying, and listening to lectures, together with what I already knew from medical school, residency, and a fellowship, would determine what went on between me and my patients in the office. And I imagined that what happened in my office would be very much like what was happening in every other doctor's office. After all, physicians are generally conscientious, dedicated professionals, and we all go through the same kind of extensive, rigorous training. I wasn't entirely wrong about this and I was definitely correct that everything I did would evolve over time. What tests I ordered and what medications I prescribed, what conditions I screened for and what preventive strategies I advocated, would all change. One reason for the changes would be the appearance of new evidence, ideally one of those randomized, double-blind controlled studies that was published in a distinguished, peer-reviewed journal like the *New England Journal of Medicine.* What I didn't appreciate when I started out, though I learned quite quickly, was that all kinds of factors other than scientific evidence determine what goes on in the doctor's office. I had no idea, and I doubt patients do either, that what I would spend time discussing with patients—their blood pressure, their blood sugar, getting a flu shot—would largely be shaped by the demands of the Medicare program. I didn't anticipate that what body parts I examined or tests I ordered would be dictated by an electronic medical record that would hound me to check off particular boxes depending on what disease I listed as the reason for my patient's visit. I didn't realize that how long I would spend with patients or whether I sent them to a nurse practitioner would be influenced by Medicare reimbursement rates. I had no idea that the medications I would find myself prescribing might have more to do with what drugs are on the hospital formulary than what I thought was best for my patient. And I was naively unaware of the influence of drug companies and insurers, as well as the hospital and device manufacturers, on the practice of medicine.

How Physicians Shape the Office Practice of Medicine

The number one source of satisfaction for physicians continues to be doing a good job taking care of patients.[1] But physicians are human. We have preferences, tastes about what we like most and what we like least about our work. We are concerned with our quality of life, and with the impact our work has on the rest of our lives. And we are interested in assuring that we have a good standard of living, which means that we do pay attention to remuneration. While not all physicians share the same tastes, the same understanding of what determines our quality of life, or the same view of how much income is appropriate or sufficient, certain strong preferences have shaped or at least influenced the way office medicine is practiced.

Consider taste: what kinds of medical problems do physicians find most rewarding to take care of? Clearly, there is tremendous variability: what Intensive Care Unit (ICU) specialists, or "intensivists," find challenging is caring for complex, tremendously sick patients who depend on a variety of life supports. I find such patients intimidating and prefer talking to patients with advanced illness about their goals of care *before* they become acutely ill. But, in the primary care setting, it's common for physicians to want some kind of intellectual excitement and that doesn't come from handling minor medical problems such as a viral upper respiratory infection or vaginitis, however bothersome these are to patients. Patients may find their hemorrhoids more disturbing than their elevated blood sugar level, since hemorrhoids hurt while high blood sugar does not, but the physician's perspective is that the former are a minor nuisance and the latter is a serious threat to health. Primary care doctors tend not to like dealing with problems we cannot do much about, which means that chronic low back pain or insomnia are not our favorite symptoms. We also don't much care for problems we know little about, which for many general internists include incontinence and cognitive impairment. And while physicians tend to like solving puzzles, we are not so excited about complex patients with multiple chronic conditions, even when they present a diagnostic dilemma. Few patients engender a greater sense of dread than the eighty-year-old who shows up with not one or two, but three or even four "chief complaints" for a four-thirty or five o'clock appointment after a long day in the office.

There's another dimension of what makes physicians satisfied, and that relates to our work environment. Physicians generally want to devote the time we are at work to practicing medicine, not to performing administrative responsibilities or carrying out the business side of medicine. We want a pleasant, collegial atmosphere with sufficient support staff so we can focus on the parts of medicine we find rewarding: diagnosing and treating disease. That means we like having a medical assistant to weigh patients and check their vital signs, an administrative assistant to book follow-up appointments, a nurse to administer flu shots, and a care coordinator to interface with the myriad of community service providers involved in a modern patient's care.

In addition to caring about the health and well-being of patients, we physicians also care about our own well-being, our personal quality of life. The truth is that physicians have always cared about their own lives—tales from another era of the selfless physician who worked night and day for his patients simply reflect the ideals of a good life in another time. What it means to lead a good life today is a bit different. As more and more women with young children go into primary care, a good life increasingly means having controllable work hours. It means keeping night call to a minimum, having few weekend responsibilities, and avoiding unpredictable hospital rounds. And it's not just women who define their quality of life in terms of "work-life balance"; men also want to have the opportunity to devote their time to things outside of medicine. Some of them are married to high-powered lawyers or tech workers at start-up companies, wives who expect them to share in child-rearing responsibilities.

Then there's money. By the beginning of the fourth year of medical school, students have to decide where to apply for post-graduate training, for residency. That means first deciding what specialty is most appealing. I couldn't imagine going into surgery, for example: I didn't have the dexterity or the visuospatial skills to remember the requisite anatomy, and I preferred my patients to be awake and talking, not anesthetized and unresponsive. I didn't much care for taking care of very sick children, either—the prospect of a child dying was too overwhelming for me. Radiology was out for some of the same reasons as surgery: I didn't have the right kind of mind to imagine how two-dimensional images corresponded to actual pathological processes, and I wanted to interact with patients, not just with pictures of their insides. The list went on: I didn't have a taste for dermatology, with its rashes and its lumps and bumps; pathology was a kind of cross between surgery and radiology. What was left, what made most sense to me, was internal medicine. Further specialization, choosing cardiology or hematology or, in my case, geriatrics, would come later.

For many of my peers, the choice of a specialty isn't just dictated by personal preferences, it also reflects earning potential. The vast majority of students graduating from medical school these days are faced with sizable debts—81 percent of 2015 graduates owed an average of $172,751, which was a combination of medical school and undergraduate college loans.[2] This mammoth debt burden surely plays some role in guiding students' choice of specialty. Orthopedists (the top of the scale) earn $421,000 a year, compared to $243,000 for a medical specialty such as nephrology, and contrasted with a low of $195,000 for family physicians.[3] Not surprisingly, medical students are strongly influenced in their specialty choice by personal preference and quality of life concerns—but students choosing high earning, non–primary care careers tend to face greater debt and to place a greater premium on higher earnings than their counterparts selecting primary care medicine.[4]

Most physicians don't think they should make more money than they do—with the possible exception of those at the lowest end of the income spectrum such as geriatricians, and a few outliers who are hopelessly greedy. Nonetheless, physicians do worry about the very real possibility that our incomes will fall. Many doctors fear that their practice will have trouble collecting co-pays and deductibles from patients. They worry about the rising cost of just doing business; the median cost of personnel (including information technology support) is a staggering $52,000 for each full-time doctor employed by the practice.[5] They are anxious about an audit—Medicare has been known to retroactively demand a refund, or even levy a fine, when an audit reveals that doctors charged Medicare either too much or too little for a visit, in light of the information contained in the record.

To promote optimal billing, many physician practices have adopted the use of an electronic medical record (EMR). These EMR systems typically have built-in templates for documenting the patient's history, the review of systems, and the physical exam. This makes it easy to record all kinds of "negative" findings that were not terribly important in the physician's evaluation but that allow additional "elements" to be counted up. It's simple to say that the skin appeared normal, with no rashes or unusual pallor, and that the patient's psychiatric status was normal, with no confusion or worrisome behaviors, even if neither the dermatologic system nor the psychiatric system was specifically and deliberately examined. All the physician needs to do is to be aware of the patient's face and demeanor and to check off the relevant boxes. The approach works—to boost revenue. Over the period 2001–10, physicians consistently used billing codes associated with high levels of reimbursement, though there is no evidence that patients had gotten sicker, resulting in upwards of $11 billion in additional fees.[6] The net effect for patients is that doctors spend an ever-growing proportion of what's supposed to be face-to-face time with patients glued to their computer screens, fanatically checking off boxes.

Perhaps the most extreme way that physicians shape the office practice of medicine is by leaving primary care altogether. High on the list of what physicians dislike most about medical practice, whether they work in a rural or an urban area, whether they are part of a large, multispecialty practice or they work in a small, single-specialty group, are the administrative burdens.[7] Physicians don't like getting "prior authorization" before prescribing a medication, but for one out of five of the brand-name medicines covered by Medicare Part D, we are required to explain in writing why only this medication and no other will do. Physicians dislike the countless forms to fill out for the Visiting Nurse Association, testifying that the patient is under a physician's care, confirming the patient's medications, and verifying that the patient is homebound.

Perhaps most annoying and intrusive of all the administrative responsibilities is the electronic medical record. Electronic medical records were supposed to save time, among other virtues, and, as indicated above, they are welcomed by physicians as a way to optimize billing. But using the electronic medical record turns out to increase the time spent documenting what happened during a visit.[8] The net effect of all these requirements is that physicians spend about one-sixth of their work day on administrative tasks. Professional satisfaction, however, turns out to be inversely proportional to the time spent on paperwork.[9] As a result, just under half of all practicing physicians say they plan to take steps to reduce patient access to their services, either by cutting back on the number of patients in their practice, retiring, closing their practice to new patients, or looking for nonclinical employment.[10]

The attitudes, wants, and needs of physicians influence the nature of the office practice of medicine. But some of the other influences on physician behavior, in particular the administrative requirements that are causing some physicians to shy away from primary care, have nothing to do with what physicians enjoy. They are external to physicians. And looming large among those influences is the Medicare program.

Medicare and the Office Visit

Medicare used to care mainly about hospital care—acute illness is what Medicare was designed from the outset to pay for, and most very sick people are cared for in the hospital, or at least that was the usual practice in 1965. In those days, patients stayed in the hospital until they were well enough to go home, with office-based medical care playing only a minimal role in treating their illness. Once chronic disease surpassed acute illness as the major source of both morbidity and costs among older people—in 2010, 68 percent of Medicare recipients had two or more chronic diseases and 37 percent had at least four[11]—much of the care of illness shifted from the hospital to the office and the skilled nursing facility. Nearly 30 percent of every dollar spent on the health care of older people goes to ambulatory care, whether it's spent in the office or in the hospital outpatient clinic, and whether it goes to primary care physicians (only a small piece does) or to the tests they order and the referrals they make. In light of the growing emphasis on the outpatient sector, Medicare began to wonder whether physicians in the office were providing "high value care." And when researchers at Dartmouth showed that primary care doctors vary considerably in the way they treat patients,[12] and that these differences cannot be attributed solely to differences in the patients' severity of illness, Medicare began to suspect that they were not.

At just about the same time that the Centers for Medicare and Medicaid Services (CMS), the agency that runs the Medicare program, became concerned with quality, it also got interested in saving money by improving efficiency. And one source of inefficiency was the needless duplication of tests that took place because physicians had no good way to communicate with each other. The office physician who ordered a chest x-ray for a patient with a cough and a fever, diagnosed pneumonia and sent the patient to the hospital for treatment, couldn't share the x-ray with the emergency room physician who evaluated the patient for admission. Medicare's solution to rooting out redundancy was the electronic medical record. The agency that recommends policy changes for the Medicare program suggested that maybe Medicare could kill two birds with one stone. Maybe EMRs, which physicians were already beginning to use in order to optimize billing and communicate with other physicians, were the key both to preventing excess test ordering *and* to promoting quality.

The way that Medicare pushes physicians in the office setting to use an EMR is straightforward—the agency reimburses more generously for their services if they have an EMR and, commencing in 2015, penalizes them if they don't. But to affect quality, Medicare does more than merely encourage physicians to use an electronic record; it prods them to use it in a clinically productive way. "Meaningful use," rather than merely "use" has come to determine reimbursement. Elaborate regulations now define what constitutes meaningful use. Reviewing the patient's medications at each visit—even if the patient was seen the previous day by the same physician—is an example of meaningful use. So, too, is providing an "after visit summary," a piece of paper for the patient to take along that summarizes what the doctor regards as the high points of the visit.

Medicare has also learned the hard way that it needs to scrutinize what goes on in the office to avoid fraud—with so much money being paid out by Medicare, there's a risk that a few bad apples will manipulate the system to their own financial advantage. Sometimes this involves flagrantly illegal behavior, such as billing for services that were never provided. Sometimes it is more subtle and entails systematically billing at a higher rate than is justified. In an effort to be fair and to reward physicians for "cognitive" work as well as for procedures, but also to protect against fraud, Medicare came up with an elaborate scheme for measuring the value of physician services—and for paying accordingly. Translating that system into practice requires that physicians go through a complicated exercise to figure out how much to bill for a visit— and to be sure they have recorded enough information to justify their conclusion. The way this works is that patients are separated into two groups: new patients and established patients. Then, the visit is broken down into three components—the history, the examination, and medical decision making— and a point system is used to grade the complexity of each of these elements. These "evaluation and management" codes are periodically revised and a new rate scale is set every year.[13] Using this system correctly places yet another administrative burden on physicians, an obstacle in the way of their spending more time interacting with patients instead of computers.

The newest development from CMS that affects office practice is its effort to incentivize physicians to promote "value" rather than volume. For a long time, physicians have been accustomed to seeing their income rise or fall depending on their "productivity," on the number of patients they see. But today their earnings are influenced by how closely they achieve a set of "benchmarks" established by organizations such as the independent, not-for-profit National Quality Forum and adopted by Medicare. These benchmarks, also called "quality indicators," directly affect what happens to patients, whether in a multispecialty group practice or in solo practice. My father-in-law had no idea why his doctor kept worrying about his blood sugar since, as far as he knew, he was not and had never been a diabetic. He didn't realize that an entire set of quality measures is devoted to recommended interventions for diabetic patients: checking their cholesterol, checking for protein in the urine, monitoring how well their blood sugar is controlled by ordering a test called the Hemoglobin A1c, and keeping their blood pressure down. Because he had once been labeled diabetic—because of a single abnormal blood sugar measured while he had been very ill in the hospital—diabetes was on his problem list, and all those quality indicators applied to him.

Medicare's focus on value seems like a good idea, an idea that should improve the quality of care delivered to older patients. Maybe it will have the desired effect, but at a cost: instead of just driving out poor care, it fosters the tendency to order tests patients don't need or expensive medications when cheaper ones would do, and supports an elaborate value-oriented system that may result in physicians neglecting those aspects of care that do matter to patients but that Medicare doesn't currently regard as a priority, such as functional assessment and advance care planning.[14] Other approaches intended to improve the quality of outpatient care, such as education around medication usage, likewise seem reasonable, but in the hands of the pharmaceutical industry, they may take on a different hue.

Pharma and the Office

My father-in-law was not Big Pharma's favorite sort of patient: he was among the small minority of older patients who took only two prescription medications, both of them for his blood pressure. His blood pressure was difficult to control, however, so there was always the possibility that one day his doctor would try him on one of the newer, more expensive blood pressure medications in the hope of finally achieving more consistently good levels. To boost the odds of that happening, the major drug companies—all of which have at least one blood pressure–lowering medication in their armamentarium—wanted to be absolutely sure that both Saul and his doctor knew all about their products. There was also the distinct possibility that, sooner or later, Saul would develop another problem amenable to drug treatment. He did, after all, still have diabetes on his problem list. The drug companies could hope that one day he would qualify for a medication to lower his sugar—the threshold for what counted as diabetes has been dropping, much like the criterion for what counts as high blood pressure. And, as an octogenarian, Saul was at risk of all kinds of other problems, from arthritis to Alzheimer's disease. No harm teaching him a little about what was available, just in case.

Traditionally, the way that pharmaceutical manufacturers have gotten the word out about their drugs is through advertising to physicians, and outpatient doctors have been a prime target. After all, while a substantial volume of drugs is used in hospitals and nursing facilities, the majority are prescribed by doctors in their offices. For years, pharmaceutical companies invested a great deal of money in sending what they call pharmaceutical sales representatives, and everyone else calls drug reps, to peddle their wares to physicians. They still do, though not to the same extent as previously. In 2014, 63,000 drug reps made direct pitches to physicians, down considerably from the peak of drug company detailing in 2007, when there were 105,000 reps and the pharmaceutical industry spent a total of $14.5 billion on marketing in the United States, with roughly one-third of that amount on detailing.[15] The script is different from what it once was—less aggressive, less focused on explicitly urging physicians to prescribe whatever drug they are selling, and more oriented to providing information, to supplying educational materials for patients.[16] But the intent is unchanged—to sell pills by influencing physician practice. And in some ways, the outpatient setting is more important than ever: hospitals increasingly restrict the prescribing choices of the physicians on their staff by limiting the "formulary," the drugs available to inpatients.[17]

When I first started out in medical practice in the 1980s, the pharmaceutical industry regularly paid physicians to attend conferences held in exotic locations, including conferences of dubious educational value, and made a habit of wining and dining physicians at fancy restaurants, speaking to them about the virtues of their latest would-be blockbuster over dessert. But outspoken critics such as Jerry Kassirer, the former editor in chief of the *New England Journal of Medicine* and author of *On the Take*, gradually changed this behavior.[18] State laws have put a stop to many such activities and have introduced public disclosure requirements. As a result, drug companies have increasingly adopted new strategies, tactics that have the potential to directly influence patients' experience when they go to the doctor.

The first of these new approaches, direct-to-consumer advertising, isn't so new any longer but it's been growing twice as fast as advertising targeting physicians. Direct-to-consumer advertising first appeared on the scene in the 1980s, but with the recent emphasis on patients' involvement in their own medical care, its popularity has soared.[19] When the FDA began regulating the advertising of prescription medications in 1969, it took for granted that such advertising would be directed toward physicians. They were, after all, the ones with the power of the pen. And, in most other countries of the world, with the exception of New Zealand, advertising directly to patients is illegal. The uniquely American conception of free speech, along with the generally permissive attitude toward large corporations, have made this form of advertising extremely attractive.

The most recent wrinkle in direct-to-consumer advertising is what the industry calls "point of care marketing." In this variant, the drug companies capitalize on the fact that patients typically spend time sitting in a waiting room before they see their physician. What they do while they wait, according to a recent study, is watch television. The drug companies have responded by putting their own infomercials on the large flat screen TVs increasingly found in physician waiting areas—along with leaving "informational brochures" prominently displayed in doctors' offices. Since 2010, the money spent on this kind of advertising in doctors' offices, hospitals, and drugstores has grown at a rate of 10 percent a year, reaching $400 million in 2014.[20] The drug companies are quite happy for patients to believe that their physicians have endorsed whatever is being advertised. What they hope will happen, and what evidently does happen, is that patients march into the office and request the latest miracle drug they learned about while they waited.

Pharmaceutical companies also hope to hook patients on a particular brand by giving out free samples, and it's physicians in their offices who get the samples to distribute. The idea is simple: the physician wants to prescribe a new medication. It's possible that after the patient has been on the medicine for a few days, he will develop a side effect and have to stop the drug. Or when he goes back to the doctor for a blood pressure check—assuming the new medication is a blood pressure pill—he'll discover that the medicine wasn't working. In either case, he'll then start yet another medication, which he will have to pay for out-of-pocket (if his insurance doesn't cover drugs) or with a co-pay (if it does). With a free sample, a week or a month's worth of pills, he won't have to pay up front for the trial and error process. But if the pills do work and they don't cause any side effects then, of course, both the patient and the doctor will want to continue that particular medicine, even if in the long run it is a more expensive and not necessarily more effective option. That, of course, is precisely why the drug company handed out free samples in the first place.

Drug companies have another ingenious strategy for influencing physician prescribing. Instead of elbowing their way into the doctor's office and using a hard sell, a technique that has faded in popularity as physicians have come to recognize that they are being conned—pharmaceutical reps are now often barred from the office entirely—the companies supply physicians with educational pamphlets for their patients. They position themselves as "partnering" with doctors to produce better clinical outcomes by promoting patient engagement in their own health care—and who could argue with that strategy? To demonstrate their commitment to patient education, they give out brochures that summarize the latest national recommendations for achieving the ideal cholesterol level, or the optimal blood pressure, or the perfect blood sugar level. And there's no reason why they shouldn't include data on their own products, studies that happen to show that their drug will work well to achieve the best possible numbers. If patients don't want to watch the infomercials on the screen while they wait for their physician, they can read the educational materials supplied by the drug company instead. The end result: physicians are happy because they have information to provide to their patients, patients are happy because they have an easy way to become informed, and the drug companies are happy because sales for their products rise.

Office medicine revolves to a remarkable degree around prescribing pills. Patients go in expecting to get medicine for whatever ails them and they come out with a prescription. The medications that older people take—and they take a great many of them—form a central part of their medical care. And just which medications they take is sometimes determined by what medications were initiated in the hospital. But the hospital cares about more of what happens in the office than just the prescription of medications.

The Hospital and Outpatient Care

Hospitals have always understood that they need outpatient physicians. They depend on them to refer patients to their emergency departments and sub-specialty clinics, to send them for complex procedures and tests, and to admit them to their beds for surgery or for the diagnosis and treatment of serious medical problems. Moreover, hospitals have always had relationships with primary care physicians; they've given them "privileges," or the right to admit patients to the hospital, and they've discharged patients to their care. But only in the relatively recent past, with growing competition among hospitals for business and with shrinking profit margins, have hospitals begun cultivating those relationships with a vengeance.

Perhaps the simplest—and most draconian—way that hospitals have gone about cultivating relationships with primary care doctors is to buy up their practices. The practices then serve as feeders for hospital services, ranging from x-rays in the hospital's radiology suite, to procedures in the catheterization lab, to inpatient care. As a result, an increasing number of physicians work in an environment in which the hospital has an ownership stake in the practice. My father-in-law Saul went to Dr. Walker Wilson who was a partner in a group practice that was "affiliated" with the local community hospital, where affiliated is a euphemism for partial ownership. In return, Dr. Wilson and the others in his group were able to rent space in a building owned by the hospital; they were able to use the hospital's billing system (which, for Saul, just meant more incomprehensible charges). Even the Palo Alto Medical Clinic (later the Palo Alto Medical Foundation), which for the first fifty years of its existence was solely a medical group practice, recognized that both its physicians and its patients would benefit from a tight hospital affiliation and therefore decided in 1993 to merge with Sutter Health, owner and operator at the time of thirty-four hospitals. All told, as many as 42 percent of all physicians practice as salaried employees of a hospital system, up from less than a quarter in 2004.[21]

Academic hospitals, those with residency programs that train young doctors, need sites where those doctors can see patients. Since the time of the earliest residencies, established one hundred years ago, the hospital has served as the primary locus for teaching physicians. Patients are concentrated in hospitals, where they are generally quite sick and where they form a captive audience. Initially, they were also the "deserving poor," patients receiving charity care—wealthier patients were generally cared for at home—who, by the mores of the time, were obligated to allow the hospital that cared for them to use them as teaching material.[22] For the last several decades, as hospital stays have shortened, more and more medical care has moved to the outpatient setting. With the switch has come a recognition that physicians in training need to learn how best to care for patients in the office, and how to diagnose and treat illness even when the patient is not constantly under the watchful eye of doctors and nurses. That implies that hospitals, the organizational home of residency programs, need to find outpatient practices in which their trainees can evaluate and manage patients longitudinally. Traditionally, the hospital's ambulatory clinic has served this function, but internal medicine and family medicine residencies have increasingly looked for more diverse training opportunities. Practices such as Dr. Wilson's—a private group practice just down the street from a community teaching hospital—suddenly became very attractive as potential teaching sites.

Primary care doctors, too, are generally pleased to partner with a teaching hospital to teach residents. Having a resident in the practice, even temporarily, means another pair of hands to take care of patients. It means the opportunity to teach, which for many primary care physicians constitutes a welcome diversion from their daily routine. Teaching isn't for everyone, however, and it can be a time sink, particularly if the resident is weak or just a beginner and in need of extensive supervision. For the patient, having a doctor in training along with the regular physician may result in more time and attention, and in having two minds thinking about his medical problems instead of one very busy mind. But sometimes the arrangement is merely disruptive, interfering further with the already fragmented and frayed doctor-patient relationship.

While the hospital's interest in the office practice of medicine grew because it is a source of patients and a site for teaching, the concern with what transpires in the examining room did not—until very recently. The Affordable Care Act (ACA) of 2010 gave hospitals a new incentive to pay attention to what exactly physicians *do* with their patients in the previously sacrosanct office. The ACA achieved this feat by encouraging the formation of a new organizational entity in health care, the Accountable Care Organization. An ACO is a loose affiliation among various health care providers, typically including hospitals and physician practices, that have an economic incentive to work together to treat an individual patient across all care settings, including the doctor's office, the hospital, and the skilled nursing facility. The way this works in the Medicare context is typically that the providers sign a "risk-bearing contract": they continue to be paid by Medicare for each service provided, in accordance with the traditional fee-for-service model, but they share in any savings they generate over a pre-specified target. These extra payments, in essence bonuses, are contingent on the group's performing well on a variety of quality indicators.

Patients in the first few generations of ACOs didn't enroll the same way they signed up for a Medicare Advantage Plan (a capitated version of Medicare, subcontracted to private health insurance companies, that combines parts A, B, and often D into a single plan). Instead, physician practices and hospitals band together to form an ACO and then notify their patients that they are now, by default, participating in an ACO. The patients may continue to see any physician they choose who accepts fee-for-service Medicare, although the ACO would prefer that they restrict their medical care to providers in the same ACO. Only if their patients see doctors and go to hospitals that are part of the ACO will there be any opportunity to truly "manage" their care. The fact that Saul's doctor belonged to a physician group that was part of Partners Healthcare, which in turn became one of the original Medicare ACOs (designated a Pioneer ACO), didn't affect any of his choices. But his experience as a patient was nevertheless shaped in part by the agreement his physician had entered into—and that agreement was just one more source of pressure on Dr. Wilson to adhere to recommended quality standards (whether or not they were relevant to Saul), and for his group to use an electronic medical record.

The penetration of the Medicare ACO model into clinical practice varies tremendously across the country. In the greater Boston area, nearly 30 percent of Medicare patients are part of an ACO, while in the greater San Francisco metropolitan area, fewer than 10 percent are. Saul's doctor was part of the Partners ACO, but the Palo Alto Medical Foundation does not participate in a Medicare ACO.[23] While patients may not even realize they belong to an ACO and it certainly doesn't affect their choice of a physician, membership can affect their experience of health care. In one survey, patients reported that not long after the date on which their doctor became part of an ACO, access to their primary care physician improved. Communication between specialists and primary care doctors got better. And older patients with multiple chronic diseases rated their quality of care more highly after their doctor joined an ACO.[24]

Now, ACOs are on the march. In January 2016, CMS announced a new type of ACO, the Next Generation Plus model, with twenty-one participants, bringing the total number of ACOs to 447, involving nearly nine million Medicare beneficiaries.[25] Over time, hospitals will increasingly regard the physician's office as an extension of itself. The growing merger of the office and the hospital means that medical procedures, and the x-ray equipment, endoscopes, and other devices that procedure-oriented specialists use, can be ordered by physicians in either site. Patients are no longer admitted to the hospital for a workup of gastrointestinal bleeding except in cases of emergency; instead, they have the upper and lower endoscopies, the CT scan, and perhaps the right upper quadrant ultrasound on an outpatient basis. As a result, the companies that make the endoscopes, the CT scanners, and all the rest have as much of an interest in the office practice of medicine as in the hospital.

Medical Devices in the Physician's Practice

Saul wasn't much of a complainer and he rarely had a bad word for anyone, but he did grumble about having his blood drawn. He didn't see why he had to have a blood test every time he went to the doctor's office—and usually an EKG as well. Once a year he also had a chest x-ray and an echocardiogram, and he definitely didn't understand the point of those tests. But from the perspective of the medical device industry, Saul had far too few tests. The companies that make the EKG and cardiac echo machines that noninvasively measure the heart's function, and the auto-analyzers and Coulter counters that process blood samples, as well as an enormous array of other sophisticated medical machines, know that their products are not confined to hospitals and ambulatory surgery centers; they also find their way into doctors' offices and free-standing facilities. And the device manufacturing industry, much like its cousin, the pharmaceutical industry, recognizes that doctors are the key: they are the ones who prescribe tests and procedures, and much of their prescribing takes place in the outpatient setting. The device manufacturers go further still. They realize that doctors might order more tests and more procedures if they benefited personally from each one.

There is just one problem with giving monetary incentives to physicians to order tests, whether through kickbacks or by encouraging them to set up their own lab or imaging facility, and then refer their patients to those labs: it's illegal. The Stark Law (technically Section 187.7 of the Social Security Act) was enacted by Congress in 1989 to put an end to the practice of physicians owning and operating their own labs. The law was expanded in the early 1990s to apply to a whole host of other domains, including x-ray equipment and pharmaceuticals. Perhaps device manufacturers need to rely on advertising and detailing to boost doctors' ordering of tests and procedures.

Device manufacturers do use marketing to influence physicians—or, as they prefer to put it, to educate them. In 2014, American drug and device manufacturers combined spent $6.49 billion on doctors and teaching hospitals, only half of which went to research. The remainder went to royalties, licensing fees, consulting fees, and food and lodging, all of which played a role in persuading doctors to use their products.[26] But some of the more creative companies found a way to circumvent the Stark Law, resulting in increased sales for them, greater income for physicians, and more tests for patients.

Health Diagnostic Laboratory (HDL), a company which at its peak reported annual revenues of close to $400 million, came up with a particularly ingenious strategy. The lab paid doctors a fee—others might say a bribe—for ordering tests from its lab. Health Diagnostic Lab transformed what sounds like a straightforward and patently illegal kickback into an apparently legitimate approach by designating the physician compensation a "processing and handling fee." What the lab did was to sell a bundle of multiple tests—as many as twenty-eight—as a single test that ostensibly measured the risk of heart disease. Performing this mix of tests, the lab argued, entitled it to compensate physicians who ordered the test twenty dollars for handling the blood specimen on which the tests were conducted, substantially more than the three dollars that Medicare normally pays for simply drawing a blood sample. The justification was the "safe harbor" exception to the anti-kickback statute, which states that the seller (the lab) can pay the buyer (the physician) for services related to their product. The twenty dollar fee, in this view, is not a bribe or an incentive to doctors to order the combination test; it is merely a means of paying doctors for expenses incurred by obtaining the test—labeling the specimen, cooling it, and coordinating the processing of the sample.[27]

The net effect of HDL's scheme was that, in 2012, the lab managed to collect $11.9 million from Medicare for one particular combination test. It was so successful in its marketing that the payments to HDL accounted for 93 percent of all Medicare payments nationwide for this unproven package of tests. Some physician practices "earned" as much as $4,000 a week from HDL in these processing and handling "fees." But that's not all. In addition, the most egregious prescriber also occupied a paid position on the lab's medical advisory board and accepted speaking fees from the company.[28] But HDL stopped its fee-paying practice after federal regulators began investigating its business. In 2015 it reached a settlement with the Department of Justice for close to $50 million and agreed to enter into a five-year "corporate integrity agreement" with the Office of the Inspector General, all the while denying any wrongdoing.[29] Shortly afterwards, only a few years after its meteoric rise from small start-up to formidable firm, HDL declared bankruptcy.

Paying physicians to order particular lab tests, including tests of no proven benefit, is not the only way that the medical device industry has found to evade the Stark Law. The law exempts simple, routine procedures done in the office. The idea is that patients benefit if they can have basic lab tests performed in their doctor's office; they don't have to travel to another site and are more likely to comply with their doctor's orders if they can act on them immediately. The challenge is defining "simple" and "routine." Some group practices have entered into unique relationships with device manufacturers that allow them to benefit financially from self-referral—and, in the process, to increase the purchase of expensive medical equipment. In one such scheme, groups of urologists buy a particular kind of radiation therapy machine needed for Intensive Modulated Radiation Therapy (IMRT), a controversial form of treatment for prostate cancer. Then the urologists hire radiation oncologists to administer the treatment using the special equipment, and refer their patients to their own staff for therapy. Intensive Modulated Radiation Therapy is an especially lucrative form of treatment, commanding as much as $40,000 per patient in Medicare fees. And it just so happens that urology practices that own their own IMRT equipment have far higher rates of IMRT use than other urology practices that refer out. One large urology group, Integrated Medical Professionals, prescribed IMRT to over half of its Medicare patients with prostate cancer in the mid-2000s compared to a rate of about 15 percent in other urology practices—for which Medicare paid them $26.7 million. Most striking, Integrated Medical prescribed IMRT for 35 percent of its prostate cancer patients who were over eighty years old, earning $3.7 million for just ninety-one patients, even though IMRT is generally not advised in this age group.[30]

Most physicians order tests because they believe they are necessary—and occasionally, because patients or their families insist on them—not because they benefit financially. They strive for diagnostic certainty and want to be sure not to miss a significant condition, no matter how rare or unlikely that disorder may be. As a result, test ordering has gone up dramatically in the ambulatory setting. At Group Health, a multispecialty group practice on the West Coast whose physicians are salaried, like those at PAMF, the number of CT scans ordered per patient doubled and the number of MRI scans tripled over a ten-year period ending in 2006.[31] The physicians could request scans to their hearts' content because, after all, Medicare would pay for them. We have come full circle: what happens to the older patient in the office is shaped by physicians, by drug companies, and by device manufacturers, each of whom, in turn, is influenced by Medicare.

Going to the Doctor, circa 2015

Patients take for granted that "going to the doctor" means traveling to an office that's often far from home and spending just a few minutes with a harried physician, or perhaps not even with a physician, but rather a nurse practitioner or other "mid-level" clinician. They know the routine: a few questions about symptoms, a physical examination perhaps targeted to particular body parts, a requisition for assorted lab tests, and maybe a referral to a specialist as well. The recent fall, the episodes of incontinence that are increasing, and the nagging problems with memory probably won't come up at all. The visit ends with a prescription for medication—as universal as favors for party guests. And if patients develop an acute medical problem and need urgent attention, they might be able to reach their physician by phone; more than likely, they will speak to someone who is "covering" for their doctor or they will be referred to the local hospital's emergency room. This is the reality for most of the older patients in the United States today. But the invisible hand that determines their experience is not the market, nor is it a divine creator; rather, it is the combined influence of powerful players in the health care system, none of which have any interest in seeing major change in the office practice of medicine.

Primary care physicians already find themselves strapped for time—busy mastering the art of coding to maximize revenue and minimize the risk of accusations of Medicare fraud—and are eager to avoid adding new responsibilities. Coordinating care and engaging in advance care planning, which are uniformly essential for geriatric patients, would eat into their day. Moreover, physicians find themselves singularly ill trained to undertake either task.

Big Pharma has no interest in persuading older patients to substitute generic medications for their expensive brand-name drugs or cut down on the number of medicines they are taking, even if the former would spare their pocketbook and the latter might prevent delirium and other perils of poly-pharmacy. Its interest is to boost the number of people taking its most recent and most expensive medications through direct-to-consumer advertising and point of care marketing. Accordingly, drug companies supply television ad-vertisements and infomercials in the hope that patients will demand the drugs they've learned about when they see their physicians. Device manu-facturers similarly benefit when physicians order more tests, not fewer, even if technological intervention might prove useless or hazardous for patients. They profit if the demand for their equipment increases, resulting in enhanced sales, and they cultivate relationships with doctors to stimulate usage, with direct subsidies, educational grants, and royalties serving as potent incentives to shape physician practice.

Hospitals don't want to foster a system that substitutes home care for hos-pital care, even if the home would be a far safer environment for some of their patients, because they need patients to fill their beds—and older patients are their principal customers. Apart from their interest in preventing untimely readmissions for patients who have been recently discharged, they have every wish to see patients come to their facility for diagnostic workups, procedures, operations, or intensive medical care.

The Medicare program is, in principle, concerned with improving the quality of care for frail patients, especially if the approach saves money. But in its approach both to promoting quality and to standardizing reimbursement, it takes for granted that an outpatient visit starts with a medical history, moves on to a physical examination, and culminates in a lab test. Medicare is having difficulty shifting gears to allow for telephonic medicine, video visits, involvement of caregivers, and delegation of crucial functions to other mem-bers of the geriatric team. The Centers for Medicare and Medicaid Services is trying to change: it now reimburses for coordination of care and pays for an advance care planning meeting, though it is not clear whether the modest sums involved will alter practice, especially when physicians have not been trained to carry out either service. Medicare rewards physicians for complet-ing an "after visit summary," a potentially useful written account of the rec-ommendations made by the physician. But it imposes an elaborate system for "coding" visits, further shackling physicians to their computers as they strug-gle to enter all the information necessary for billing.

Physicians, hospitals, drug companies, device manufacturers, and Medi-care each exert a force on the complex system that constitutes American medicine today. But, with the exception of Medicare, which only came into existence in 1965, all the players have been around for a long time, raising the question of why the office practice has evolved as it has over the past fifty years. The answer requires an understanding of the social, scientific, and policy factors that have, in turn, altered physicians, Medicare, drug companies, hospitals, and device manufacturers.

CHAPTER FOUR

The March of Time, 1965–2015

When the residents of Markle, Indiana, lost their only physician in a tragic accident in the early 1960s, they set out to find a replacement. They knew what they were looking for, and after scouting out some possibilities at the nearest medical school (one hundred miles away in Indianapolis), they found just what they wanted. In fact, they found a pair of new doctors. Gerald Miller and Lee Kinzer were young, eager, idealistic, and fresh out of internship. They were a perfect fit for Markle, a town of just under 1,000 located twenty-five miles from Fort Wayne, the closest urban center.[1]

The two physicians proceeded to set up what they considered a dream practice and the community, by all accounts, shared their view. Sporting the slightly grandiose name of "Markle Medical Center," the practice cared for everyone in town and, as its reputation grew, in neighboring towns as well. Miller and Kinzer worked hard seeing patients six days a week, with evening hours once a week—at least for a time—and rarely got home to their wives and children before seven on the remaining days. They saw patients in the office, they visited patients in their homes, and they made rounds on patients in three nearby community hospitals, until they finally consolidated their hospital work in the thirty-three-bed Welles County Hospital, twelve miles down the road from Markle.

Markle Medical Center was for children and old people and everyone in between; its physicians delivered babies, diagnosed and treated pneumonia, referred patients with heart attacks or cancer to specialists, and patched up local farmers when they came in with an injury. They relied on their wives to serve as nurse, bookkeeper, and receptionist until they earned enough income and had sufficient volume to hire a full-time staff. In their first years, they charged four dollars for an office visit, adding another dollar for a urinalysis. They dispensed medications themselves, billing at cost. The two doctors lived, worked, and participated in the life of their community. Dr. Miller joined the local Lions Club, volunteered as team doctor for high school sports teams, and attended the school's football and basketball games. His wife was active in their church and the local chamber of commerce, and wrote for the town newspaper.[2]

When Drs. Miller and Kinzer made house calls, toting the black bags universally supplied by Eli Lilly Company to medical students in that era, they brought with them a stethoscope and a blood pressure cuff, a reflex hammer, sterile gloves, bandages, a thermometer, tongue depressors, and some basic medications: aspirin, an antacid, penicillin, digoxin, and nitroglycerine. When they returned to the office, they jotted down a few notes in the office medical record—no doubt a manila folder filed alphabetically on a bookcase in the backroom.

Of course, not all doctors in practice fifty years ago were like Gerald Miller and Lee Kinzer. But their practices were far more likely to resemble the Markle Medical Center than to look like the San Carlos Medical Center site of PAMF or even the hospital-affiliated suburban group practice where my father-in-law received his care. Primary care medicine in the immediate pre-Medicare era tended to be small and intimate; a survey conducted by the American Medical Association (AMA) in 1965 found that 89 percent of all doctors were engaged in solo practice.[3] Among general practitioners, the rate was even higher—the group model appealed principally to anesthesiologists, radiologists, and other non-direct care specialists. Moreover, the 11 percent of physicians who then worked in groups tended to work in small groups. Three-fourths of groups operating in 1965 consisted of between three and five doctors (partnerships comprised of two doctors were not considered groups). Subsequent AMA surveys found that by 1983, 41 percent of doctors were in solo practice, and by 2012, the rate was only 18 percent.[4] Group practices today are not only more common, but they are larger, with over half comprised of at least five doctors, 16 percent made up of ten to twenty-four doctors, and 12 percent made up of fifty or more doctors.[5]

Who the doctors are has also changed significantly. In 1965 physicians were overwhelmingly white and male. Only 4 percent of American medical school graduates were female, compared to 47 percent in 2014.[6] As a result, it's not surprising that the majority of the physicians who provide "adult primary care" (internal medicine or family practice) at San Carlos Medical Center are women.[7] The complexion of primary care doctors has changed as well. In 1965 fewer than 2 percent of graduating medical students were black; by 2014, 42 percent were nonwhite, with 6 percent being African-American.[8]

What doctors *do* in the outpatient setting has changed as well. In the early 1970s, one-third of office visits made by older patients were for acute conditions—problems such as a sore throat, cough, burning on urination, fever, or chest pain. The remainder were for chronic conditions such as emphysema, arthritis, or high blood pressure.[9] By 2007, only one-fourth of office visits were for new, acute problems, with most appointments focused on the management of chronic conditions.[10] Fifty years ago, 25 percent of patients left the office with an order for a lab test, and fewer than 10 percent with an order for an x-ray or an EKG. But today, fully 30 percent of outpatients have an imaging procedure ordered, mostly for studies that didn't exist in 1965, such as CT scans, MRIs, and PET scans.

Where patients go for primary care has also changed. House calls were already on their way out in 1966, accounting for only 3.3 percent of all physician visits.[11] By 2006, house calls had almost entirely vanished, except in rural areas where geriatricians in solo practice continue to see patients in their homes.[12] Care has shifted away from free-standing offices to care in the hospital outpatient department or in large centers like the San Carlos campus of PAMF.

Physicians' fees have changed enormously as well. In the first year of the Medicare program, 1966–67, the average charge for a physician visit was $7.80. There was a slight surcharge for house calls: they cost, on average, ten cents more.[13] Adjusting for inflation, that comes to $59 in 2015 dollars.[14] By comparison, the base rate at which Medicare reimbursed physicians for a new patient office visit was between $86 and $164 in 2015, depending on the level of complexity, and the base rate for a follow-up visit ranged between $16 and $115.[15]

How did we get from the small, intimate low-tech practice of the 1960s to the multiphysician, rule-driven, computerized practice of 2015? Office practice has changed in part because medicine has evolved to incorporate the tremendous growth in scientific knowledge. But while scientific advances help explain the shift in what doctors actually do to patients, they don't account either for changes in the delivery of medical care or for the style of physician practice. To understand the evolution of the organization of outpatient practice, we need to consider social trends as well. Figuring prominently are feminism and corporatization, both of which had profound effects on all aspects of society, and health care was no exception. But while these forces influenced the broad outline of medical practice, we need to look elsewhere to understand the intricate workings of the health care system. And it turns out that the Medicare program has played a leading role in determining the texture of ambulatory practice. Acting through its rules, regulations, quality indicators, and economic incentives, Medicare has consistently played a pivotal role in affecting the hospitals, device manufacturers, pharmaceutical companies, and other groups that determine the patient's experience in the office.

Scientific Advances in Medicine

Office visits all begin the same way: someone—it used to be the doctor or perhaps a nurse, now it's likely to be a medical assistant—checks the patient's blood pressure and records the result. The majority of office visits end the same way: with a trip to the lab for a blood test. One of the blood tests the doctor typically orders is for blood sugar and, if the patient is a known diabetic, the Hemoglobin A1c, a measure of average blood sugar control. In between those two iconic events, the physician, or perhaps the nurse practitioner or physician assistant, spends much of the remaining time reviewing whether the patient should take medications for blood pressure and diabetes, what specific medications to take, and how to take them. The intense focus on the optimal management of these two chronic diseases had its origin in new developments in medical science over the last fifty years.

Advances in the Treatment of Hypertension

When I attended medical school in the 1970s, the elevation of systolic blood pressure (the pressure generated when the heart contracts) that is common in older people was assumed to be good for them. Given the presumed inevitability of atherosclerosis, or hardening of the major arteries, the only way adequate blood flow to crucial organs like the brain could be achieved, or so physicians reasoned, was by raising the pressure. Conversely, without that extra force to propel the blood through the circulation, the heart and brain would suffer from ischemia—or lack of oxygen—resulting in heart attacks and strokes, respectively. But then a major clinical trial upended the prevailing view. The Systolic Hypertension in the Elderly Program (SHEP), a large, carefully conducted comparison of different approaches to stroke, found that keeping blood pressure below 160 reduced the risk of stroke by 36 percent and the risk of a cardiac event by 27 percent.[16]

I was in practice at a community teaching hospital outside Boston, caring exclusively for geriatric patients, when the article came out. I remember reading the issue of the *Journal of the American Medical Association* that featured the landmark study—and changing my approach to high blood pressure almost overnight. Strokes, in my view, were one of the worst of the many terrible conditions that could afflict my patients. Sometimes they were lethal but, if they didn't kill you, they left you impaired, often profoundly, inevitably diminishing your quality of life. They transformed robust older individuals into frail and dependent people. If systolic hypertension didn't protect people from strokes, as I had been taught, but instead *caused* strokes, and if an inexpensive and innocuous pill or two could bring the blood pressure down, surely this was important for the health and well-being of my patients.

There were, of course, skeptics. The mean age of the study participants was only seventy-two. Was it fair to conclude that treating high blood pressure was equally as important for octogenarians as for people in their fifties, six-ties, and seventies? How about for nonagenarians? Just how low should blood pressure go? Was there a point beyond which treatment was actually danger-ous? And the SHEP trial was just one study. It has become commonplace in medicine to expect that just about every statistically significant result must be confirmed by duplicating the findings in a subsequent study, however strong the temptation to take the tantalizing findings as fact.

Then in 1997, the *Lancet*, a premier British medical journal, confirmed SHEP's findings in a mammoth trial carried out in twenty-three European countries from Belgium to Bulgaria. The Systolic Hypertension in Europe Trial reported even more dramatic results than the American study. Using a similar approach to treatment—starting by prescribing a diuretic and then adding a second drug if necessary—but with a different choice of medi-cations, the Europeans found a dramatic 42 percent decrease in stroke. Non-fatal cardiac events, principally heart attacks that did not result in death, were down by 33 percent.[17] Questions remained about how low to go and what drugs to use, and with each new antihypertensive that appeared on the mar-ket in the ensuing years, the recommended practice changed. But the consen-sus was overwhelming: systolic hypertension in older patients was well worth treating. For the 72 percent of people aged sixty-five and older with high blood pressure, antihypertensive treatment would become a key part of the office visit.[18]

Many other medical advances reshaped office practice, but few were more important than changes in the scientific understanding of diabetes, which af-flicts over a quarter of people over age sixty-five.[19] The treatment of diabetes—and even the definition of who has diabetes—has been revolutionized by medical science over the past several decades.

Advances in the Treatment of Diabetes

The modern era of diabetes treatment began with the discovery and isolation of insulin by Banting and Best in 1922. As soon as insulin could be produced in the lab—by grinding up animal pancreases and laboriously separating out the life-giving hormone—diabetes was transformed from a uniformly fatal disease to a chronic illness. Traditionally, diabetes had been divided into two types: juvenile diabetes, which, as the name suggested, started in childhood and then entirely destroyed the insulin-producing capacity of the pancreas, and adult-onset diabetes, which developed in middle-aged or older people who were overweight and whose pancreas could still make some insulin, though not enough to keep blood sugar levels normal. Juvenile diabetes was treated with insulin injections; adult onset diabetes was typically treated with diet until it became severe enough to warrant the use of insulin.

This situation changed in the 1950s with the discovery of oral medications that could lower blood sugar in the large population who were not insulin dependent. Many older adults with diabetes could be spared injection therapy and instead take pills. And so the state of diabetes care remained for the next twenty years until the 1970s, when some physicians questioned the wisdom of using hypoglycemic drugs. They were responding to a highly controversial study that suggested not only that the oral agent used in adult-onset diabetes was ineffective compared to insulin, but also that it actually caused heart attacks.[20] After a decade of wrangling, some of the former luster of hypoglycemic agents was restored, aided and abetted by the appearance of a new generation of drugs with an as yet untarnished reputation.

Throughout the seventies, the prevailing wisdom was that juvenile diabetes was a very serious illness that led both to complications involving large blood vessels (coronary artery disease, cerebrovascular disease, and peripheral vascular disease, which in turn cause heart attacks, stroke, and intermittent claudication) and to complications involving small blood vessels (nephropathy, neuropathy, and retinopathy, which lead to renal failure, loss of feeling in the extremities, and poor vision). Adult onset diabetes, by contrast, was thought to be a mild disorder that was chiefly a problem because high blood sugar causes people to urinate frequently, predisposing to dehydration. Only in the relatively rare circumstances in which the blood sugar becomes extremely high, precipitating coma, was it thought to be dangerous. But then a series of scientific discoveries overturned that view.

Over the next ten years, juvenile onset diabetes would be renamed type 1 diabetes and adult onset diabetes renamed type 2 diabetes, based on whether the patient had lost all insulin producing capacity (type 1) or just had diminished insulin producing capacity (type 2). Type 2 diabetes would be upgraded to a serious illness that had the same capacity as its better recognized counterpart to cause mayhem in blood vessels and therefore to inflict "end organ disease" such as stroke or heart attack. Both types of diabetes would be treated with insulin, although a new set of alternative oral medicines would be introduced to treat type 2 patients.

Perhaps the single most important study that would affect office visits for diabetic patients was the Diabetes Control and Complication Trial, which demonstrated that intensive treatment of diabetes, either via multiple insulin injections a day or with an insulin pump, was far more effective in preventing the long-term complications of the disease than the usual, more casual approach to care.[21] Heart attacks and stroke deaths, however, remained stubbornly resistant, even to the most vigilant control of blood sugars.

A second study transformed the view of type 2 diabetes: instead of being seen as the harmless cousin of type 1 diabetes, it came to be regarded as a dangerous disease in its own right. The United Kingdom Prospective Diabetes Study Group trial, the first installment of which was published in the *Lancet* in 1998, was widely hailed as showing that patients with this disorder suffered from the same kinds of problems as others with the disease: heart attacks or strokes, poor circulation in the legs, kidney failure, eye problems, and neuropathy.[22]

Drug development kept pace with epidemiological studies, and a second generation of oral medication for diabetes was inaugurated in 1984 with FDA approval of the drug glipizide. Glipizide was followed some ten years later by the introduction of a whole new class of diabetes medication, the biguanides, the best known of which is metformin. The device manufacturers did their share in revolutionizing treatment of diabetes as well, coming up with nifty ways for patients to measure their own blood glucose, including a method that requires just a drop of blood, and later another method that obviates entirely the need to prick the skin.

Based on the prevailing cut-off for normal blood sugar, 11 million older people were labeled diabetic in the mid-1990s. But the American Diabetes Association was concerned that millions more suffered from what it called "pre-diabetes." Without some kind of intervention, and assuming they lived long enough, they too would develop diabetes. The society estimated that 50 percent of people over the age of sixty-five would qualify as pre-diabetics using its new definition. It concluded that all older people should be screened for diabetes, and it proposed using the Hemoglobin A1c, the test that measured average blood sugar over time, for this purpose.[23] The expectation was that a majority of those screened would qualify for advice about diet and exercise as well as intensified ongoing monitoring and, in some cases, medical treatment: metformin was found to be helpful in prodromal diabetes as well as with full-fledged disease. And everyone categorized as diabetic was then subject not only to treatment with the latest glucose lowering medication, but also intensified treatment of high blood pressure and cholesterol (the combination of risk factors increases the chance of heart disease by far more than the sum of each individual risk factor), exhortations and medication to stop smoking, and aggressive efforts at weight reduction.

New knowledge about medical conditions common in old age, of which diabetes is a leading example, radically changed what doctors do during primary care appointments. But science does not fully explain the changes in the way health care is delivered today. To understand how the delivery system evolved, we need to turn to social trends.

Social Trends and the Evolution of Ambulatory Care

The health care system reflects and is shaped by the wider society of which it is a part, and the office practice of medicine is no exception. It should come as no surprise that two of the forces that have had some of the most profound influences on the way ambulatory care changed over the last fifty years are feminism and the ascendancy of the market. The rise of feminism, which opened the doors of opportunity to women, led to changed definitions of job satisfaction for both women and men in medicine. The triumph of neoliberalism, with its enthusiasm for the market as the solution to all of society's problems, led to the commercialization of the practice of medicine. Both movements gathered steam in the late sixties, took off during Ronald Reagan's presidency, and continue to affect the patient's experience to this day.

The Women's Movement and the Practice of Medicine

The women's movement of the 1960s sent a growing stream of female applicants to medical school until at last the trickle became a deluge. Women made up just under 23 percent of the applicants to medical school in 1975; in 2003, the proportion would peak at just over 50 percent.[24] And those women, when they graduated from medical school, tended to go into a small number of specialties. They did not hammer down the doors of the male orthopedic sanctuary or the even more heavily fortified door to neurosurgery with anything like the vigor with which they knocked down barriers to entry for psychiatry, pediatrics, and general medicine. The result of the influx of women into these areas was that by 2010, fully one-third of the doctors actively practicing family medicine or internal medicine were women, as were just under half of the small number of doctors who became geriatricians or who undertook combined residencies in both medicine and pediatrics.

As women became primary care doctors—and also wives and mothers—they adopted new role models and styles of practice. By and large they rejected figures such as Marcus Welby, the family physician portrayed on television in the early seventies as one who always knew what was best. The genial Welby was regarded by his patients as a demigod; he made house calls; and he worked all the time. The women entering medicine wanted to make patients better and they were willing to work hard, but in their view, there was more to life than medicine. They wanted to have time for hiking or jogging. They wanted to use the income from their work to go to concerts or to travel, and they had no intention of completely outsourcing the care of their children to a nanny. They wanted control over their work lives: a predictable schedule with only a small amount of weekend or night call, and days that began and ended at a fixed time. As a result, many women were drawn to careers in dermatology and radiology, where emergencies were few and the demands on their time manageable. But they were also attracted to careers in primary care, both adult medicine (internal medicine, family medicine and, to a lesser extent, geriatrics) and pediatrics. Once they completed residency training and started looking for a job, these women found life as a primary care doctor in a community health center or a large multispecialty group practice far more attractive than life as a solo practitioner or with just one partner.

It wasn't just the women for whom lifestyle mattered. Male doctors were increasingly married to lawyers or professors or to other doctors, most of whom expected their husbands to be involved in child-rearing. These wives weren't interested in singlehandedly running every aspect of their household, in providing the kind of emotional and domestic support a man needed if he was working all the time. And many men were inspired by the example of their female colleagues to allow themselves to view extra-curricular activities in a new light; suddenly, they too discovered they didn't have to give up playing tennis or the piano just because they were physicians. They, too, rejected the absentee parent role.

If physicians were to practice medicine but also see their children and enjoy other aspects of life, something had to give. For many doctors, the part of medical practice they were more than grudgingly willing to give up, the part they were in fact delighted to delegate, was practice administration. They didn't want to worry about billing ten—or fifteen or twenty—different insurance companies for their services. They wanted to have a competent receptionist and a medical assistant, but they didn't necessarily want to spend time hiring them. They would even be willing to use an electronic medical record (EMR) since it promised better coordination of care, improved communication, and reminders to do all the screening tests they were supposed to do. But using an EMR wasn't the same as choosing which one to purchase and contracting with a vendor to supply the hardware, the software, and the information technology support required to actually use the system.

Feminism had a profound effect on moving ambulatory medicine from its 1965 version to the 2015 incarnation, changing the complexion of the medical profession, altering the public's image of the good doctor, and modifying the organization of practice. The unprecedented ascendancy of the corporation in the seventies and eighties would have a similarly transformative effect on outpatient medicine, dramatically altering the patient's experience.

The Corporatization of Medicine

Boundless faith in the capacity of the market to solve all social problems became the dominant American political ideology in the 1980s. Disillusioned with government after the debacles of the Vietnam War and Watergate, and the failure of Great Society programs to usher in an era of universal prosperity, college graduates sought careers in investment banking rather than science. Congress turned right, reaching new heights in the Reagan era with the passage of legislation that deregulated industry and deferred to big business.[25] In the medical arena, the enthusiasm for the market led to medical practices that were increasingly run as profit-maximizing, efficiency-promoting businesses.[26]

The most overt way for corporations to affect the office practice of medicine was to buy medical practices outright. And in the 1980s and 1990s, that's exactly what happened. Physician practice management companies built whole medical empires made up of medium and large multispecialty and single-specialty physician practices. They acquired all the tangible assets of the practice and then took charge of their operations. For a brief period in the late 1990s, these organizations fizzled, collapsing under mismanagement after they had overextended themselves. But they are once again on the rise, offering help with marketing, hiring staff, providing the information technology infrastructure that practices increasingly need to survive, and even promoting "best practice guidelines" among sometimes unruly, notoriously individualistic physicians.[27] Even practices that are not acquired by a physician practice management company, including those that are nominally physician-owned and operated, typically find they need someone with business expertise to provide administrative oversight. Those administrators make up the growing world of practice managers who effectively run many of the private group practices, hospital-based practices, and integrated delivery systems where physicians work and older patients get the majority of their medical care.

In addition to facing the challenge of burgeoning regulations and a complex reimbursement system determined by third-party payers, practice managers have to deal with the special financial challenges posed by practices composed of salaried physicians. What the managers who run these groups worry about is low productivity. From the perspective of administrators who assume the profit motive is the driver of all economic activity, why would physicians see many patients, generating greater revenue for the group, if they earn the same amount by seeing fewer patients? The recognition that physicians are professionals who are driven by the desire to provide high-quality care is foreign to the managerial ethos. Efficiency, the ultimate goal of practice management, can best be achieved by standardization, and that translates into fifteen-minute visits for all patients. But this fundamental tenet of good business practice collides with the clinical reality that, as patients become older and sicker, and as medical care increasingly moves away from the hospital and into the office, physicians have to spend more time with each patient. It does not readily allow for physicians to spend time on the many uncompensated activities essential to the care of complex patients—writing referral letters to specialists, filling out forms to authorize a visiting nurse, or rewriting prescriptions when the patient changed to a new health insurance plan. One strategy for improving efficiency and increasing the number of patients that doctors see every day is to use productivity incentives.

Common productivity incentives seek to push physicians to see as many patients as possible in the shortest time conceivable by tying their compensation to "patient volume." Such incentive systems entered the practice of medicine in force in the 1980s; by the 1990s, they had become commonplace, and today almost all group practices use performance incentives, though now "performance" often includes achievement of quality targets as well as volume targets.[28] The nonprofit integrated delivery system Geisinger Health, which has a history of attracting talented, dedicated physicians who want the best for their patients, is one of countless examples. Geisinger, which owns and operates about sixty community practices along with both tertiary and community hospitals and provides care for nearly 300,000 people, uses performance incentives for its physicians. The way this works is that Geisinger guarantees its primary care physicians a specified salary each year that is an estimated 80 percent of the total they *could* earn. If they participate in certain special projects over the course of the year, they have the potential to earn another 8 percent of that target amount. The remainder, or potentially a little over 13 percent of the total, is incentive pay that is allocated according to a mixture of factors: performance on clinical quality indicators, good citizenship (as defined by the physicians in the practice), and the group's overall financial performance. According to Geisinger's internal evaluation, their doctors see more patients, are paid higher salaries, and are more satisfied with such a system than without one.[29]

Physician surveys tell a different story. They indicate that physicians are fed up with employers who believe they need to be manipulated to be good doctors; they feel their autonomy is being eroded, and they regret that they are spending less time than they want in true doctoring.[30] Patients also have a different perspective. They may come away from a medical appointment feeling that their doctor doesn't really know them. They feel like widgets on a production line.

Practice managers are well aware that the model of the well-oiled machine may not be what patients have in mind when they go to the doctor, and they don't want discontented patients. Unhappy patients might go somewhere else, they won't recommend the practice to their friends, and they might even write complaint letters to the local newspaper. They are definitely bad for business. Practice managers have tried to remedy the problem, but they have approached it by regarding patients as consumers and doctors as "providers" of a product known as "health care." They treat the erosion of the patient/doctor relationship as a customer service problem. And the path to improving customer service, in the contemporary business world, starts with a survey.

Satisfaction Surveys and the Commodification of Medicine

Characterizing the patient's experience and using the information to make that experience better has the potential not only to enhance business but also to improve the quality of care. When patients and doctors communicate well, and patients get the help they need to navigate increasingly complex systems, they are more likely to take their medications correctly, monitor their chronic diseases assiduously, and generally be more effective in caring for themselves. This was the starting point for the Picker/Commonwealth Program for Patient-Centered Care, which spent years in the late 1980s studying how patients experienced medical care.[31] But the endeavor was quickly taken over by the hospitality industry which, as discussed previously, took as its ideal the five-star hotel. Some of the consultants hired to teach physicians how to provide better service even came from the hotel world. Typical questions included in patient satisfaction surveys deal with how helpful the office staff is and how easy it is to speak with a doctor. The effect of such surveys, paradoxically, is to further transform the encounter between a doctor and a patient into an interaction between a salesperson and a customer.

A recent study showed just how demoralizing and counterproductive patient satisfaction surveys can be for physicians. Researchers found that half of all doctors believed that the pressure to obtain good scores on these surveys promotes inappropriate care, including unnecessary use of antibiotics, inappropriate use of opioid pain medication, unjustified procedures, and unwarranted hospital admissions. Physicians said that the survey mentality caused job dissatisfaction and even encouraged them to leave the medical profession.[32] What began as a sincere attempt to make medical care more effective by incorporating the perspective of the patient has been hijacked, transformed into a strategy for commercializing medicine. And one of the forces pushing physician practices to adopt satisfaction surveys is Medicare. Medicare hopes that transparency will drive up quality—as the results of the surveys, whether of hospitals, skilled nursing facilities, or physician practices, are made public and constitute one component of the government's overall rating system. But measurements of patient satisfaction are not the only way that legislation in general, and changes to the Medicare program in particular, have shaped the development of the modern office practice.

Legislative Milestones and the Office Practice of Medicine

From the moment that Medicare enrolled its first patients, the program had a profound influence on the practice of medicine. Initially, the transformation occurred through the massive infusion of funds into health care as the entire medical enterprise grew to accommodate the expanded market of older people. New hospitals were built, existing hospitals expanded, new companies sprang up to make the devices that Medicare paid for, and drug companies ballooned to produce medicines for older people. In the outpatient arena, Medicare influenced practice at its inception by stimulating physician manpower—or, in response to the ethos of the time, woman power.

In 1966, the year that the Medicare program went into effect, the United States had eighty-eight medical schools, as it had had for years. By 1971, the number of medical schools had jumped to 103 and the size of the entering class had gone from 8,759 to 11,348. Ten years later, the number of medical schools reached 126, where it would remain for decades, and the size of the entering class had swelled to 17,320.[33]

With more seats to fill, the dramatic growth in the number of female applicants was easier for the largely male, very traditional medical school faculty to accept. After all, even with the influx of women, the absolute number of entering male students went up, reflecting the overall increase in class size. What the medical school admissions committees that opened their doors to women may not have fully realized was that, as women entered medicine in growing numbers, often going into primary care, the nature of medical practice would change. And while the women's movement was an essential ingredient in the shift, as was the growth and aging of the American population—the Surgeon General had already recommended expanding the number of physicians in 1959 in anticipation of the impending demographic transition—it was only with the arrival of Medicare and the resultant surge in the demand for medical services that the expansion of medical education took off.

The Growth of Home Care: OBRA '80

Medicare would be repeatedly tweaked and occasionally substantially overhauled during the next fifty years, and many of those changes would affect ambulatory medicine. One of the first major modifications came in 1980, with the passage of the Omnibus Budget Reconciliation Act of that year (OBRA '80). The legislation expanded the home care services available through Medicare and abolished the requirement that a patient be hospitalized prior to initiation of those services. What this meant was that patients could have a visiting nurse, a home health aide or—since Medicare had already been expanded in 1972 to cover speech therapy and physical therapy—rehabilitative therapy at home. What the legislation did not do was facilitate a physician's care in the home. Patients continued to have to travel to the office to see their doctors, even if the office was further away from the patient's home and increasingly inaccessible with the passage of time.

Physician Reimbursement: OBRA '89

Even more far-reaching than OBRA '80 would be OBRA '89. This law would change how doctors were paid, including in their offices. Until then, Medicare hadn't been particularly concerned with physician services. Its focus was predominantly the hospital. As far as Medicare was concerned, doctors saw patients, billed for their services, and Medicare paid the "reasonable, customary, and usual" fee for the local geographic area—essentially, whatever doctors asked for. Medicare worried about the big spenders, which were hospitals. But having brought hospital costs under control by payment reform in 1983, Medicare turned its attention to the office setting. Expenditures on this sector were growing by leaps and bounds, just as hospital costs had earlier, and cost control seemed essential. To solve this problem, Medicare asked faculty members at the Harvard School of Public Health to come up with a way of fairly and equitably measuring the value of a physician's services. The system they proposed allowed comparisons between different types of specialists by using what they called a Resource-Based Relative Value Scale, codified in OBRA '89 though not fully implemented until 1992.

The way this works in practice is that physicians have to the select the "Evaluation and Management code" that corresponds to what they did in their visit with a patient. These five-digit codes are submitted to Medicare, which converts them into dollar amounts based on another complicated system called Relative Value Units (RVUs). These RVUs are supposed to reflect the time required to perform the service, the technical skill required, the amount of mental effort and judgment needed, and the stress associated with the riskiness of the service. Relative Value Units are determined with a proprietary algorithm patented by the American Medical Association for the exclusive use of Medicare. Further adjustments are made based on the cost of living in different geographic areas.[34]

The effect of the system on the office practice of medicine has been twofold. First, it has transformed billing by physicians from a simple, albeit often inaccurate, process of billing by time (inaccurate because studies indicate that physicians, who never adopted the "billable minutes" approach used by lawyers, underestimate how much time they spend with patients) into a cumbersome, time-consuming process of billing based on complexity. Second, it has reinforced the prevailing preponderance of subspecialists over generalists in medicine by institutionalizing higher payment for specialty medicine—even though the initial intent was to compensate "cognitive" as well as "procedural" care, the disproportionate representation of specialists on the rate-setting committee produced the opposite effect.[35]

Quality Indicators and Patient Care

Throughout its history, Medicare has been concerned about cost. But as the principal health insurance company paying for medical care for older people, it has also worried about quality. And the theoretical concern with quality became a concrete concern, with specific tactics for measuring and improving quality, after the seminal Institute of Medicine study, *To Err Is Human*, documented the alarmingly high rate of adverse events in hospitals.[36] The way Medicare began promoting quality was to come up with quantitative ways of assessing it; later, the program began paying extra when those measures are achieved—or paying less when they are not. The use of quality indicators dates to the early 1990s when the Agency for Healthcare Research and Quality came up with a series of measures to evaluate hospital quality. These were gradually introduced into Medicare's reimbursement to hospitals. But while hospitals were a particularly attractive target for Medicare monitoring since they accounted for the largest single share of the budget, physicians increasingly came under scrutiny as well. With the Physician Quality Reporting System, Medicare moved gingerly into the doctor's office. First introduced as a voluntary program in 2005, it enabled physician groups that agreed to report their performance in a variety of domains to reap rewards if they met prespecified targets. The bonus paid out wasn't very generous and not many groups signed up. But then in 2010, Congress passed the Patient Protection and Affordable Care Act which mandated, among other things, that physicians report quality indices. Starting in 2015, they stand to lose up to 1.5 percent of reimbursement fees if they fail to meet the expected standards, rising to 2 percent the following year, and continuing to go up in subsequent years. And the program is no longer voluntary: Medicare decreed that in 2015, any solo physician or very small group would be penalized 4 percent for not reporting their data, and groups of ten or more doctors would be penalized 6 percent.

The quality indicators include some very reasonable measures of performance. Getting on the list of indicators requires careful vetting by multiple distinguished and thoughtful authorities. Even after this intense scrutiny, a proposed indicator can be modified or thrown off the list after the "public comment period" that allows interested parties of all stripes to make their case to the Centers for Medicare and Medicaid Services (CMS) explaining just why the indicator should not stand as drafted. After all this study and debate, not many indicators remain that apply exclusively to older people. There's the percent of patients over sixty-five who have received a pneumonia shot. There's the percent of people over sixty-five who are screened for the risk of falling and the percent who have engaged in advance care planning, chosen a surrogate decision maker in the event they lose capacity, or specifically said they are not interested in doing so. And there are several other indicators that apply to all adults, including at least some of those who are over age sixty-five: diabetics between the ages of eighteen and seventy-five are considered to be poorly controlled if their Hemoglobin A1c is more than 9 percent, and patients up to age eighty-five should have a blood pressure of below 140/90. Few would quarrel with these standards for most patients—except very frail older patients with multiple medical problems and those who are in the final months of life, for whom these issues may be moot. But office visits are typically short. To be assured that their Medicare reimbursement won't suffer, physicians will prioritize those domains that Medicare cares most about. That means cramming in questions about falls and advance care planning and checking blood pressure and diabetes control, whatever the reason for the patient's visit. The system is tantamount to a medical version of teachers teaching to the test—it makes perfect sense for average students or typical patients, and for below average teachers or physicians. But if physicians do what the quality indicators recommend, they will be less responsive to the needs of some of their sickest, most vulnerable patients.

How We Got Here

What happens in the physician's office today is the end result of many scientific developments, social trends, and legislation—principally affecting the Medicare program—of the last fifty years. And how we reached the current reality is even more complicated than suggested by the handful of examples in this chapter: other scientific, social, and public policy developments have put their stamp on outpatient practice as well.

Advances in the understanding of high blood pressure and diabetes were important, but so too was a new understanding of cancer, which made the office a principal site for cancer treatment. Until the 1960s, physicians relied almost exclusively on surgery and radiation to treat cancer, with both modalities provided exclusively in the hospital setting. The results were disappointing, with very high relapse rates for most cancers. Medical scientists gradually realized that the reason was that many cancers had already metastasized by the time of diagnosis, although the metastases were often too small to be detectable on x-rays. But remission rates for a disease such as advanced Hodgkin's lymphoma went from near zero to 80 percent when a few daring and visionary physicians used a combination of four different drugs to attack the disease. A similar approach would soon be extended to solid tumors such as breast cancer, and the field of medical oncology was born.[37] No longer was treatment restricted to the hospital. In fact, most chemotherapy regimens were administered in the office. For the many older individuals who develop cancer—people over age 65 account for 60 percent of newly diagnosed cancers and 70 percent of cancer deaths—going to the doctor is all about getting intravenous chemotherapy.

Feminism played a major role in reshaping the landscape of the office by bringing women's sensibilities and capitalism's imperatives into the examining room, but women were not the only newcomers to the medical profession. What in the pre-Medicare era had been a field overwhelmingly dominated by white, Anglo-Saxon men became far more diverse. Jews, who had been excluded from the nation's medical schools in large numbers by explicit quotas and implicit policy, found their path to medical school opened up in the aftermath of World War II. Asian-Americans flocked to medicine, reflecting the large immigration of Chinese, Korean, and Vietnamese combined with a tradition of valuing education. And African-Americans increasingly sought medical training in the wake of the civil rights movement. As a consequence, by 2011, nearly half of all applicants to American medical schools were nonwhite, with African-Americans representing a little over 7 percent and Asian-Americans slightly over 20 percent.[38] Older patients, who were themselves an increasingly diverse group, found that the aged white man in the white coat whom they had long associated with doctoring was rarely old, white, or male.

Medicare had a major effect on the older patient's experience: first Congress created Medicare, then it went on to expand the program to encompass select types of home care and hospice care, and subsequently it reformed the program to modify the way doctors are paid as well as the incentives that shape their practice. But other legislation affected office practice as well, including laws that had little to do with the Medicare program. The Stark Law, for example, prevents financial conflicts of interest from shaping the test-ordering behavior of all physicians. The Health Insurance Portability and Accountability Act of 1996, which seeks to protect patients' privacy but also impedes information sharing, applies to all areas of medicine.

Despite the multiplicity of factors shaping office practice, it is the outsized role of Medicare that is particularly striking. Medicare influenced all the other actors in the drama: physicians, the device industry, Big Pharma, and hospitals, not just one or two of them. And it consistently affected developments over the past half century. Each new amendment or regulation sent ripples throughout the world of health care—when Medicare instituted the use of quality indicators to measure performance, it affected what physicians spent their time on in the office, it affected how drug companies marketed medications, and it spurred the development of technology to monitor the conditions on which Medicare chose to focus. The profound effect of past changes in Medicare on medical practice suggest that, in the future, we just might be able to look to Medicare for help in modifying medicine to adapt to the needs of the oldest, sickest, and frailest patients. But I am getting ahead of myself. First we need to continue to follow patients as they embark on the health care journey. "Going to the doctor" is just the beginning. The next stop is the hospital, where most older patients find themselves, sooner or later.

Part II
The Hospital

CHAPTER FIVE

Entering the Palace of Technology

As a medical student, I was awed and intimidated by the hospital. There was so much equipment—small stuff like IV poles, big machines like CT scanners, and in-between paraphernalia such as defibrillators. There was so much activity and so much noise: nurses wheeling their medication carts down the corridors, teams of doctors rushing to respond to a "code red," alarms ringing, loudspeakers broadcasting, pagers beeping. And the patients were so very sick. There were the gaunt ones who had lost thirty pounds as their cancers greedily grabbed whatever nutrition their hosts were able to ingest; the pale ones who suffered from profound anemia; and the comatose ones who had sustained devastating strokes. But by the time I was an intern, I had learned to love the hospital. All that equipment was what gave me the power to look inside my patients and see the pancreatic tumor that was making them jaundiced, or to administer potent medications that killed bacteria thereby eradicating pneumonia, or that neutralized stomach acid, curing an ulcer. I regarded the nurses and lab technicians and unit secretaries as my allies; we were a team and together we would prevail over disease and suffering—at least some of the time. And nowhere else in the hospital was there a greater concentration of machines, nurses, and extraordinarily sick people than in the Intensive Care Unit (ICU).

If the hospital is a palace of technology, then the ICU is its throne room. I remember as a medical resident the anxiety I felt when a patient's blood pressure began to plummet, and the thrill I experienced when I "dialed up" his dopamine drip, a potent medication that constricts the blood vessels, raising the pressure within their walls. The patient had an "arterial line," a catheter in the artery of his wrist that was hooked up to a blood pressure sensor and provided continuous blood pressure readings. Within seconds after I had increased the drip rate ever so slightly, I saw the dial show the blood pressure creep up. If it rose too high, I turned down the drip rate. That immediate feedback conferred a sense of power, of control. Even if the patient ultimately died—and most of those in the ICU of the public hospital where I trained did, whether from overwhelming infection, a massive heart attack, or widespread metastatic cancer—at least I had been able to act. I was following the dictum of the surgeon or the "intensivist" (specialized ICU physicians): *Don't just stand there, do something.* It would be years before I came to appreciate that for many frail, older patients, it was far better to adopt the palliative care maxim: *Don't just do something, sit there.*

For patients, the hospital is likewise a palace of technology. It's where doctors produce miracles, where cancerous growths are excised, life-giving kidneys transplanted, anemic blood rejuvenated, and dangerous microbes vanquished. The hospital figures prominently in the lives of old people not just because of its death-defying powers, but also because it's such a common destination. Over the course of a year, just over one-fifth of Medicare beneficiaries are hospitalized at least once, and a third of those are admitted more than once. For people over age eighty-five, the chance of being hospitalized is 34 percent, and if they have limitations in their daily activities, it's higher still, at 43 percent.[1]

For some patients, death-defying technology fails. Among hospitalized patients in the age bracket 65–74, 3 percent die during their hospital stay. And even if they live to be discharged, they are not yet out of the woods. Close to 15 percent of them will be readmitted within the next thirty days.[2] For those who apparently do well, the ones who aren't readmitted and don't die, there are other problems. About one in three will develop a "hospital-associated disability," and they will have more trouble taking care of themselves after the hospitalization than before.[3] The ultimate outcome of the hospitalization runs the gamut from cure to death, with most people lying between these two extremes; what actually happens to people in the hospital also varies considerably, but with a number of common themes.

Just Your Average Hospital Stay

At age seventy-five, Barbara Ellis didn't expect all her parts to be in tip-top shape, but she wanted to feel better than she did. Her legs were so swollen that she sometimes imagined she had ten-pound weights strapped to each ankle. She got short of breath just going from the living room to the bathroom—and her one-bedroom apartment wasn't exactly spacious. She'd had to downsize after her husband died, but she was still independent: she did her own cooking and cleaning, though food preparation tended to mean zapping a prepared meal in the microwave, and she couldn't remember the last time she'd vacuumed.

Barbara wasn't sure what she expected her primary care doctor to do about the fluid buildup. Probably give her a stronger diuretic or maybe another heart medication. She already took a beta blocker and a blood thinner along with a mild diuretic. She knew that regulating her heart was tricky since her kidneys weren't working very well, and every time her primary care doctor or her cardiologist adjusted her heart medicines, her kidney function seemed to get worse or her blood pressure dropped to dangerous levels. Barbara figured her doctor would order blood tests and maybe an electrocardiogram and a chest x-ray. It seemed doctors needed to have test results before they prescribed anything, though Barbara was pretty confident that her problem was the same as it had been the last few times she'd gone in complaining of shortness of breath. What she hadn't anticipated was that her doctor would insist she be admitted to the hospital.

Admitting Diagnoses

Despite the high frequency of hospitalization among older people, the rate has actually been falling as an ever-growing proportion of acute medical problems are handled in the outpatient setting. But some issues continue to warrant hospital-level care, and the single most common precipitant is congestive heart failure (CHF), a condition in which the heart does not pump properly and the lungs fill with fluid. Pneumonia, an infection of the lungs, whether bacterial or viral, is a close second, and then come a series of three different cardiac problems: coronary atherosclerosis (producing symptoms such as angina), cardiac dysrhythmias (irregular electrical activity in the heart resulting in very fast or very slow heart rates), and acute myocardial infarction (a heart attack, which is usually the result of coronary atherosclerosis). The next ten diagnoses include chronic obstructive pulmonary disease (number six), stroke (number seven), and osteoarthritis (number eight), which is the diagnosis underlying knee and hip replacement surgery.[4]

Infection is another leading reason for hospitalization: either urinary tract infection, which is number twelve on the list, or sepsis, at number fifteen, which means bacteria in the bloodstream, regardless of the source. A final category worth mentioning is hip fracture (number thirteen), the only condition that is a surgical problem. That matters because the way patients are cared for on a hospital surgical service is often very different from the way they are cared for on a medical service. In many hospitals, physician assistants or other "advanced practice clinicians" handle most of the day-to-day issues since the surgeons are in the operating room. On a typical medical service, by contrast, the attending of record—the doctor officially in charge—is more apt to play an ongoing role in care. And in all hospitals, much of the actual hands-on care is provided by registered nurses.

Getting in the Door

Barbara Ellis traveled by ambulance from the physician's office to the emergency department of her local community hospital. She didn't much care for the emergency room, and she was disappointed that she had to wait over an hour to be seen when the reason she had traveled by ambulance in the first place was to assure that she received urgent attention. Then she waited another three hours until the harried emergency room doctors finished their assessment, at which point they concluded that Barbara would be better off at a major medical center. She might need another cardiac catheterization—she'd had one years ago, when her cardiologist determined she needed a triple bypass operation, and then again a few years later, when one of the grafts had become blocked and she'd had a stent placed to pry it open. Or she might need dialysis to get the extra fluid off. So, the emergency room doctors reasoned, she may we as well be in a place that was equipped to do all those things. Never mind that Barbara Ellis was adamant that she didn't want dialysis—she'd already had that discussion with the kidney specialist and concluded that spending five hours hooked up to a machine to cleanse her blood three times a week was not a life for her. Never mind that she'd already said she didn't want another cardiac catheterization, or that the local community hospital was much more convenient for her son, who would be visiting her once she actually had a bed. A second ambulance transported her to the Beth Israel Deaconess Medical Center, the big downtown Boston teaching hospital with which the community hospital was affiliated.

Barbara Ellis spent the next six hours in the second emergency department perched on the singularly uncomfortable stretcher that passed for a bed, located in a noisy cubicle that was euphemistically called a room. She told the parade of young doctors and nurses who serially took a history from her and examined her that her primary care doctor had already done these things and decided she needed to be admitted. She couldn't understand why they hadn't sent her directly to a room on the inpatient unit. They explained, with varying degrees of patience, that they wanted to start treatment immediately, though as far as Barbara was aware, it was two hours before she got a single shot of furosemide, the same medication she took at home, and she didn't get any other treatments while in the ER. One male doctor with a ponytail—who reminded Barbara of her nineteen-year-old grandson—told her that they needed to figure out whether to send her to a medical floor or a cardiology floor or even the Coronary Care Unit. Barbara didn't see why that decision took six hours to make, but she had no choice but to wait.

When Barbara was finally wheeled by stretcher to the medical unit, her home for the next week, she was greeted by a young woman who introduced herself as her doctor. Barbara looked at her skeptically, shook her head, and told her there must be some mistake, she wasn't her doctor. She had a doctor, an internist who'd been her physician for the past twenty years. In fact, she'd seen him earlier that day—though it felt like weeks ago—and he had sent her to this circus in the first place. Barbara glared at her and tried to decipher her nametag. "Marianne Charon, MD," she read. She looked at her dark, wavy hair and the long white lab coat that narrowly concealed the shapely figure underneath. "My doctor's a man. And he's got about thirty years more experience than you," Barbara said.

Dr. Charon assured her there had been no mistake. Her regular doctor was affiliated with the hospital but that didn't mean he actually took care of patients there. No primary care doctors saw their own hospitalized patients anymore, she explained. They transferred the job to a new breed of physician called a hospitalist, a doctor who specialized in treating patients who were sick enough to be hospitalized. "I'm the captain of the team," Marianne Charon went on. "I work with two interns and a medical resident who will also be involved in treating you while you're here."

Barbara was too tired to argue. Over the next forty-eight hours she just did whatever the team—or, as she called them because they traveled in a group of five, "the Celtics"—asked. She meekly extended her arm when the phlebotomist came to draw blood, initially three times in one day. She let "transport," as she learned to call the sullen orderly who moved her from her bed to a stretcher, bring her to the radiology suite for yet another chest x-ray. She swallowed whatever pills her nurse handed her, no questions asked. She didn't quite trust Dr. Charon or the Celtics, but she knew better than to protest too strongly.

The Hospitalist System

Marianne Charon, the hospitalist caring for Barbara Ellis, had not planned on becoming a hospitalist. When she applied to medical school, she expected she would be a primary care doctor, working in a group medical practice with a large panel of adult patients. She'd never heard of hospitalists and didn't encounter any until she did her medical rotation as a third-year student—a several-month-long stint at a teaching hospital where she learned the practical fundamentals of being a physician.

Marianne Charon still planned on becoming a primary care doctor when she began her three-year medical residency. But, along the way, she got married and began imagining raising a family. She thought about the primary care doctors she knew who worked long hours and talked more about their "difficult patients" and their conflicts with health insurance companies than about the joys of patient care. She began to think perhaps she should specialize in a less stressful branch of medicine, maybe dermatology or radiology. But those options would require her to spend another three years as a resident, a physician-in-training. They were also difficult programs to be accepted into since a great many other young physicians had the same thoughts about wanting a stimulating but manageable career. She considered doing a fellowship but wasn't sure in what subfield of medicine to specialize—maybe endocrinology, perhaps rheumatology. While she figured out what to do next, she needed a job. She saw an advertisement for a hospitalist at a major local teaching hospital and decided to apply. One thing led to another, and now she and her husband were both working in the same city, he as a lawyer, and she as a hospitalist.

It wasn't just the hours that made the job appealing to Marianne, though that was an important factor. Hospitalists in her institution had twelve-hour shifts, with seven days on followed by seven days off, for a total of twenty-six weeks a year. They worked hard while they were in the hospital but, when they went home, they turned off their pagers and all those sick patients became someone else's responsibility. The hospitalist role appealed to Marianne because it offered the excitement and challenge of treating very sick patients, just the sort of patients she had spent three years learning to care for during residency. The viral syndromes and vaginal infections of a typical primary care population, by comparison, sounded boring, not what she'd spent seven years—four in medical school and three in residency—preparing to treat. And the job Marianne landed offered a special attraction: the hospital was a teaching facility, which would give Marianne the opportunity to work with the next generation of physicians.

Surveys corroborate Dr. Charon's experience: hospitalists are among the most satisfied group of physicians. They like their work more than many other specialists, including doctors who are considerably better paid.[5] They also are associated with efficient medical care—hospitals with hospitalists have shorter lengths of stay and lower average costs than hospitals that rely on primary care doctors to take care of their own patients, with no measurable difference in quality.[6]

For patients, the hospitalist system is a mixed blessing. They benefit from having their attending physician on site many hours a day. They benefit from the greater familiarity that hospitalists have with the latest, most sophisticated inpatient treatments, compared to primary care physicians who have plenty of work keeping up with the latest developments in ambulatory care. And hospitalists have a good record in the quality arena, though they are not necessarily any better at avoiding iatrogenic complications than other physicians. Whatever their faults, hospitalists are now the attending physicians of record in one-third of Medicare hospital admissions to a medical service nationally.[7]

The Tests They Have

Regardless of why they were admitted, patients are going to undergo tests. Tests include the ubiquitous blood draws—typically, a phlebotomist makes rounds every morning and extracts at least one tube of blood from just about every patient. With electronic ordering and the availability of "order sets," or whole groups of studies that can be ordered in conjunction with a particular diagnosis or suspected diagnosis, the number and frequency of blood draws has increased. Only when physicians are provided with information about the cost of each test as they enter their orders does lab test ordering fall, but the results are not necessarily sustained over time.[8] Tests also refer to x-ray procedures—simple black and white, two-dimensional pictures, and CT scans, MRIs, and most recently, PET scans. Tests may include measures of lung capacity (pulmonary function tests) or of liver performance (liver function tests). And they include procedures in which a substance is injected or a tube inserted such as with vertebroplasty (the injection of cement into a spinal fracture) or colonoscopy (the examination of the large intestine using an endoscope).

By far the most common procedure that older adults experience in the hospital is a blood transfusion. Now that blood donors are screened for human immunodeficiency virus (HIV) and other diseases transmissible via blood, serious complications from transfusions are rare, though patients are still at risk of a transfusion reaction if the donor's blood is not entirely compatible with that of the recipient. The next most common procedure is a cardiac catheterization, in which a needle is threaded into an artery and dye is injected into the heart, looking for narrowed coronary arteries or a malfunctioning heart valve. This is a much bigger deal than a transfusion. Complications are relatively uncommon but, when they occur, they are significant. Injecting the dye can dislodge atherosclerotic plaque, precipitating a heart attack—precisely the condition the test was intended to prevent. The dye can also cause the kidneys to shut down, especially when given to patients who already have some degree of kidney malfunction. After cardiac catheterization in frequency comes upper gastrointestinal endoscopy, a procedure in which a tube is passed from the mouth into the stomach so the examining physician can peer inside in search of an intestinal or stomach ulcer, irritation of the lining of the stomach, or cancer. This procedure, too, is fairly safe relative to other procedures. And next on the list is intubation and mechanical ventilation, in which a tube is inserted through the nose or mouth, passed into the lungs, and connected to a machine to breathe for the patient. It is used to support patients during surgery but also for patients with severe pneumonia or a worsening of chronic obstructive pulmonary disease.[9]

Sometimes all these procedures go smoothly and sometimes they don't. How the patient fares during testing is one of the main determinants of their hospital experience.

Rough Waters

On the third day Barbara was in the hospital, she didn't greet her nurse with her usual polite and cheerful "good morning." Instead, she barked at her nurse that "room service is awfully slow in this place." The nurse thought she was joking, but when she told the terrified woman from the dietary department who came to collect her menu that she hadn't ordered anything because "they're out to poison me," the staff became alarmed.

One of the "Celtics," the intern on the team of doctors caring for her, came to check on Barbara, and quickly concluded that she had delirium, or an acute confusional state, a serious and all too common condition complicating hospitalization. The young doctor ordered more blood tests, another chest x-ray, and a urine test looking for the cause of the delirium. And after the urinalysis showed white blood cells, raising the possibility of an infection, the physician started an antibiotic.

When Barbara's son came to visit later that evening, he was horrified to discover that his usually lucid mother, who was methodical and rational about everything, would only speak to him in a whisper because she said the patient in the adjacent bed was a spy. Her son tried asking his mother what interest a spy could possibly have in a retired high school teacher, but Barbara insisted her roommate had been sent by the hospital to make sure she was sick enough to justify occupying a bed. Bob Ellis Jr. got in touch with one of the Celtics and demanded an explanation. He'd heard that sometimes old people got confused from medications and wondered just what drugs his mother was getting. It turned out that, in addition to diuretics and other heart medications, and the antibiotics that had just been initiated for the presumed bladder infection, Mrs. Ellis had been started on an antidepressant because she seemed listless and apathetic. It also turned out that Barbara Ellis had been on the same medication in the past and had, as her son put it, "gone bonkers on it."

The antidepressant was discontinued and Barbara's other medications remained unchanged. Finally, on the fifth hospital day, Barbara Ellis's mental status began to clear.

Delirium

Delirium is one of the most dreaded complications of hospitalization in older people—and among the most common. Just how frequently it occurs varies depending on the hospital, the population studied, and the methods used to figure out whether patients are delirious, but the most conservative estimate is 20 percent of all patients over age sixty-five. For older patients in the ICU, the rate is upwards of 75 percent.[10]

The problem with delirium is that it's not just unpleasant for patients and their families, which it invariably is, and not only costly because it extends hospitalization—on average, delirious patients stay in the hospital eight days longer than comparable patients without delirium—but it's also dangerous. The symptoms of delirium persist long term in as many as one-third of the patients who develop acute confusion in the hospital. The result is that patients have more disabilities when they leave the hospital than when they came in, and are more likely to end up in a nursing home for long-term care. They even are at substantially greater risk of death.[11]

Delirium is just one form of *iatrogenesis*, of problems that develop related to the treatment of disease. Physicians have known for a long time that hospitals are rife with iatrogenesis: already in 1964, an insightful physician documented the "hazards of hospitalization," including reactions to procedures and drugs.[12] I became interested in this phenomenon when I was a medical resident, and carried out a study at the hospital where I was in training. What I found was that the adverse consequences of hospitalization were far more common in older people than in younger ones: problems such as confusion, falling, not eating, or incontinence, even when not directly attributable to the acute medical problem for which a patient had been admitted, were five times as common in people over age seventy as in younger adults.[13] Not only did older people suffer unfortunate complications during their hospitalization, but these new problems led doctors to intervene with another round of procedures or medications, which in turn could lead to other symptoms. Patients with delirium, for instance, might be put in physical restraints or medicated with sedatives, which predisposed them to falling. An entire cascade of untoward events was often the result. The net effect of hospital-based complications is that older patients often leave the hospital unable to carry out the basic activities of daily life. Overall, 30 percent of people over age seventy are discharged from the medical service of a hospital with at least one such difficulty that they didn't have before they became acutely ill.[14]

Another Setback

Just when Barbara Ellis was pronounced ready to go home for the second time, she developed fulminant diarrhea. The diarrhea was so severe and the bouts came on so precipitously that she could not always make it to the bathroom in time. She was mortified; she'd always been a neat and tidy sort of person, and that extended to her demeanor. The discharge was called off. The Celtics came to evaluate her. They concluded that she most likely had developed an infection with the notorious bacterium, *Clostridium difficile*, a common complication of treatment with antibiotics.

For the next two days, her physicians treated Barbara Ellis with a different antibiotic, this one for her diarrheal infection. She still had to go to the bathroom every few hours, and on one of her forays to the bathroom, she fell. The Celtics were summoned again. Her blood pressure was low and it became even lower when she stood up. Her heart was racing. Barbara Ellis was dehydrated, which was not altogether surprising in someone who had first been vigorously treated with diuretics and who next developed diarrhea, each in their own way leading to loss of fluid. It didn't help that her appetite was poor, thanks to the *Clostridium difficile*, so she neither ate nor drank very much. Her doctors instructed the nursing staff to put Mrs. Ellis to bed and give her intravenous fluids.

The house staff—the interns and residents who comprised the Celtics— were eager to discharge Mrs. Ellis. She had already been in the hospital four days longer than the norm and they had twenty-two patients on their service, three more than the average. Any minute they would be called to the emergency room to admit another sick patient. They were impatient to see this particular patient get better, so they decided to increase the rate at which the intravenous fluid entered her veins, hoping to rehydrate her quickly. But Mrs. Ellis's heart could not process so much fluid so fast and she went into heart failure, precisely the condition that had brought her to the hospital in the first place.

Hospital-Associated Infections

A number of the complications that occur during the hospital are related to the patient's disease or to its treatment, not to the hospital itself. Those complications might have arisen even if the patient had been treated at home. Without carefully comparing similar patients with similar conditions, some of whom are treated at home and others in the hospital, it's impossible to know. But some complications are unique to the hospital setting. Hospital-acquired infections, now more properly called "health care–associated infections," are bacterial illnesses that a patient didn't have on arrival at the hospital and that they weren't already incubating. Within forty-eight hours of arriving in the hospital, a patient's flora—the bacteria that normally coat the skin and inhabit places such as the gastrointestinal tract—begin to mirror the types found in the hospital. Some of these bacteria may be transmitted from patient to patient by inadequate hand washing, and some are passed to patients through contaminated equipment. In older patients, whose immune systems are often not working at full capacity, the new microorganisms don't just take up residence, they also produce disease. These include blood-borne infections, pneumonia (typically associated with the use of a ventilator), urinary tract infections (commonly associated with use of a catheter inserted into the bladder to monitor urine output), or an infection at the site of a surgical incision.

The number of health care-associated infections occurring in U.S. hospitals every year is stunning. In 2007, hospitals documented 1.7 million health care-associated infections—and 99,000 related deaths.[15] And older patients are the hardest hit: elderly patients with bloodstream infections acquired in the hospital have a 50 percent mortality rate and spend 50 percent longer in the hospital than patients of the same age without such infections.[16] The cost of their hospital stay is about one-third greater than their uninfected peers.

Journey's End

Ten days after Barbara Ellis first reluctantly entered the teaching hospital, she was discharged. Because she was too weak and deconditioned to return home, she first went to a nursing home for short-term rehabilitation. But she didn't improve in the rehab facility. Every time she seemed to get a little stronger, her lungs once again filled up with fluid. The physician at the facility increased her diuretics, much as the physicians in the hospital had, and she became dehydrated, dizzy, and unsteady on her feet. Barbara called this cycle "the merry-go-round" and concluded she wasn't ever going to get well again. The rehab staff proposed sending her back to the hospital, but she declined, saying she just wanted to go home. Her son didn't think she would be able to manage at home, so the SNF staff held a family meeting with Barbara, her son, her nurse, her physical therapist, and the facility physician in attendance. In the end, they agreed to send her home with hospice services. Barbara signed a form indicating she didn't want to be resuscitated, she didn't want intravenous medication, and above all, she did not want to return to the hospital. She went home, enrolled in hospice, and died peacefully in her own bed a month later.

If Barbara Ellis had not insisted first on treatment in the SNF and then on care at home with hospice services, she almost certainly would have been re-hospitalized within a month after her discharge. She would have been one of the 20 percent of older people discharged from an acute hospital who end up right back where they started, often for the same problem.[17] The problem is so widespread—within three months, a third of patients will have been readmitted—and so costly both to patients, as measured by suffering and disrupted lives, and to the health care system, as measured by cost, that hospitals all over the country have been trying to do something about it.

The Readmission Problem

Hospital readmissions can be due to new problems, unrelated to whatever the patient had gone to the hospital for the first time. Sometimes patients become sick again, sick enough to warrant hospitalization, because they are very frail or dying and not a whole lot could be done to prevent the natural deterioration of their condition. But sometimes it's the transition from the hospital to home that accounts for the repeat admission. As a result, an enormous number of programs have sprung up that offer "transitional care," often in the form of a nurse who makes telephone calls to see how the patient is doing, occasionally in the form of a nurse who makes a home visit, and sometimes utilizing other strategies. The hope—and from time to time the reality—is that if patients have a prompt follow-up visit with their primary care physician, or if there is a careful "medication reconciliation" process to make sure the patient is actually taking the pills prescribed at discharge and only those medicines, then they won't get sick again so soon.[18]

The risks of iatrogenesis in the hospital and of readmission after discharge are related. The problems that lead to repeated hospitalization are often complications of treatment, complications that did not play out until *after* discharge. Barbara Ellis developed *Clostridium difficile* diarrhea while in the hospital only because her discharge had been delayed thanks to delirium. If all had gone according to plan, she would have come down with profuse diarrhea once she got home, potentially precipitating a readmission because of dehydration and dizziness, perhaps leading to falling or even fainting. This has been dubbed "post-hospital syndrome," but it is not substantively different from iatrogenesis during the hospitalization.[19] With the much shorter length of stay commonplace today compared to thirty years ago, acute illness often does not fully resolve until long after discharge, so hospital care, rehabilitative care, and home care *together* constitute the "illness episode."[20]

Not only are frail older people at risk of leaving the hospital more disabled than when they were admitted, not only are they at risk of readmission once they go home, but they are also at risk of dying in the hospital. Death isn't a common outcome of hospitalization, but it is the final pathway for between 3 and 6 percent of older people, depending on whether they are the young old or the oldest old.[21] Everyone has to die sometime and somewhere, and fully one-quarter of older people do their dying in the hospital. This is down from just ten years earlier, in 2000, when one-third of older people died in the hospital.[22] It's way down from ten years before that, when 41 percent of all patients died in the hospital, and dramatically down from 1980, when 54 percent of patients died in the hospital.[23] The hospital is no longer where you go to die, as it was a century ago, and it's no longer feared as a place you only go to if you are expecting to die, but it is nonetheless the site of death for a substantial number of older people.

The experience for those patients who die in the hospital, while on average better today than it was ten or twenty years ago, is rarely a peaceful one with loving family in attendance. More commonly, patients have pain, shortness of breath, nausea, or other symptoms in their final days, and feel anxious and alone. They have invasive procedures—intubation, feeding tubes, dialysis, and attempted cardiopulmonary resuscitation—in a sometimes desperate effort to stay alive. They spend time in the intensive care unit. And after all that, they still die.

This scenario, still all too common today, was documented back in 1995 by a group of researchers at five different American hospitals who were interested in elucidating the kind of care that patients with advanced illness receive. When they looked at patients who died in the hospital, they found that a substantial proportion spent time in an intensive care unit and many of those patients who were conscious reported moderate to severe pain in the last week of life. When they examined what kind of care those very sick patients actually wanted, they discovered that just under half of them did not want aggressive treatment such as attempted CPR—but their physician was typically unaware of their preferences. And even after a second phase of the study introduced an intervention to inform patients of their prognosis and inform physicians of their patients' wishes, the results were the same.[24]

The situation for patients with advanced illness in the hospital has improved in recent years, but not much. Medicare patients with advanced cancer who died in 2010 were often hospitalized in their last month of life, and many were admitted to the ICU.[25] Many of these older patients received invasive and burdensome treatments in the hospital at the very end of life.[26]

The Hospital Experience

The hospital is a wondrous and perilous place for older people, and the frailer and older they are, the riskier it is. Barbara Ellis, while she managed to avoid readmission and death in the hospital because she chose home hospice care instead, had what in many ways was a typical experience. She encountered care provided by a hospitalist, someone whom she didn't know and who wasn't familiar with—and didn't have access to information about—her medical history. She developed several forms of iatrogenesis: delirium, probably related to a medication she was given; and diarrhea due to a hospital-associated infection, which was triggered by the antibiotic she received to treat bacteria in her urine that most likely did not need to be treated. These two new, hospital-acquired problems stretched out her hospital stay. At the end of it, she was so deconditioned and weak that she could not return home but instead was transferred to a rehabilitation facility. If she had not then opted for hospice care, she would no doubt have been readmitted to the hospital one or more times, eventually taking her last breath within its walls.

Ideally, Barbara Ellis would not have been hospitalized in the first place. She could have received a dose of intravenous furosemide, a potent diuretic, in her doctor's office instead of waiting hours until she got precisely the same medication in the emergency department. She could have gone home after her treatment, armed with instructions to double her oral furosemide. Her doctor could have arranged for a visiting nurse to check on her daily, recording her weight, listening to her lungs, checking for swelling in her ankles, and reporting the findings to the primary care physician for further instructions. At home, nobody would have administered an antidepressant, both because she wouldn't have seemed depressed and because they would have known she'd taken the same drug in the past with unfortunate consequences. No intern would have ordered a urinalysis to determine if a bladder infection was the culprit behind her delirium because she probably wouldn't have become delirious in her familiar home environment. The principal justification for hospitalization was the ready availability of a cardiac catheterization lab—but Barbara Ellis had been abundantly clear that she would under no circumstances undergo another cardiac catheterization.

Home treatment might have failed, perhaps because Mrs. Ellis needed more monitoring than a once-a-day nursing visit provided. Perhaps it would have failed because she didn't have anyone to take care of her at home, and she was anxious as well as unsteady on her feet. But she could always have been hospitalized later, once the need had been more clearly demonstrated.

The hospital stay, if one had actually proved necessary, could have looked very different. Barbara Ellis might have stayed in the community hospital where she was first seen, a location convenient for her son, rather than being transferred to the downtown teaching hospital, a facility that was inaccessible to those among her friends who didn't drive. Her doctor could have written her "admission orders" in the office (assuming he had admitting privileges at the hospital), and arranged for a "direct admit," circumventing the long wait in the emergency department. If her primary care physician had served as her attending, he would have had access to his office records—and his memory—and would not have prescribed a drug to which she'd previously had an adverse reaction. A geriatrically trained physician would probably not have ordered a urinalysis unless his patient had specific bladder symptoms such as burning with urination. And a geriatrically oriented hospital would have had a special Acute Care for the Elderly (ACE) unit to provide acute care for her. The ACE environment would have minimized the chance of developing delirium—the trigger for the fateful urinalysis that led to antibiotic treatment, which caused *C. difficile* diarrhea.

Barbara Ellis was a patient at one particular hospital, the Beth Israel Deaconess Medical Center. This hospital is an academic teaching facility of Harvard Medical School, a training site for young physicians and medical students. It is a mid-sized, not-for-profit urban institution. While much of what happens to patients is due to the acute condition for which they were hospitalized, and some of what happens relates to the particular individuals involved in their care, other aspects of what happens might well be affected by the organization of the hospital itself. Some hospitals are small and intimate; others are huge and bureaucratic. Some are for-profit; most are not-for-profit. Some hospitals rely exclusively on physicians for medical care; others make extensive use of physician assistants and nurse practitioners to provide medi-cal care—along with the registered nurses, physical therapists, occupational therapists, technicians, and countless other employees. A look inside other hospitals is crucial in order to figure out which forces are most important in shaping the patient's experience.

CHAPTER SIX

The Varieties of Hospital Experience

My first "rotation," as the intense, one-to-three month hospital stints of medical students are known, was at the Beth Israel Hospital in Boston, which one merger later became the Beth Israel Deaconess Medical Center—the same hospital where Barbara Ellis would one day be a patient. The new version of this venerable institution (Beth Israel first opened its doors in 1916 as a forty-five-bed hospital serving the Yiddish-speaking Jews of Boston) spans two campuses, boasts 672 beds, incorporates an equally venerable Methodist hospital, and is a major teaching hospital of Harvard Medical School. But already in the 1970s, the BI, as we called it, was a sophisticated, modern academic hospital. Medical care was delivered by teams made up of three interns—newly minted physicians in the first year of a three-year residency—and a couple of junior residents, slightly more seasoned physicians in the second year of residency. The teams were supervised by a community-based doctor or sometimes by a specialist on the hospital staff who agreed to spend a month "attending" on one of the medical floors as part of his or her—mainly his, at the time—responsibilities. I remember that the senior physician during one month of my medical clerkship (another name for a rotation) was a primary care doctor who practiced at Harvard Community Health Plan, a newly formed multispecialty group of physicians, and the other was a gastroenterologist on staff at the BI who spent most of his time peering through endoscopes and colonoscopes. And then there were the medical students, one for each of the three interns.

We medical students spent our time shadowing our intern mentors. We were charged with replicating much of what they did, which involved performing a comprehensive admission history and physical examination and writing up our findings—by hand—in the medical record. The medical students also did the scut work, the lowest status busy work: we chased down lab results, drew blood samples, and looked at urine specimens under a microscope. What was striking about the Beth Israel Hospital, as I would come to appreciate when I rotated to one of the other hospitals in the Harvard Medical School orbit, was that it had its own culture.

Some hospitals, such as the BI, are known for being academic, which means the medical students are expected to look up journal articles pertaining to the diseases for which their patients were admitted and report the principal findings. But within the designation "academic" was considerable variability. At Massachusetts General Hospital, another of the major Harvard teaching institutions, with its moniker "Man's Greatest Hospital," students were rumored to be required to make their presentations of journal articles without relying on notes. The BI, by contrast, was reputed to be a genial hospital, and its friendliness took many forms in addition to gentleness with students. Long before the term "patient-centered" entered into common usage, the BI had invented "primary nursing," a model of care in which patients are assigned the same nurse every day of their stay, at least during the day shift. And the BI was generally felt to be to the Peter Bent Brigham Hospital, another major Harvard teaching hospital just a few blocks away, much like Boston was to New York: smaller, more intimate, more manageable, but still a first-class destination. For the BI, that meant the members of its medical staff were every bit as smart and its technology as cutting edge as the competition's.

Mount Auburn Hospital, where I had taken my introductory course in physical diagnosis during my second year of medical school—before entering the dizzying world of clinical rotations—had a very different culture. It was fundamentally a neighborhood hospital that catered to the surrounding community, but unlike most such institutions, it boasted a small residency training program and hosted occasional medical students. With some notable exceptions, Mount Auburn's physicians did not perform the most elaborate operations or utilize the most sophisticated technology; the complex patients who stood to benefit from those modalities were transferred to a "tertiary" referral hospital such as Mass General or the Brigham or, for some procedures, the BI. What the Mount (as we called it) was best at were the more commonplace conditions—pneumonia, angina, hip fractures. Its staff physicians were held to a high standard and were expected to know about the latest treatments and the newest guidelines. But interns and residents cited Harrison's textbook, *Principles of Internal Medicine*, on rounds, not last week's issue of the *New England Journal of Medicine.* The hospital had only a couple of medical floors, a small ICU, and an equally small coronary care unit (CCU). The nurses knew all the doctors and the doctors knew all the nurses, as well as many of the other support staff. Many of the staff members had worked at Mount Auburn for years—they'd been born there, they lived in the vicinity, and they were employed there. The hospital looked like a diminutive version of Beth Israel: it had the same two-bed patient rooms flanked by long corridors, the same central nursing station where doctors wrote their notes and their orders, and the same x-ray machines tucked away in the basement. But it felt different. If a hospital, with its polished floors and institutional décor, could feel homey, then Mount Auburn was homey.

When it was time for me to embark on my residency in internal medicine, I went to a very different kind of institution. I spent most of my waking hours and some sleeping hours at Boston City Hospital, a moderately large municipal hospital. Although it was a public hospital, it was also an academic teaching facility originally affiliated with all three Boston medical schools, but in my day, exclusively associated with Boston University School of Medicine. Boston City had its own culture too, featuring a pioneering, do-it-yourself spirit that arose initially out of necessity—public hospitals are not known for their amenities—and later by self-selection. There were teaching attending physicians, but it was the residents who ran the show. The residents, along with their interns and medical students, evaluated the patients, collected test results, read the medical literature, synthesized the information, made a diagnosis, and instituted a plan. The next day, after we'd already ordered the tests and procedures that comprised our plan, we informed the attending physician what we'd been up to. There were phlebotomists to draw blood, but more often than not they couldn't get anything out of the scarred veins of drug addicts or didn't dare approach the alcoholic patients in the throes of delirium tremens, leaving the job for the intern. There were a few IV nurses, nurses whose job was to put in an IV and check on its status every day or two, replacing it if needed, but I don't remember seeing them around very often. If the team wanted to treat a patient with intravenous medication, the intern started the IV. At Boston City Hospital, we didn't expect interns to quote chapter and verse of standard texts or to have read the latest journal article; what we valued was getting things done.

American hospitals come in a variety of flavors: teaching and non-teaching, for-profit and not-for-profit, large and small, government and private, urban and rural. Their different cultures translated into varying experiences for me as a medical student and then as a physician; surely those cultural differences affect what happens to patients as well. But how much the differences matter in terms of clinical outcomes, personal satisfaction, and actual care is not so clear. Would Barbara Ellis's experiences—the unfamiliar and alien surroundings, a new doctor, delirium, a hospital-associated infection—have been any different at another hospital?

The Academic Teaching Hospital

Of the roughly 5,000 general hospitals in the United States, only 400 call themselves academic medical centers. To qualify, a hospital has to be affiliated with a medical school and engage in teaching and research along with patient care. They are considered tertiary referral centers and are usually in urban locations. Not all major cities have an academic medical center—and some, such as Boston, have several.[1]

What the teaching mission means for inpatients at the hospital is that they will have an entire team participating in their care, typically comprised of medical students, residents, and another category of physician-in-training: fellows. Fellows have already completed a residency, whether in medicine, surgery, or something else—there are also separate residency programs in psychiatry and neurology in addition to fields that are irrelevant for older patients such as pediatrics—and are specializing further. In the case of internal medicine, that entails developing additional expertise in oncology, nephrology, cardiology, or any of a host of other subspecialties. In surgery, it involves acquiring special skills in a particular region of the body—thoracic surgeons operate on the heart and lungs, and otolaryngologists operate on the head and neck. Being cared for by a team creates built-in redundancy since each member of the team takes a history, performs a physical examination, and reviews the laboratory data as it trickles in. The system is supposed to provide a series of checks and balances—any time one member of the team finds something interesting, such as a new heart murmur or a new test result, all the others verify the finding and debate its significance. But it also stimulates extensive test-ordering since all those trainees don't want to leave any stone unturned. They haven't yet developed the finely honed clinical judgment that will allow them to focus on the most likely diagnoses and only seriously consider the more unlikely ones if the more plausible ones don't pan out. Being a patient in a teaching hospital also means an increased chance of treatment with a new or experimental therapy that may not yet be available anywhere else.

At the same time that patients in a teaching hospital are surrounded by people who are eager to develop their clinical skills, who *want* to take care of patients, the more complicated the better, they are also surrounded by research physicians who may be more interested in what happens in their research lab than at the bedside. Physicians on the staff of teaching hospitals, at least of the major teaching hospitals, which are generally the largest academic institutions, spend a good deal of their time designing studies, writing grant applications, and carrying out their research. The Beth Israel Deaconess Medical Center (BIDMC) for example, where Barbara Ellis was a patient, is regularly among the top five hospitals in the country as measured by the amount of grant money its researchers are awarded by the National Institutes of Health: in 2015, BIDMC received a total of $116 million, though this was overshadowed by two other Harvard affiliates, the Brigham and Women's Hospital, with $334 million, and Massachusetts General Hospital, with $353 million.[2]

The crucial question is whether any of this affects what happens to patients. It certainly affects the day-to-day experience of hospitalization in small ways: perhaps patients will have their blood drawn daily rather than every other day, maybe when they go to the radiology suite for an x-ray, the test they have will be a PET scan rather than an MRI. But do teaching hospitals have any larger or more durable effects? Will patients go home with different medications when they are discharged from a teaching hospital rather than from a non-teaching hospital, or will they have more—or fewer—hospital-associated complications? Are they any more likely to improve clinically?

Most physicians who practice at teaching hospitals are convinced that the quality of care they provide is superior to what is available anywhere else. For some technically complex procedures—quintuple coronary artery bypass surgery or a Whipple's procedure, in which the pancreas is removed and new connections established among the intestinal organs—it's true that teaching hospitals usually perform better. Many small community hospitals won't even undertake these challenging operations. But for the bread-and-butter problems such as appendectomies, pneumonia, and gastrointestinal bleeding, the outcomes at community hospitals are at least as good as at their academic counterparts.[3] And in some of the areas that matter most to older people, teaching hospitals aren't quite as good as they are cracked up to be.

For patients with advanced illness who may be in their final months of life, the nation's teaching hospitals, even the most prestigious of them, offer varying approaches to care. That's the conclusion drawn by researchers who examined the performance of those hospitals that *U.S. News and World Report* ranked among the best hospitals in the country in cardiology, pulmonary medicine, or geriatrics. Evidently somebody thought those seventy-seven hospitals were top-notch places for people with the kinds of medical problems that lead to serious illness. Next, the researchers identified a group of patients who were "loyal" to this group of hospitals, patients who got their care at those institutions on a regular basis. Finally, they asked what sorts of health care resources these loyal patients of the country's best hospitals used in their last six months of life and how intensively they used them. What they found was tremendous variability across the seventy-seven hospitals, variability that couldn't plausibly be explained by differences in how sick the patients were. And since the hospitals couldn't *all* be providing ideal medical care, given that what they provided varied so much, they couldn't *all* be first-rate.[4]

The study's authors were at great pains to say relatively little about what they thought constituted good care. But they made an exception for referral to hospice, which most authorities believe constitutes optimal care for dying patients. A low rate of hospice enrollment among patients who died, according to this standard, would imply that many patients didn't get the best possible care—and in fact, hospice enrollment varied among the seventy-seven hospitals from 11 percent to 44 percent. The researchers also recognized that most people say they would prefer to die at home rather than in the hospital, and accordingly ranked care for terminal patients who died in hospitals as inferior to that for patients who stayed at home. It turned out that, in some of the hospitals, only 16 percent of patients died at home whereas in others, 56 percent did. Lastly, the researchers thought it was at least possible, and maybe even likely, that patients who were dying would prefer not only to die at home, but also to spend the months before their death at home rather than in the hospital. And perhaps not surprisingly, the amount of time that patients who ultimately died typically spent in the hospital during the six months prior to death could be as low as nine days or as high as twenty-seven days.[5]

The For-Profit Hospital

If academic affiliation does not predict what happens to patients in the hospital, maybe ownership status does. The majority of American hospitals are nonprofit institutions, but a substantial and growing number are for-profit, with the remainder publicly owned. These proportions vary tremendously by geography, with far more hospitals in the South owned and operated by for-profit corporations than in the Northeast. Nevada and Florida are essentially tied for having the highest rate of for-profit hospitals, with just over half of their institutions in this category. Four states, Hawaii, Minnesota, New York, and Vermont, don't have any for-profit hospitals at all, and another three, Connecticut, Maine, and Maryland, have just a handful.[6] While ownership might differ, in actuality all these hospitals seek to make a profit; the difference between them lies in what they do with the profit. For-profits use the income they earn to distribute to shareholders, while not-for-profits plow it back into the facility in the form of new or enhanced technology and services. But even that distinction is not quite accurate since a growing number of for-profits are owned by private equity firms. In 2010, Nashville, Tennessee-based Vanguard Health Systems, which is owned by the private equity firm Blackstone Group, purchased Detroit Medical Center. A year later, St. Louis, Missouri-based Ascension Health took investment from Oak Hill Capital Partners, another private equity firm. In such cases, both the hospital's earnings and also capital from the parent company can be invested in upgrading the facility, at least over the short run.[7]

Not-for-profit hospitals are supposed to provide a public good in exchange for which they don't have to pay taxes. For-profits don't operate under the same constraints, but you'd never know it from their mission statements. Memorial Hospital in Jacksonville, Florida, is a 418-bed community hospital that is part of the giant, for-profit hospital system Hospital Corporation of America (HCA). Its patients are drawn from the residents of Jacksonville, the largest city in Florida, a city where 11 percent of the population is over age sixty-five. All in all, it's an average hospital in an average American city. Its mission is to "deliver high quality compassionate healthcare to all in our community." Travel west for 2,000 miles and you will reach the Banner Estrella Medical Center in Phoenix, Arizona, a 305-bed community hospital that is part of the large, not-for-profit hospital system Banner Health. Its patients are residents of Phoenix, the largest city in Arizona, where 8.4 percent of the population is over age sixty-five. Banner Estrella is another typical hospital in a typical American city. Its mission statement is "to make a difference in people's lives through excellent patient care."[8]

The real question is whether what happens to patients at Memorial Hospital is substantively different at Banner Estrella Medical Center. In general, for-profit hospitals are more likely to offer relatively lucrative medical services such as open-heart surgery, and are less likely to offer money-losing services such as emergency psychiatric care than are nonprofits.[9] But, while some studies have found that for-profit hospitals have higher mortality rates and more complications than not-for-profit hospitals, other studies fail to bear this out. Whether there's a difference depends on geography and on what diseases the patients were admitted for, as well as on the era in which the study was conducted.[10]

To try to tease out whether ownership matters for clinical outcomes, researchers at the Harvard School of Public Health looked at what happened when hospitals were acquired and changed from a not-for-profit status to a for-profit status. The buyouts regularly improved the hospital's financials but

had no impact on either mortality or clinical outcomes of Medicare patients.[11] If ownership matters, independent of hospital size, location, and the
type of patients, it's awfully hard to prove that it does.

The Veterans Administration Hospitals

Maybe private hospitals are all alike, whether they are for-profit or not-for-
profit, but perhaps public hospitals are different. A sizable number of older
people, primarily older men, receive health care through the Veterans Administration (VA) system, and some of these veterans, though not all, use VA
hospitals for inpatient care.[12] The VA is a fascinating anomaly in the United
States health care system: it's totally run by the federal government, unlike
Medicare, which is just a government-operated health insurance program.
And despite the 2014 scandal over prolonged wait times for appointments,
the VA system overall provides high-quality medical care. It has offered
first-rate care since its transformation in the 1990s, when it made managers
more accountable, improved the coordination of care, introduced quality improvement measures, and upgraded its information systems.[13]

The VA has a long history of innovating in the arena of geriatric care. It has
a network of Geriatric Research and Education Clinical Centers that conduct
cutting edge research in how to care for older patients. The earliest study of
an inpatient geriatric service was carried out at the Sepulveda VA Medical
Center in Los Angeles, California; it showed dramatically better outcomes
for those frail older people cared for in this special environment compared to
those getting usual care. Patients went home with better function and, after
one year, they had experienced less mortality and fewer admissions to nursing homes.[14] The improvement in survival was not borne out in subsequent
studies, but another examination of the VA's "Geriatric Evaluation and Management" units, this one focusing on frail older patients and conduced at
eleven VA centers, confirmed that patients didn't decline nearly as much during their hospital stay if they had the benefit of a specialized geriatric unit.[15]

The VA also has a model home visit program and an Extended Care
Program, its name for a service that provides care in long-stay nursing facilities. Both options offer an alternative to hospitalization for selected patients. These special programs and services translate into a unique hospital
experience for VA patients, and the VA regularly outperforms Medicare on
quality indicators.[16] But not many older patients get medical care in the VA
system. Only those with a "service-related condition" qualify, and since older

people who qualify for VA benefits are also eligible for Medicare, many of them use the private system of health care. Even among patients who make use of various outpatient VA facilities, a substantial proportion seek care in hospitals outside the VA system.

What Shapes the Hospital Experience?

Big or Small

Perhaps what primarily determines the patient's hospital experience is simply the size of the hospital. Large hospitals are inevitably more confusing for older people to navigate; they're by definition less intimate. They feel different, too: the employees don't all know each other and they certainly don't know all the patients. But size is intimately intertwined with geography and with academic affiliation. A hospital in the rural Northeast is categorized as small if it has fewer than fifty beds, but in the rural West it is deemed small if it has less than twenty-five beds. Similarly, an urban teaching hospital in the Midwest is designated large if it has more than 375 beds, but it's considered large only if it has more than 175 beds if it's an urban, Midwestern non-teaching hospital. And in the South, urban teaching hospitals are large if they have more than 450 beds but urban non-teaching hospitals are categorized as large if they have over 200 beds.[17]

Intuitively, size ought to affect the patient experience. Large hospitals do more of everything, including surgical procedures, and it's well established that mortality rates among Medicare patients are inversely associated with surgical volume for all kinds of procedures, including colectomy, coronary artery bypass surgery, and prostate surgery.[18] Larger hospitals can afford to purchase the latest, most expensive high-tech equipment, confident that their investment will pay off because they have the necessary patient volume to support its use. Some hospitals operate their scanners around the clock, and not just for inpatients—outpatients will have appointments scheduled at nine in the evening or six in the morning to keep the machines whirring. But technology is like housing—as the saying goes, if you build it, they will come. When a patient like Barbara Ellis developed delirium, the temptation was great to send her for a CT scan just to make absolutely sure that the cause of her confusion wasn't a stroke or bleeding in the brain, even though the doctors had a perfectly good explanation for her condition—the new medication they had prescribed for her. If they had had to arrange to send her across town to another facility for the scan, suddenly the test wouldn't have seemed so important, but at the large urban hospital, all it took to order a scan was a click of the mouse.

A single extra scan might not dramatically alter the patient's experience— unless, of course, the sedative the patient gets in order to stay still for the scan leads to other problems, such as trouble swallowing, resulting in further complications, such as pneumonia. But when the tests add up, when they include very invasive techniques, and when they are carried out in the last months of life, at which point they are very unlikely to be beneficial, they do affect quality of life in important ways. Certain procedures in particular, including use of a ventilator for breathing, or more generally ICU care, in which testing is a way of life, are generally acknowledged to be burdensome for patients. If they have a reasonable chance of conferring benefit—of curing disease or prolonging life—many patients are willing to accept the extreme discomfort of these procedures. But if they don't have much likelihood of benefit, then they're best avoided. And it turns out that in hospitals all over the country, patients like Barbara Ellis with advanced heart disease, as well as patients with advanced dementia, advanced cancer, and other similarly dire conditions, are getting just this kind of care, whatever the facility's size.

Among older patients with very advanced cancer, by way of example, 29 percent are admitted to the ICU in what will turn out to be the last month of their lives. A smaller, but still significant, percentage gets some kind of life-sustaining treatment in their last month, whether it's attempted CPR, a respirator, or a feeding tube. Six percent of them even get chemotherapy just days before death.[19]

Extensive use of high-tech treatment isn't limited to cancer patients in their final weeks. Medicare patients who died in 2012 spent an average of 3.6 days in the ICU at some point during their last six months of life, with the amount of time ranging from one day in some areas to nine days in cities such as Miami and Los Angeles. And patients with dementia who died continued to have feeding tubes inserted to supply nutrition during the last six months, even though the procedure is widely held to confer no advantage to such patients. The risk of having a needless surgical procedure to insert a tube in the stomach varied considerably from 2 percent in Portland, Oregon, to 12.8 percent in Los Angeles, California. The exact reason for the variability is uncertain, but hospital size was largely irrelevant.[20]

Geography as Destiny

Maybe what determines both patients' degree of satisfaction and their clinical outcomes in the hospital is whether they happen to be in a rural area, where only 38 percent of U.S. hospitals are located, or an urban area, where the majority are found.[21] Figuring out whether the urban/rural distinction matters proves to be rather tricky since rural hospitals differ from urban hospitals in two important ways: they are rarely teaching institutions and they are almost always small. Once these factors are taken into account, there's not much that distinguishes rural from urban hospitals.

Geography does turn out to matter, but sorting out its precise role is a good deal more complicated than just whether the hospital's location is rural or urban. Since 1996, researchers at the Dartmouth Institute (which used to be called The Center for Evaluative Clinical Sciences) have been tracking how much and what kind of care Medicare enrollees receive in their last two years of life. What they find, no matter whether they are looking at the number of different doctors that patients see—they are particularly interested in patients who see ten or more physicians over the course of a year—or the number of days they spend in an ICU in their last year of life, or the proportion of patients who die in the hospital, is mind-boggling geographic variability. When they correct for regional differences among patients, such as differences in the average age or in racial makeup or in socioeconomic status, the distinctions persist. But the phenomenon isn't purely regional: there is no one pattern that describes all Midwestern hospitals and another that describes Southern hospitals. There is variability between cities within the same state. There is variability between hospitals in the same city. As long as there's no absolutely, unequivocally optimal treatment for a particular condition—say, surgery for a hip fracture—whenever the treatment is "preference-sensitive," or affected by the values and attitudes of patients, physicians, or both, there is geographic variability. And different kinds of treatment translate into vastly different experiences for patients.[22]

Whether a chronically ill older patient will spend any time at all in a hospital depends as much on where he lives as on what he has wrong with him. Manhattanites as recently as 2007 spent an average of 20.6 days in the hospital in the six months before they died; residents of Ogden, Utah, spent 5.2 days. When patients did end up in the hospital, whether they were admitted to a regular hospital floor or the ICU, with its beeping alarms, perpetual daylight, and sophisticated technology, was also a function of where they lived. In Miami, Florida, they spent 10.7 days in the ICU; if they lived in Bismarck, North Dakota, they spent 1.1 days in the ICU.[23]

Hospital Systems

Perhaps the patient's hospital experience is shaped by whether or not the hospital is part of a health care system. Over the past twenty-five years, a growing percentage of hospitals have joined some kind of larger umbrella organization, fueled in part by hospital executives' efforts to improve efficiency through mergers and acquisitions. The first wave of hospital consolidation occurred in the 1990s; the merger fever subsequently subsided, but since the passage of the Affordable Care Act (ACA) in 2010, with its new incentives promoting efficiency, mergers and acquisitions have again been on the rise. Those hospitals that weren't already part of a system hastily sought to join one or create a new system by developing a business relationship with other solo hospitals. Existing hospital systems went on a buying spree, snapping up small community hospitals, and in some cases converting not-for-profit hospitals into for-profit hospitals.[24]

Hospital CEOs, anxious about what they regard as inadequate reimbursement by Medicaid, promote geographic expansion for another reason—to gain access to better-insured patients. Sometimes this approach involves building a new, full-service hospital outside their usual jurisdiction; in other cases, hospitals buy or merge with existing community institutions in areas with a high proportion of the privately insured—patients who don't have government insurance such as Medicare or Medicaid. At the same time, hospitals buy up or occasionally form physician practices to serve as referral sources for their hospitals.[25]

Hospital systems are not confined to the for-profit world. One system that was born during the first wave of mergers and that underwent a second growth spurt during the post-ACA era is the non-profit Massachusetts heavyweight, Partners HealthCare. Partners burst onto the Boston scene in 1994, when the two largest and most prestigious Harvard Medical School teaching hospitals, Massachusetts General Hospital (MGH) and the Brigham and Women's Hospital (BWH), announced they were forming an alliance. In their first decade, they acquired five community hospitals extending from Martha's Vineyard, an island off the coast, to the Pioneer Valley in the western part of the state. Included were two small neighborhood hospitals in their own backyard, one in the affluent western suburbs and another just one mile from BWH. As a result, Partners could shunt patients with routine medical problems such as pneumonia or appendicitis to one of its smaller facilities, whether the patients liked it or not. The idea was that the medical issue would be dealt with relatively inexpensively in the small community hospital, thus freeing up beds in the tertiary care center for more complex patients. In addition, the network facilitated the transfer of patients from a low-tech to a high-tech facility if their condition warranted it—cardiac catheterization and open-heart surgery were done at BWH and MGH, but not at the lesser community hospitals. For patients, the net effect of the expansion is that they often start out at one hospital near home and end up downtown; the result for Partners was that by 2012, the chain collected nearly one-third of the money spent by Massachusetts commercial insurers on acute care.[26]

Having made major inroads into the markets east and west of Boston, Partners was eager to have a presence north and south of the city. As a result, when the 378-bed South Shore Hospital showed signs of financial instability in 2012, Partners swiftly stepped in with a plan to buy it, hoping to extend its empire south of Boston. The following year, it set its sights on two small hospitals comprising the Hallmark Health System, which would facilitate expansion north of Boston. Both deals were challenged on the grounds that the cost of health care in Massachusetts, already one of the costliest states in the country, would have risen further if Partners gobbled up additional hospitals. The Health Policy Commission, appointed by the governor to help constrain costs after Massachusetts passed its universal health care law in 2006, agreed, estimating that the deal would increase health care spending by $23 to $26 million per year.[27] Subsequently, the Commission revised its estimate upwards. Even with the settlement proposed by the Massachusetts attorney general, which would have limited price increases across the network until 2020 and allowed insurance companies to bargain with the constituent hospitals individually rather than with the Partners behemoth, prices were predicted to rise considerably. Partners, by virtue of its size, exercised enormous bargaining clout with third-party payers. It was in the enviable position, from the perspective of hospital CEOs, of being able to extract generous payments from insurers—or it would refuse to care for the insurer's members. With strong political winds threatening to topple the agreement, Partners agreed to put its proposal on hold. It was a proposal that would have affected costs for every patient in the Commonwealth and that might have forced patients to change doctors or hospitals for insurance reasons.

At the same time that Partners was flexing its muscles, another hospital system arose to provide some competition, Steward Healthcare. Steward represented a new departure for Massachusetts, its first major foray into for-profit medicine. While states such as Tennessee, home to HCA, have long been dominated by for-profit hospitals, other states such as Massachusetts have a tradition of not-for-profit medicine. In a bold move, the private equity firm Cerberus Capital Management bought the ailing Catholic hospital chain Caritas Christi Health Care, which owned two financially troubled Boston hospitals. Cerberus immediately converted Caritas to a for-profit company which it named the Steward Healthcare System. Within two years, Steward had transformed itself into a network of eleven hospitals with roughly 2,100 beds. Every year it operated at a loss, plowing millions of dollars into construction projects (including a new cardiac catheterization laboratory at one hospital and new emergency departments at two others), as well as into information technology. Steward gambled that it could provide lower cost care than Partners without requiring patients to travel to Boston for complex treatment.[28] Ultimately, it would have to stop relying on infusions of funds from its private equity progenitor and become profitable—typically, private equity firms buy companies, restructure them, making them more efficient, and then sell them within eight years.[29] Constrained to some extent from closing critical but money-losing services such as mental health by its agreement with the Massachusetts attorney general, Steward nonetheless engaged in other cost-cutting activities. It repeatedly cut nursing staff, leading the Massachusetts Nursing Association to file a complaint against Steward, since quality of care has been shown to be directly related to the ratio between nurses and patients. In fact, the nurses filed over 1,000 complaints against Steward, alleging that its practices impair quality. In addition to firing nurses at several of its hospitals, it eliminated the geriatric psychiatry unit at one of them, Quincy Medical Center, leaving older psychiatric patients without any comparable facility in the area. Then it closed down the hospital almost entirely, retaining only an urgent care center and a freestanding emergency room, leaving thousands of residents of the area without a community hospital.[30]

Steward also affected patients' choice of doctors and hospitals. It aggressively recruited physician practices to join its network in order to keep the pipeline to its hospital chain full. Its tactics sometimes backfired, as when it signed on the 200-physician Whittier Independent Practices Association, luring them away from the third major hospital system in the Boston area, CareGroup, only to have the group turn around and rejoin CareGroup two years later. Whittier then sued Steward for withholding the incentives contractually owed them, a step taken by Steward, or so the physicians argued, to punish them for having withdrawn from the system.[31] Patients, in the meantime, had a choice between switching doctors to keep their ties with the hospital they had been using, or keeping their doctor and switching hospitals.

More Alike Than Different

The older patient's hospital experience varies depending on the type of hospital—a little bit. At an academic teaching hospital, patients are more likely to get lots of tests than at community hospitals, but they can count on having plenty of diagnostic tests and procedures wherever they land. They are more apt to receive the latest therapies at a teaching hospital, but they are also less likely to be cared for by a physician who knows them, sometimes leading to their getting a treatment they've had—and that failed—in the past. If patients are at a large hospital, they are on average more likely to receive technologically intensive medical care than at a smaller facility with fewer resources, but they may simply be transferred from one site to another if they could potentially benefit from more elaborate interventions.

Similarly, whether the hospital is for-profit or not-for-profit can affect the patient's experience—sometimes. The for-profits are more likely to cut money-losing services such as mental health and to build up lucrative ones like invasive cardiology (that's actually the name that cardiologists use for performing procedures such as cardiac catheterization). But if you have a common condition that just about any hospital is well-equipped to manage, such as pneumonia, you will probably fare just as well—or as poorly, if you develop a hospital-associated complication—at either type of institution.

Size matters to the extent that small hospitals seldom provide all possible services. But that doesn't mean that for rarer or more complex conditions patients get poorer care at small facilities; it just means they are likely to be transferred elsewhere. And geography makes a difference for the patient's experience, but not so much for clinical outcomes; the amount done to patients suffering from a heart attack or colon cancer or a hip fracture varies enormously from one part of the country to another, with some patients getting 60 percent more interventions than others, but mortality, patient satisfaction, and the ability to function independently are unaffected.[32]

The only type of hospital that consistently makes a difference in the lives of older patients is a VA hospital. The VA offers a more comprehensive package of services for frail older patients than other hospitals. It is a pioneer in geriatric assessment, home care, and long-term care for its oldest, most vulnerable patients.

All hospitals could be improved to better address the needs of older patients. The basic principles required—avoiding medications that often precipitate delirium, promoting a good night's sleep, providing input from the primary care physician or, better yet, assuring that the primary care doctor is the attending physician, and tailoring treatment to conform to the patient's goals of care—are not esoteric knowledge, they are not the carefully guarded secrets of an arcane cult. They constitute the fundamentals of geriatric medicine. But hospitals only rarely implement these principles. Powerful forces—the now familiar litany of physicians, drug companies, device manufacturers, and Medicare itself—all have a vested interest in maintaining the status quo, an arrangement that functions reasonably well for younger or more vigorous patients. How they manage this feat requires looking at the role of each one in the modern hospital.

CHAPTER SEVEN

The Hospital through Other Eyes

When I was a member of the Public Health Council, an advisory group to the Massachusetts Department of Public Health, the Council often considered proposals for new hospital construction or for the acquisition by hospitals of expensive technology. The group was charged with approving or, in rare cases, failing to approve, the granting of a coveted "Certificate of Need" that would allow the expansion to proceed. We didn't have much of an effect on technological proliferation—our hands were tied by laws that spelled out exactly what a hospital had to do to win approval, with no provision for discretion on our part, and hospitals almost always followed the rules—but we did learn a great deal about how important hospitals are to their communities, and not just in terms of patient care.[1]

At one meeting, when we were considering the addition of a new wing to a hospital in Springfield, Massachusetts, the room was packed. The meetings were always open to the public and how many people attended varied depending on the level of interest in the agenda, but a full house was rare. What struck me about this meeting was that the most vocal spokespeople favoring the expansion of Bay State Medical Center, beyond the hospital's administrators, weren't current or prospective patients complaining about how long they had to wait in the emergency department or about the Coronary Care Unit being out of date. They weren't staff physicians pleading for a more modern facility. The most eloquent proponents of the expansion were the construction workers who spoke of all the jobs the project would bring to the community. It was a compelling demonstration that what goes on in a hospital is important to all kinds of people because of the institution's critical role in contemporary society. Springfield had been hit hard by the recession of 2008; its unemployment rate was higher than the state average, and the community hadn't been thriving even in better times; but still, I was surprised to see there was greater interest in jobs than in medical care.

The trade organization for hospitals, the American Hospital Association, likes to point out just how much of a contribution hospitals make to the United States economy, quite apart from their effect on the nation's health. In 2011 hospitals directly employed just under 5.5 million people. Adding the indirect labor—the workers in the outside laundry services that hospitals contract with, and the suppliers who provide the food hospitals cook for their patients—brings the total to 15 million. And the value of the economic activity generated by hospitals, including the indirect activity, has been estimated at $2 trillion.[2] With so much on the line, it's understandable that the business of a hospital is not just of great concern to the doctors and nurses who work there, but also to the device manufacturers and drug companies for whom hospitals are the major customers, to the health insurance companies that underwrite it all, and to the administrators and boards that run them.

Physicians and the Hospital

Hospitals, probably even more so than medical schools, are where physicians actually become doctors. It's in hospitals that young people who have been awarded the MD degree but have never actually had the responsibility for caring for sick people, and who have not truly put their classroom learning into practice, begin to function independently. They are still supervised during their internships and residency—and the Libby Zion regulations, instituted in the aftermath of the tragic death of a young woman misdiagnosed in the emergency room because of inexperienced physicians with inadequate oversight, assure they are supervised—but the degree of monitoring wanes as the physician's competence and confidence increase. Given the intimate relationship between hospitals and doctors, it's not surprising that, as with parent-child relationships, the interaction should at times be respectful and appreciative and at others tense and troubled.

Interns, residents, and fellows view the hospital as the center of their lives. It's not just that they practically live there; it's also that they depend on the hospital for their education, they rely on it for patients and for the mentoring that will lead to their functioning as qualified, independent physicians. If you are an intern, you want broad exposure to all kinds of medical (or surgical) problems. You want the opportunity to perform procedures, to demonstrate technical competence. But you also want your patients to get well enough soon enough for a quick discharge, otherwise you will accumulate a large "service": fifteen or twenty people to round on daily and to examine, people for whom you need to check labs and write progress notes.

Patients, on the other hand, want their medical problems addressed regardless of whether their doctor has seen ten other cases of the same disease in the past month or has never seen an analogous case in his or her young life. They want procedures done competently and efficiently—if they have to be done at all. And they want to be discharged when they are good and ready, preferably when they are strong enough to go home directly without stopping off at a skilled nursing facility, and not whenever the intern and resident on their team need to devote more time to other patients.

Interns and residents want to have cooperative, satisfied patients and families, patients who adapt well to the hospital routine of early morning awakening and bloodletting, rounds with five or six doctors and assorted students, a separate visit by the attending physician whom they may never have met before, summonses to the radiology department at seemingly random times, visiting hours that end at eight P.M., and, throughout it all, alarms ringing and public address systems sputtering, doors slamming shut, and televisions blaring. Patients, especially those with dementia or hearing loss or delirium, may find the regimented order of the hospital—a world that was designed for the convenience of doctors and nurses—confusing and frightening.

Physicians-in-training have one goal in common with their patients in addition to their mutual desire for resolution of whatever problem precipitated the admission: they are concerned about safety. Physicians want to protect their patients from hospital-associated infections, falls, and delirium as much as the patients want to be protected; for the doctors, the development of these problems is a blot on their record and may have the additional effect of prolonging the patient's hospital stay. But young doctors often don't know how to keep their patients safe. They use side rails and restraints to prevent falls—even though these measures have been shown to be largely ineffective, and may even promote more injurious falls if patients climb over the side rails to get out of bed or pull the entire chair down on top of them as they struggle to get up when tied to a chair.[3] And physicians may experience a conflict between the desire to keep patients safe and the equally strong desire to sleep during the night and not be called by a nurse to handle irksome problems such as a patient who can't sleep. To avoid what interns consider nocturnal nuisance calls, they may well prescribe a sleeping pill—even though sedatives are associated with an increased risk of confusion and falls in older hospitalized patients.

What interns and residents want for themselves, what makes their lives easier, are IV nurses, lab technicians, transport services, secretaries on the medical units, and a good information technology system. They want cheap meals in the cafeteria, available at all hours of the day or night, and a comfortable place to sit and do "paperwork," which is now primarily electronic. These services aren't bad for patients; arguably, they can improve their hospital experience by promoting efficiency; but they aren't what patients would focus on if they were telling the hospital CEO how to improve the hospital experience.

Outpatient doctors have entirely different needs and interests. They want the acute care hospital to take the sickest, most complex patients off their hands. They don't want to spend time arranging for Visiting Nurse services, intravenous medication at home, and a lab to monitor blood levels of potentially toxic medications, which is what they have to do if patients are to be treated at home instead of the hospital. As far as office-based physicians are concerned, it's much easier just to send the patients to the hospital. For frail, elderly patients, however, that may be far from the best approach to dealing with an acute medical problem. If they are able to stay out of the hospital in the first place, they don't run the risk of hospital-associated infections or falls from being in an unfamiliar place, or delirium from sleep medication.

Office-based physicians are also generally quite happy to have a hospitalist take care of patients who are admitted. Otherwise, they have to break up their day to go in to round on their patients and they may need to respond to multiple telephone calls over the course of a day to give medical orders to the hospital nursing staff. Patients aren't quite as happy with the hospitalist system, as Barbara Ellis discovered; they would generally prefer to have their own physician when they are at their sickest and most vulnerable.

The primary care physician wants good communication from the hospital. At the very least, he or she wants to be notified that a patient has been admitted; there is little that's more embarrassing than getting a call from a family member with a question about some test or procedure that's been scheduled and not even knowing the patient is in the hospital. Primary care doctors want a discharge summary after the patient leaves the hospital that includes a correct medication list, information about what happened in the hospital, and any follow-up appointments that were scheduled. In this one area, patients and their doctors are aligned.

Hospital-based senior physicians have needs and interests that differ from those of either office-based physicians or residents, and they do their best to influence the hospital administration to assure they get what they want. Doctors who practice primarily or exclusively in the hospital tend to prefer complex, intriguing patients, which does not bode well for the patient with a more routine problem such as pneumonia or a flare of chronic congestive heart failure. They want the resources to diagnose and treat, which means all the basic services such as a good radiology department and a well-equipped operating room, as well as the fastest scanners and newest medications. And if patients don't really need the latest and greatest scan, but it's available, they'll get it anyway, even if it results in finding a small nodule in the lung or a growth in the kidney that will in all likelihood never cause any trouble but that the hospital-based physician feels obligated to pursue—with yet more tests.

Hospital-based senior physicians, like their junior colleagues, the interns and residents, want adequate support staff. If they are not practicing in a teaching hospital, they want nurse practitioners or physician assistants to help care for their patients. Increasingly, hospital administrators oblige since these "advanced practice clinicians" are a good deal less expensive to hire than additional physicians, but substituting NPs for physicians may add to patients' confusion about just who is in charge.

Finally, physicians who work in hospitals are interested in having good colleagues, specialists and subspecialists and sub-subspecialists who can help with patient care. Surgeons depend on good anesthesiologists; general internists rely on oncologists, nephrologists, and other medical specialists. In principle, patients, too, feel that the more good doctors on staff, the better. What they don't know is that there is a direct correlation between the number of specialists they see and the number of tests they will have, with no discernible improvement in outcomes.[4]

Physicians influence what happens to patients in the hospital by shaping the hospital to meet their own needs. They affect what happens by writing orders for medical consultation by other physicians, for lab tests and x-rays, and for procedures. They also have a significant influence on the patient's experience because they order the medications that their hospitalized patients receive. But along with the power of the prescriber, there is another formidable influence on the drugs patients take, and that's the pharmaceutical industry.

Big Pharma and the Hospital

Americans spent an impressive $373.9 billion on prescription medications in 2014. Most of that total, close to three-fourths, went to retail and mail-order businesses. But $30.2 billion went to hospitals.[5] While that's a mere 8 percent of the total, it's a sufficiently sizable chunk for drug companies to be very interested in influencing what medications hospitals purchase.

The relatively modest share of total medication use attributable to hospital patients actually understates the true influence that drugs prescribed during a hospital stay have on overall drug prescribing. Hospital doctors feel free to change the medicines a patient has been taking at home when the patient arrives at the hospital—whether because the drugs aren't working, there's something better available, there's a different medication that the prescribing physician prefers, or simply because the hospital pharmacy stocks a different but comparable medication. But when the patient goes home, considerable effort is expended on "medication reconciliation," or making sure that the patient is taking exactly what was prescribed on discharge and *not* whatever he was on before. The new medicines are presumed to be the right medicines; after all, the patient was admitted sick on the old regimen and sent home cured (or at least better) on the new one. Never mind that the patient was taking a proton pump inhibitor as prophylaxis against a gastrointestinal bleed or "stress ulcer" in the ICU, but he isn't in the ICU anymore so he doesn't need to continue taking the medicine. Forget the fact that oral hypoglycemic agents were started to lower blood sugar when the patient developed elevated sugars in the setting of the high-dose steroids he was given for his acute asthma attack, but now that the steroids have been tapered, his sugars are close to normal and medication to lower them is unnecessary, if not downright dangerous. And, of course, the patient might be taking a certain medicine because the hospital pharmacy negotiated a good deal with the manufacturer of that particular brand. But the patient's Medicare Part D plan, which will cover medications after discharge, may regard that brand as a tier three drug, the drug with the highest co-pay, since other, less expensive brands or even generic versions are available and Medicare, unlike the hospital pharmacy, is not legally allowed to negotiate prices with manufacturers. The selection of medicines in the hospital directly determines the 8 percent of drug company revenue derived from hospitals, but it indirectly exerts an effect long after the patient goes home.

In light of the importance of hospital decision making on medication use, we know surprisingly little about just how many and what kinds of medications older patients take while in the hospital. Prescription drug use by the hospitalized elderly is just one of the components of their care and Medicare pays a lump sum for each admission, regardless of what medicines patients take. We do know that 41 percent of older patients are sent home on between five and eight medications, and another 37 percent go home on nine or more medications. By some estimates, 60 percent of elderly patients are taking at least one unnecessary prescription medication when they go home.[6] Another report calculates that the average number of medications taken by hospitalized patients over age sixty-five is 4.9—and that excludes over-the-counter medicines such as acetaminophen, antacids, and antihistamines.[7]

What is clear is that which medications are prescribed for hospitalized patients depends on what medications are available in the hospital pharmacy. That is dictated by the hospital's formulary, which in turn is selected by the hospital's Pharmacy and Therapeutics (P&T) Committee. This body is typically composed of physicians and nurses who are on the hospital staff as well as hospital pharmacists and a host of other interested parties, including administrators and quality improvement managers. Since the P&T Committee is responsible for choosing the drugs that go on the hospital formulary, along with other functions such as keeping track of medication errors and adverse drug events, drug companies are very interested in influencing this committee. As one drug rep put it, "Nothing in pharmaceutical sales compares to having your product added to a hospital formulary. Imagine the throb of winning a therapeutic interchange, so that every time a physician orders a competitive product, the order is filled with yours. Envision boxes of your pharmaceuticals being stocked at the pharmacy. . . ."[8] To counteract any baleful influences, hospitals generally require committee members to disclose their financial relationships with pharmaceutical manufacturers; some ban professionals from committee membership altogether if they have a conflict of interest. They also develop guidelines for when and under what circumstances drug reps can interact with P&T members, and whether they may fund educational programs or provide free drug samples.[9]

The P&T Committee has been growing in importance in parallel to the waning influence of private physicians. At the height of pharmaceutical company detailing, companies dispatched over 100,000 drug reps to individual physicians in their offices. By 2014, the army of drug reps had been whittled down to 63,000.[10] In part, the change is due to a growing movement to eliminate or at least vastly reduce the influence exerted by detail men pitching their wares to individual doctors. After a series of muckraking articles and books appeared documenting drug company tactics such as providing all-paid expenses to island resorts and ghostwriting articles extolling their products in medical journals,[11] drug reps gradually became persona non grata at major medical centers. Medical schools issued codes of conduct for their faculty. States passed laws requiring physicians to disclose "gifts" from pharmaceutical companies. Forty-four medical schools had prohibited their faculty from participating in pharmaceutical speakers' bureaus by 2013.[12] Some academic medical centers prohibited doctors from holding drug company-sponsored lunches or taking trips on Big Pharma's tab. As individual physicians became more elusive targets for drug company marketers, the hospital P&T Committee became an ever more attractive alternative.

The P&T Committee is also alluring because the hospital formulary undergirds prescribing for physicians who work for the hospital in any of a variety of capacities—as hospitalist, in an outpatient clinic, or as part of a satellite group practice—and fully 42 percent of physicians today are salaried employees of a hospital system. This remarkable development is recent—in 2004, only 24 percent of doctors were employed by a hospital system.[13] Pharmaceutical companies have also begun hiring "key account managers" to try to influence hospitals, targeting an administrator on the P&T Committee.

However important the P&T Committee is in determining what medications hospitalized patients will receive, and however influential the drug companies are in peddling their wares, it is the patient's physician who has to prescribe medicines. The attending physician, the doctor officially designated as the one in charge (as well as interns and residents in those hospitals with a teaching program), is clearly a major force behind the patient's hospital experience. Drug companies, physicians, and hospitals are intertwined—together, they determine the medicines that older people take. The way Big Pharma operates in the hospital is similar to the way that device companies sell their products.

Device Manufacturers and the Hospital

Hospitals are where the most technologically sophisticated procedures are performed, and older patients are on the receiving end of the lion's share of those procedures. When I looked at a list of the most commonly performed procedures in patients over the age of sixty-five for 2011, I was intrigued that upper gastrointestinal endoscopy was number one, with hospitals reporting 619,000 cases in older patients; number two on the list was cardiac catheterization, with 563,000 people between the ages of sixty-five and eighty-four undergoing this procedure. Number three was knee surgery, with 374,000 older people leaving the hospital with a new artificial knee.[14] To perform an upper endoscopy, the gastroenterologist needs an endoscope, a device that's passed from the mouth into the stomach. To do a cardiac catheterization, cardiologists need a special device that can be threaded all the way into the coronary arteries, and if they are going to perform angioplasty or insert a stent at the same time then they also need a catheter with an inflatable balloon at its tip or a wire stent, respectively. And to provide an artificial knee, orthopedists need to have available a knee prosthesis. It's the hospital that supplies the necessary equipment to its physicians including, commonly, an assortment of different types of stents and artificial joints. With all this procedural activity, it's no accident that hospitals are among the big medical device manufacturers' best friends. Firms such as St. Jude Medical—maker of pacemakers, implantable cardiac defibrillators, and other cardiac devices including artificial heart valves and cardiac catheters—sell almost exclusively to hospitals. Medical imaging companies such as Philips sell their CT scanners, MRI machines, mammogram technology, and PET scanners to ambulatory surgery centers and freestanding imaging centers as well as to hospitals, but hospitals are their top customers.

Device manufacturing companies may need hospitals, but hospitals need them as well: hospitals compete with other hospitals for patients, and having the newest, fastest, most amazing equipment is a major selling point. As a result, today's hospitals are in the midst of a medical arms race over devices. One of the first skirmishes in the war involved surgical robots, devices that cost upwards of $1.5 million, with another $140,000 going to their upkeep each year. The FDA approved the technology as safe and effective in 2001, and by 2008, about one quarter of American hospitals in some regions had invested in it. Just which facilities bought a robot was determined in large measure by whether their neighbor already had one.[15] Though hospitals assert that robots ensure fewer complications and a shorter hospital stay, the evidence that they are superior to conventional surgical approaches is lacking. A large study of elective colon cancer surgery, for example, found no difference in either complication rates or mortality with robotic assisted surgery compared to laparoscopic surgery, but substantially higher costs: $14,847 versus $11,966.[16]

Robotic surgery has been joined in the medical arms race by proton beam radiation therapy, a technique that promises outstanding results but which does not quite deliver. It does, however, cost much more than the available alternative. As of mid-2013, the United States had eleven proton beam therapy centers, another seventeen were being built, and other medical centers were hoping to acquire one.[17] Investing in proton beam technology does not merely entail money; it also requires space: the recently completed Maryland Proton Treatment Center in Baltimore is the size of a football field and the building housing the device is encased in cement. Its cost exceeded $200 million. Its principal use is in the treatment of prostate cancer, where it is touted as comparable to conventional radiation treatment but with fewer side effects—although no studies have borne out the claim that it results in fewer side effects.[18]

The major device manufacturers are obviously eager for hospitals to buy their technology, and if they can anticipate a multiplier effect from local competition, the first sale they make in a given market is especially valuable. One particularly effective strategy for achieving diffusion of a new device is to establish a special relationship with the most influential doctors in the hospital.

These "thought leaders" affect the decisions made by individual physicians about what device to implant in their patients. The choice of what type of pacemaker to use and what hip prosthesis to provide is critical to device manufacturers. The industry has developed and refined the process of making friends and influencing hospital doctors. And just as important a target as physicians is the hospital administration. Outlays for capital expenditures are typically part of the hospital's annual budget, and it's the hospital CEO who has ultimate responsibility for setting the budget.

The Hospital Administrator's Perspective

Hospital CEOs worry about a great many things, but what keeps them up at night more than anything else is anxiety about the bottom line. They worry about the institution's reputation and whether the hospital is equipped to handle a case of Ebola or a new strain of influenza or whatever public health crisis the community is facing. But whether the hospital is for-profit or not-for-profit, urban or rural, teaching or non-teaching, the CEO's number one anxiety is the hospital's finances. And some of the leading financial challenges in recent years, in addition to the rising cost of providing care, are Medicare reimbursement and the decision by insurers, principally Medicare, to pay based on the outcome of care, not just on what was done. The strategies the CEO deploys to deal with each of these problems has a profound effect on the patient's experience.[19]

The giant conglomerate HCA (Hospital Corporation of America), with its 163 hospitals spread across twenty states, has come up with a series of interventions to improve its bottom line, strategies it expects the CEOs of all its hospitals to implement. By all accounts, HCA has been strikingly successful: at the height of the 2007–09 recession, when hospitals were teetering on the edge of bankruptcy and sometimes falling over the cliff, HCA reported impressive profits. The conglomerate's executives promulgated a two-pronged approach to improving their financial picture: billing aggressively for their services, and lowering the costs of their medical staff.[20]

Aggressive billing doesn't sound like something that would directly impact Medicare patients since Medicare, not individual patients, pays the extra charges. But it affects them by raising the overall cost of health care. When Medicare's total expenditures go up, so do Medicare premiums and deductibles. In 1997, the hospital deductible under Medicare Part A was $760; by 2016, it had risen to $1,288. Similarly, Part B premiums, which older patients have to pay to cover physician fees, including charges generated during a hospital admission, went up from $44 to $105.[21] And there's no question that aggressive billing translates into greater revenue. At one HCA hospital, Memorial Hospital in Jacksonville, Florida, Medicare pays 10 percent more for each episode of care for an older patient than the national average.[22] One way that Memorial, along with its other HCA cousins, achieves this feat is by introducing a new set of "billing codes" for patients in the emergency departments to jack up reimbursement.

The billing codes went into effect in 2006 and reflected a new philosophy at HCA, or perhaps a resurgence, suitably modified, of an old philosophy. Six years earlier, the organization had pled guilty to a whole slew of charges, including fraudulent Medicare billing practices, and had agreed to pay a penalty that ultimately totaled $1.7 billion and to sign a "Corporate Integrity Agreement" dictated by the Department of Justice. But that contract expired in 2006 and HCA immediately thereafter introduced its new billing regime. The organization insists that the new practices, which revolve around the way emergency room physicians measure how sick and complicated their patients are, complies with official Academy of Emergency Medicine recommendations. Nonetheless, after the new approach to billing went into effect, the sickest, most complex patients suddenly accounted for 76 percent of HCA's emergency room reimbursements, up from 25 percent six years earlier—without any change in the kinds of patients for whom care was provided. Some HCA hospitals were affected particularly dramatically by the new billing codes: Riverside Community Hospital in California earned $949,000 for its sickest patients compared to only $48,000 four years earlier, without a corresponding rise in the overall number of patients seen in the emergency department.[23]

The second strategy invoked by HCA to shore up its bottom line has a more direct effect on the patient experience—and that's flexible staffing. Assuring sufficient nurses to provide three shifts a day, 365 days a year is costly, especially when hospital occupancy rates fluctuate. If a hospital depends exclusively on full-time employees for its staffing needs—technicians, therapists, and aides, as well as registered nurses and licensed practical nurses—it has no way to adjust its manpower to reflect actual need. By resorting to the use of part-time staff with flexible hours and per diem personnel, HCA realized it could lower its fixed costs. But lower nurse-to-patient ratios and greater use of part-timers can translate into a reduction in the quality of care.[24]

The Service-Line Model

In their quest to improve the bottom line, CEOs often lend their strongest support to those departments or activities that produce the greatest amount of profit, the ones that are the most generously reimbursed by third-party payers. Conversely, they provide less support—or no support at all—to those areas that don't show a profit, in the spirit of "every boat on its own bottom," even if their services save money for the hospital as a whole. In one survey, fully one-fifth of hospital executives reported they had closed services that were losing money, with geriatric patients often bearing the brunt of these financially motivated decisions.[25] Cedars-Sinai Medical Center in Los Angeles, for example, a 931-bed hospital, shuttered its psychiatric service in 2012.[26] And the Beth Israel Deaconess Medical Center in Boston, where Barbara Ellis would be admitted for heart failure, closed its inpatient palliative care unit in 2000, the only hospital-based facility of its kind in the city.

At the same time that both for-profit and not-for-profit hospitals close money-losing services, they open new ones that they expect to be more profitable. One strategy currently in vogue is to adopt new "service lines" that allow the institution to build "world-class capabilities in a few areas."[27] For the model to be most effective, and to reap the greatest financial rewards, business mavens argue that the CEO should take the lead in aligning the new area with the hospital's strategic plan.[28] Memorial Hospital in Jacksonville, Florida, has pursued this approach, adopting several "premier service lines," one of which is gastric bypass surgery.

Bariatric surgery (the other name for weight loss-promoting gastric bypass) is a good candidate. With obesity rates soaring nationwide, it has become a big business, going from a mere 37,000 procedures per year in 2000 to 222,000 in 2013.[29] It's the "gold rush in medicine," as one senior RAND economist put it, and "no hospital or doctor wants to be left behind."[30] To attract patients to its Bariatric Surgery Center, Memorial Hospital had to carve out space for the new program and make a number of investments in both physicians and technology. One investment was the purchase of the DaVinci Gastric Bypass System, a form of robotic surgery. Using this technique, the hospital's surgeons offer minimally invasive weight loss surgery, an attractive alternative compared to the older, more burdensome technique. Bariatric surgery is now handsomely reimbursed by insurance companies—including Medicare, although a far smaller percentage of older obese people take the risk of the surgery compared with younger patients.

A second premier service line at Memorial is its heart unit. Heart disease is another good choice: it's the leading cause of death in adult Americans, both under and over age sixty-five. And the bedrock of the service, cardiac catheterization, is so lucrative that, in some hospitals, cardiac catheterizations are performed in people who don't need them, with insurance companies footing the bill. Two hospitals, Lawnwood Regional Medical Center in Fort Pierce and Regional Medical Center Bayonet Point in Hudson, were among ten HCA hospitals that came under investigation by the United States attorney's office for overuse of cardiac catheterization.[31]

Just as important as the service lines that CEOs support are those that they reject. And special units for vulnerable geriatric patients are exactly the kind of intervention that CEOs tend not to like: labor-intensive, multidisciplinary, and complicated, even though they offer the best shot at preventing the kind of decline in the ability to function that is all too common in hospitals.

Acute Care for the Elderly (ACE) units have been around for some time. Built on the successes of the VA's Geriatric Evaluation and Management Units, they are special, geriatrics-friendly units. They have certain standard features such as carpeted floors and raised toilet seats to prevent falls, and a communal dining room that doubles as a place to visit with family members. They have daily, interdisciplinary team rounds to make sure that patients aren't on any medications that are apt to cause problems. Early discharge planning, along with regular communication between members of the team and the attending physician, as well as with patients and family, are also standard. And ACE units work. They worked to help patients maintain their independence when they were first evaluated in the 1990s, and they still work today.[32] But at last count, there were only about 200 ACE units in the entire country. They are high touch, low tech. And while they may result in decreased costs for the hospital as a whole, they are seldom self-sufficient.[33]

Hospital CEOs have other concerns beyond the exclusively financial. Their priorities shift a bit year to year, but consistently ranking among the top ten are worries about implementing health care reform, government mandates, and patient safety and quality.[34] One of those mandates is to use an electronic medical record.

Just as in the outpatient setting, electronic medical records are supposed to make hospitals more efficient by avoiding needless duplication of resources. They are supposed to facilitate integration of care by allowing physicians to share information, both between various hospital-based specialists and between hospitalists and primary care doctors. They are expected to improve the quality of hospital care by preventing medication errors and promoting adherence to treatment guidelines, much like in the office. And while they require a large upfront capital investment, they are alleged to save money over the long run. With all these potential benefits, the Affordable Care Act includes provisions to ensure that hospitals switch from paper to computerized records. It's one of the many "government mandates" that hospital CEOs obsess about implementing. But whether or not electronic medical records are actually all they are cracked up to be—there's now considerable evidence that the cost estimates of widespread introduction of electronic records were vastly underestimated and the benefits hugely overstated—they do affect the patient's hospital experience. They result in all hospital personnel, from physical therapists to nurses to physicians, spending a sizable fraction of their time gazing at computer screens, not at patients—analogous to their effect on physicians who see patients in the office.[35]

The reality is that many of the quality and safety issues that CEOs care deeply about are closely linked to reimbursement. They're connected to reimbursement because Medicare increasingly links them to reimbursement, and Medicare is the payer for a disproportionately large share of hospitalized patients. Understanding what matters to the hospital CEO requires looking at what motivates Medicare.

Medicare and the Hospital

The Centers for Medicare and Medicaid Services is deeply concerned about what goes on in hospitals because they account for the largest slice of the Medicare pie. Reimbursement for hospital services accounted for 30 percent of Medicare's spending in 2014, or $179 billion.[36] And the most expensive part of hospital care is inpatient treatment.

Medicare aims to keep the time patients spend as inpatients as short as possible. The major way it achieves this goal is by using prospective payment, which is based on "diagnosis-related groups." Medicare pays hospitals a predetermined amount for a given medical problem, which in turn presupposes a typical length of stay. Whatever the actual length of time a patient stays in the hospital, the hospital gets the same amount of money (adjusted for geographic differences in the cost of living). If patients overstay their welcome, the hospital loses money; if they leave early, the hospital profits. The net result is that the average length of stay for patients sixty-five and older is only 5.2 days.[37] And for the frailest, oldest patients, the push for early discharge means they often go to a SNF instead of back home, and wherever they go, it's often before they feel they are ready.

Hospitals do have one way to extract additional money from Medicare for hospitalizations, and that's by adjusting for "clinical complexity." If a patient doesn't just have a heart attack but also develops pneumonia, the hospital is paid more. Medicare realizes that some of the high complexity for which they are paying extra is related to the multiple chronic conditions that so many older patients have when they come in, but some of it is related to things that happen after they are admitted. And thoughtful people at CMS wondered whether some of the complications should never have occurred in the first place. Surely everyone would agree that surgeons should never remove the wrong kidney or amputate the wrong limb, and that they shouldn't ever leave anything inside a patient that didn't belong there, such as a gauze pad or an instrument.

Other adverse occurrences are also unfortunate but perhaps not quite so unequivocally avoidable, such as a fall that results in a broken bone or an infection that develops in the hospital. Medicare incentivizes hospitals to avoid what were first called "never events," then "serious reportable events," and now simply "hospital-acquired conditions" by using what, on paper, is a very simple strategy: it doesn't pay for them.[38] What this actually means is that Medicare reduces its payment for these hospitalizations, but no hospitalization goes unreimbursed. What Medicare doesn't do is grant hospitals an enhanced rate to cover the cost of the complications. As of 2015, there are fourteen different categories of problems for which Medicare simply pays the basic, unembellished rate, withholding any extra payment.[39]

Whether reporting serious events and reducing payments for hospitalizations in which they occur has had an impact is not clear.[40] If the policy makes hospitals more careful, if it stimulates use of techniques such as surgical checklists, then it improves the patient's experience. But short hospitalizations may do more than put patients at higher risk of complications; another side effect of the rush to discharge has been a high rate of readmissions: as many as 20 percent of fee-for-service Medicare patients are readmitted within thirty days.[41]

Preventing Readmission

Convinced that repeated hospitalizations are both costly and bad for patients—some estimates put the price tag for "potentially preventable readmissions" at $12 billion a year—Medicare has launched a frontal attack on readmissions, once again using the technique of incentivizing the behavior it wants to see by threatening to withhold reimbursement.[42] The specific policy, authorized by the Affordable Care Act, puts the onus on hospitals to develop a transitional care program—and penalizes them financially if what they come up with fails to produce results. As a consequence, hospitals whose adjusted thirty-day readmission rate is above a specified threshold for patients with any one of a handful of admission diagnoses see their reimbursement for *all* Medicare admissions decreased. As of 2014, the number of diagnoses used to determine if the readmission rate is too high went from three (heart attack, heart failure, and pneumonia) to five (the original three plus total hip or knee replacement and chronic lung disease). As of 2015, the penalty rose to a 3 percent cut in the standard rate. The effect of the new strategy on hospital finances is substantial. Three-fourths of general hospitals were penalized in 2015. In New Jersey, all hospitals except one had cuts in reimbursement, as did the majority of hospitals in thirty other states. The amount of revenue lost by hospitals because they exceed the target readmission rate is expected to climb in future years.[43]

It's far from clear that the penalties have improved the quality of care. With Medicare revenues decreasing at America's hospitals, administrators across the country have been cutting expenses. That may mean employing fewer nursing assistants to help older patients with mundane but crucially important tasks like opening the milk container on their lunch tray or removing the utensils from their almost impenetrable plastic casing. A report by the Robert Wood Johnson Foundation found that, in 2010, one in six patients were readmitted within thirty days after a hospitalization on the medical service, unchanged since 2008. The risk depended on geography, with readmission rates as low as 11 percent in parts of Utah and as high as 18 percent in parts of New York City.[44]

One of the core features of many of the transitional care programs that have sprung up to address the readmissions problem is better communication between doctors in the hospital and doctors in the community. Superior transmission of information is undoubtedly desirable, and one of the favorite strategies for enhancing communication, as in so many other domains, is use of the electronic medical record. But Medicare realizes that electronic records alone aren't going to help unless they are used intelligently, so today's hospitals are incentivized not only to have a medical record, but also to report high levels of "meaningful use."

Electronic Health Records and "Meaningful Use"

The strategy Medicare uses to promote optimal use of electronic health records is to pay out incentive payments for achieving a high degree of "meaningful use," much as the agency does in the outpatient setting. The list of all the steps that hospitals must take to qualify for Medicare's incentive payments is long and it grows yearly. And as with meaningful use requirements for outpatient practices, most of the responsibility for implementation falls on physicians. Clinicians are required to order drugs as well as lab tests and x-rays using computerized provider order entry; they are expected to maintain and update a list of active medications and medication allergies; they must acknowledge and respond to notifications of potential drug-drug interactions; they must prepare a discharge summary that is accessible to both patients and outside providers; and they must record immunizations and certain medical conditions to enable the hospital to report complete epidemiologic data to the government. All told, hospitals must meet sixteen "core objectives" plus another three to be chosen from a list of six optional objectives to qualify for their bonus. To achieve this end, doctors and nurses in the hospital, like their counterparts in the office, must spend a considerable part of their workday sitting in front of a computer. From the perspective of patients, that means less time for direct care. Whether the result is a net improvement in quality of care is unclear.[45]

All these approaches to improving quality and decreasing costs, what Medicare calls "value-based care" or "pay for performance," target the hospital staff. But Medicare has another strategy aimed at patients and their families. By rating hospitals, Medicare hopes that patients will vote with their feet, pressuring hospitals to improve.

The Rankings

Medicare believes that if patients have access to data about hospital performance, they can choose wisely which facility to use for their care. And ideally, once the information is public, hospitals will be shamed into improving their performance, or at least they will make changes so as to improve their ratings, thereby retaining patients. The way Medicare provides public access is through its website, *Hospital Compare*, which includes information ranging from readmission and mortality rates to the results of patient satisfaction surveys to the cost of care.[46] To make it easier for patients and families to process all this data, Medicare amended its system in 2015 to mirror Michelin's five-star system for rating restaurants and hotels.

Patients in Jacksonville, Florida, can look up Memorial Hospital on *Hospital Compare* and see how it stacks up compared to other facilities in town. What they see first are the results of the patient survey, a series of eleven questions that Medicare poses to every patient who is discharged from a hospital. Memorial didn't fare so well in this arena—it is one of the 13 percent of American hospitals that have a two-star rating (with the vast majority earning either three or four stars, and 9 percent earning five). Next, patients come to the arena of "timely and effective care," which includes separate evaluations of how well the hospital performs in treating heart attacks, congestive heart failure, pneumonia, and other common conditions. Memorial does very well in this domain, as do almost all Florida hospitals. As for the next domain, hospital-acquired infections, Memorial is no different from the national average for six of the infections that are measured for the report, it is better in one case, and worse in another. Readmission rates at Memorial are about the same as the national average except for patients with heart failure or stroke, who do less well. Use of medical imaging is comparable to the rest of the country. Finally, in terms of the cost of care, Medicare pays 10 percent more for each episode of care for an older patient at Memorial than the national average, where "cost" includes the costs incurred in the three days leading up to the admission and in the month following discharge.[47]

Most patients are not going to choose what hospital to go to when they are acutely ill, and they certainly are not going to pore over ratings provided by *Hospital Compare* when they are in the throes of a crisis. More likely, they first choose a physician and then go to the hospital that their physician is affiliated with or, in the case of a true emergency, whichever hospital is closest. And what they actually experience once they get to the hospital may bear little relationship to either the descriptions on the hospital's website or the report cards issued by ranking organizations. Public reporting, while a nice idea in principle, has only a limited role in spurring hospitals to do better, and it's difficult to imagine how the situation could be otherwise.[48]

Palaces of Medicine

Patients who see the hospital as the place you go for a tune-up, to get the oil changed or a part replaced—and I've had many patients who regard hospitals this way—are often oblivious to a more complex and sometimes more sinister reality. The people and the institutions that will hold their lives in their hands are not always single-mindedly dedicated to the well-being of patients. Physicians aren't mechanics who diagnose and treat in accordance with a straightforward algorithm; rather, they are actors in the health care drama with their own tastes and predilections. Hospital administrators are not focused exclusively on patients; rather, they focus on tending to the bottom line and hope that strategy will automatically result in good patient care. Pharmaceutical companies and the device manufacturers honestly believe their products improve health, which is often true, but their natural inclination is to focus on selling their wares as widely as possible, not on assuring that the right people will have the right product at the right time. And Medicare's quest for quality and what it deems "high value care" occasionally backfires when its efforts have unintended adverse consequences for hospitalized patients.

The unfortunate reality is that, while selfish pursuit of stakeholders' own best interests sometimes does result in astonishingly good outcomes for particular classes of patients, it more often militates against optimal geriatric care. The ACE unit, for instance, is a proven way to enhance hospital care for frail older patients, but it has few champions. One of the primary ways that ACE units work is to review the medications that patients are taking, removing those with potentially adverse effects such as delirium, substituting generic medications for brand-name drugs to save money for patients after discharge, and sometimes using non-pharmacological approaches altogether, such as hot milk and a massage instead of a sleeping pill. None of these strategies is likely to endear the ACE model to pharmaceutical corporations. Effective units use an interdisciplinary team of nurses, social workers, pharmacists, and geriatricians, a labor-intensive, time-consuming approach that runs counter to the top-down way that physicians, especially hospital-based physicians, have traditionally worked. One of the aims of the ACE unit is to assure that patients undergo tests and procedures only if they are unequivocally consistent with the patient's goals of care—which means thinking carefully about the pros and cons of every imaging examination, every biopsy, and every operation. That usually translates into fewer x-rays, fewer procedures, and less surgery, hardly an outcome likely to please the device manufacturers who supply the scanners, instruments, and surgical robots that make technological intervention possible. And hospital administrators are skeptical of investing in a unit that is complicated to operate and that will probably lose money if evaluated with the "every tub on its own bottom" philosophy—even if it improves patient outcomes and has the potential to save the hospital money by preventing readmissions.

Other strategies for enhancing the geriatric inpatient experience, such as hiring more nursing assistants, establishing better systems of communication with primary care physicians or perhaps even jettisoning hospitalists, are likewise either unpopular with the forces that shape hospital life or of no interest at all to them. Without a powerful champion, there is little impetus to pursue any of them. And an approach to geriatric care that seeks to keep patients out of the hospital altogether by substituting home or skilled nursing facility care for hospital treatment is decidedly unpopular with the drug companies, device manufacturers, physicians, and hospital administrators who are dependent on a steady stream of sick, elderly patients to fill their beds.

The complex web of interlinking forces that drives the modern hospital care system seems resistant to change. But the patient's experience today is substantially different from what it was fifty years ago. If all those forces are such powerful determinants of reality, it remains to be explained how the hospital became what it is.

CHAPTER EIGHT

The Transformation of the American Hospital, 1965–2015

Memory is a tricky business. Our natural tendency, or at least mine, is to take the current reality for granted, to assume things have always been the way they are now. Even though at the time I began my training as a physician, the personal computer did not exist and doctors and nurses sat at long tables and wrote up their progress notes, when I conjure up an image of a hospital today, I imagine dozens of computers, each with a physician or nurse seated or standing in front of it, busily entering or retrieving data. Even though when I was an intern, lab test results were either telephoned to the ward secretary or written on small slips of paper, I literally cannot remember what those slips looked like now that I've seen nothing but computer printouts and screen displays for years.

To understand how the hospital of the early 1960s, the immediate pre-Medicare era, has been transformed over the last fifty years, we need to begin by going back in time and looking at what hospitals were actually like then. But because doctors and patients at the time presumably also took their institutions for granted and assumed they were more or less the same as they had always been, and probably exactly the way they had to be, they didn't leave much in the way of a detailed record. To be sure, there were gripes, some features of hospitals that people could conceive of improving, and those gripes were sometimes published in medical journals or as op-eds. And we have a statistical record of hospitals: the United States government has for decades collected reams of extraordinarily valuable data about all sorts of aspects of American life. We know, for example, how many hospitals existed in 1965 and what sorts of medical problems brought patients into the hospital. We know what the average length of stay was at an American hospital in the year before Medicare went into effect. But, for a description of how a hospital looked from the perspective of what people at the time regarded as important, we have to turn to a journalist's account of the opening of a new hospital. Quite fortuitously, a new hospital opened its doors in New York City in January 1966.

The American Hospital on the Eve of Medicare

New York City hospitals have been around for a long time. New York Hospital has the distinction of being one of the oldest in the country. It was established in 1771, just twenty years after Philadelphia founded the first American general hospital, Pennsylvania Hospital. Most of the city's other hospitals had their beginnings in the nineteenth century: Presbyterian Hospital in 1868, along with several hospitals in the Bronx including Lincoln Hospital in 1839, and Bronx-Lebanon Hospital Center in 1890. There were a few mergers and the creation of several small facilities in the first half of the twentieth century, but it had been a while since a brand new hospital had been built anywhere in New York. When the Hospital of the Albert Einstein College of Medicine opened in January 1966, it was news.

The *New York Times* ran a column about the hospital, calling it "sturdy" and "majestic," a place you could trust to provide the best health care. It was a "brick-finished, concrete reinforced structure" that stood on a knoll adjacent to Albert Einstein College of Medicine. But it was more than just an elegant building rising above the one- and two-family homes of a working class neighborhood of the Bronx, a borough of New York widely associated with urban blight. The hospital, the *Times* asserted, was a truly comfortable place for patients. "All 12 stories are air-conditioned," the reporter enthused. Closed-circuit television and radio were available in patient rooms. And the patient experience would be enhanced through "electronic devices for patient-nurse communication," or the now ubiquitous nurse call buttons.[1]

By contemporary reckoning, the hospital was both large and sophisticated. When completed, it would have 375 beds along with a parking lot that could accommodate 300 cars, and it would cost $10 million to build. Of paramount importance, it would boast all the most up-to-date technology, many housed in a three-story "Diagnostic Center," which included such sophisticated services as a radiology unit and a laboratory. The hospital would be different from neighboring, possibly competing institutions, the journalist added: it would offer a variety of "special services," presumably not available at all general hospitals, such as radiation therapy for cancer patients and rehabilitation for those with strokes or fractures.

The Hospital of the Twenty-First Century

Forty-two years later, the Brigham and Women's Hospital, a Boston teaching hospital affiliated with Harvard Medical School, opened a new hospital building on its main campus. The Shapiro Cardiovascular Center portrayed itself as large, technologically cutting edge, and equipped with numerous amenities designed to maximize patient comfort. It touted many of the same virtues as its cousin in New York back in 1966, adding only that it was "environmentally sophisticated." But the definitions of large, high-tech, and patient-centered had changed dramatically.

The Shapiro Center is a 350,000-square-foot facility spanning ten floors devoted exclusively to the treatment of cardiac and vascular disease. It has 16 operating suites, 9 procedure rooms of various kinds (such as a cardiac catheterization laboratory), and 136 patient rooms. Technological sophistication is built into the facility's design: each operating suite has its own scanner (currently a sixty-four-slice CT scanner) and ultrasound equipment. Not only are the suites designed to integrate imaging into surgical procedures, to provide real-time information to physicians to help guide them through a procedure, they are also built to accommodate "robotic surgery." Never mind that no study of robotic surgery has been shown either to improve outcomes or decrease costs; it is clearly "cutting edge technology."

These two portraits, of the Hospital of the Albert Einstein College of Medicine and the Shapiro Center of Brigham and Women's Hospital, to be sure, reflect a public relations perspective. The *New York Times* article about the Einstein hospital sounds like marketing literature, and the description I provide of the Brigham and Women's Hospital cardiovascular center is from its website, which is essentially marketing literature. Both descriptions leave out a great deal: the Brigham does not tout its hospitalist system or short length of stay; Einstein did not divulge statistics on the proportion of its residents who are foreign medical graduates. But their imagery highlights what was probably important to patients. In seeking to understand how we got from there to here, how over the last fifty years the hospital was technologized, corporatized, and bureaucratized, we have to look at critical demographic, political, economic, and scientific developments, much as we did to explore changes in office practice.

Scientific Developments

A New Approach to Heart Attacks

In the early 1960s a heart attack, or myocardial infarction, was considered a "wound to the heart." The treatment, as with most wounds, was tincture of time. Patients who were lucky enough to make it to the hospital were consigned to a quiet room as far from the hustle and bustle of the nurses' station as possible. Unmonitored and with few interventions available to treat them, 30 percent of patients admitted with a myocardial infarction died in the hospital.[2] That dismal statistic would change dramatically with the introduction of the Coronary Care Unit.

The Coronary Care Unit burst onto the hospital scene in 1961 and spread like the common cold. Instead of being dispersed throughout the hospital, patients were grouped together in an environment where vigilant nurses could respond promptly to warning signals emitted from the monitors that were now routinely applied to each patient. Using the newly available technology of external defibrillation and closed chest massage (cardiopulmonary resuscitation was first shown to be effective in reversing otherwise fatal electrical abnormalities of the heart in 1960) cut the in-hospital mortality rate in half.[3]

At just about the same time—in the years immediately preceding the introduction of Medicare—early results from the Framingham Heart Study upended the traditional view of what caused heart attacks in the first place. This comprehensive longitudinal study initiated by the fledgling National Institutes of Health in 1948 sought to shed light on how heart disease develops by studying the lifestyles of people living in a representative community, Framingham, Massachusetts. What the study discovered is so widely acknowledged today that it is difficult to believe it was once a startling revelation: high blood pressure and high cholesterol levels are associated with coronary artery disease. For the first time in human history, treatment other than rest was on the horizon.

Along with the recognition that heart attacks are triggered by lifestyle factors came a new understanding of atherosclerosis itself. In work that would garner a Nobel Prize, research scientists came to understand that atherosclerosis is an inflammatory process that ultimately produces symptoms (either transient ischemia, or an episodic loss of blood flow manifesting as angina, or prolonged ischemia, causing a heart attack). What that meant was that treatment could effectively intervene in the process, either with drugs that promoted blood flow despite narrowing of blood vessels, or with a procedure that opened up blocked vessels. That procedure could be coronary artery bypass surgery or it could be a stent that compresses the offending plaque and holds the coronary artery open.

In 2015, what happened to a patient with a heart attack was totally different from what happened in 1960. In the ambulance on the way to the hospital— and most heart attack victims do come to the hospital—paramedics initiate treatment with an aspirin and nitroglycerin. In the emergency department, physicians immediately obtain an electrocardiogram. If it shows a particular pattern (ST-elevation, in electrocardiographic parlance), the patient is whisked off to the cardiac catheterization laboratory for urgent stent placement. He—or, with increasing frequency, she—is then sent to the Coronary Care Unit for close monitoring and treatment with other drugs, including a beta-blocker and an angiotensin-converting enzyme inhibitor to make it easier for the heart to pump. Barring further complications, the patient will go home within days.

Advances in Imaging

Whatever else happens to patients in the hospital, they can expect to undergo procedures. Among the most common procedures is imaging—from the lowly plain x-ray, not so different from what Roentgen designed in the late nineteenth century, to a PET scan or a functional MRI. But before 1971, there was no such thing as even a head CT scanner; it hadn't yet been invented. When a prototype scanner was released in 1971 and physicians saw the images it generated for the first time, they were stunned. Conventional radiographs are good for looking at bones. They can also show an enlarged heart or fluid in the lungs, but they cannot delineate soft tissues. Firing x-rays at a target from multiple different angles and then reconstructing what looks like a three-dimensional image is an entirely different process—and the results are astonishing.

Computerized tomography scanning technology had its beginnings with Godfrey Hounsfield, a self-taught British engineer who began his career at EMI Laboratories in 1951, where he initially worked on radar and guided weapon systems. To conduct this work, he made use of radar, scanning an area of interest and trying to detect patterns that would allow him to tell missiles where to go. It was a bold but, in retrospect, obvious leap from this approach to directing x-ray beams into the body from various angles, and then calculating what was inside based on the different rates of attenuation of the beams. Step by step, beginning in 1967 and culminating in the first demonstration of a prototypical machine four years later, Hounsfield turned his ideas into a working prototype.

Physicians immediately recognized the enormous clinical potential of the new technology, and by the end of 1973, six scanners had been installed in the United States. Five years later, there were over 1,000, with at least one in every state. The diffusion of the technology proceeded with unparalleled speed— long before any improvements in diagnostic acumen or health outcomes had been established, and despite the objections raised by health policy mavens about its high cost. Every hospital, or at least every teaching hospital, insisted on having one of the new machines.[4] But the first generation of CT scanners was slow, which meant both that patients had to remain motionless in an enclosed machine for long periods of time (sometimes necessitating sedation), and that certain tissues such as the beating heart or blood vessels could not be satisfactorily imaged. Technological breakthroughs led to the creation of 64-slice scanners, then 128-slice scanners, and now 256- or even 320-slice machines. Together with other theoretical advances, this led to the development of CT-angiography, a remarkable technology that provides views of the blood vessels within minutes after a simple injection of dye into a vein in the arm. The technique has partly replaced the far more invasive technique of injecting dye directly into an artery and following its progress through the vasculature with fluoroscopy.

Godfrey Hounsfield was awarded the Albert Lasker Clinical Medical Research Award for his contributions to diagnostic radiology in 1975; four years later, he would be one of the few scientists to receive a Nobel Prize as well. He shared the prize with Allan Cormack, who had simultaneously created the mathematical algorithms underlying scanner design.

Despite the tremendous contribution of computerized tomography to the diagnosis of disease, there were parts of the body, structures such as ligaments and tendons and the spinal cord, that proved difficult to visualize. Enter Paul Lauterbur and Peter Mansfield, who would share a Nobel Prize in Medicine in 2003 for their work developing magnetic resonance imaging.

Lauterbur was an American chemist and Mansfield was a British physicist—neither was a medical doctor. And while some of the inspiration for exploring nuclear magnetic resonance as a means of imaging the human body derived from a physician—Raymond Damidian of the State University of New York in Brooklyn published a paper in the journal *Science* demonstrating that cancerous tissues behave differently from healthy tissues in vitro when exposed to a magnetic field[5]—it was more basic scientific expertise that was required to launch the experiments that would ultimately lead to the MRI machine.

Since the 1940s, chemists understood that because atomic nuclei behaved differently in a magnetic field, spectroscopy could be used to determine the molecular composition of chemical compounds. Dr. Lauterbur, an expert in nuclear magnetic resonance spectroscopy, had the fundamental idea that subjecting parts of the body to magnetic fields of varying strength could be used to collect spatial information about human tissues. Dr. Mansfield, a professor of physics at the University of Nottingham, England, developed a way to accelerate the process of interpreting the data, allowing rapid reconstruction of an image. A prototype was developed and the first commercial MRI appeared in 1980.

As with CT scanners, the appetite for the new imaging technology proved voracious. And MRI had one major advantage over CT: because it used magnetic fields and radio waves, not x-rays, it was safer. Not only did MRI avoid exposure to potentially carcinogenic radiation, its earliest MRI images were also much sharper than the earliest CT images. As a result, MRI was *"the growth industry"* in diagnostic imaging in the 1980s, with twenty-seven companies entering the market for the machines by 1986.[6]

Magnetic resonance imaging technology continued to advance. Thanks to larger, faster computers, the power to manipulate ever-growing amounts of data grew exponentially. Images became sharper and the time required to process the data shrank. By 2014, the United States would have 38 MRI scanners for every million people, far more than other developed nations such as France with 10.5 per million and Germany with 11.6 per million, though not quite as many as Japan, with its nearly 47 scanners per million.[7]

Advances in science and technology clearly had an enormous impact on hospital care in general, and on the care of older patients in particular. But some of what happened to the elderly—the great enthusiasm for using the available technology and the willingness to use it with even the oldest and frailest patients—had as much to do with sociological factors, with attitudes and expectations, as with knowledge and know-how.

Social Factors Affecting the Development of the American Hospital

The Demographic Shift

A striking demographic shift took place in the United States during the second half of the twentieth century. Birth rates fell, life expectancy rose, and while immigration increased as well, bringing a new population of young people to the country, its effect was dwarfed by longer life expectancies. The net result was a transition from a young society to an aging one. As people live longer, they tend to develop chronic diseases. They suffer from diabetes, arthritis, heart failure, and degenerative neurologic conditions such as Alzheimer's disease and Parkinson's disease. Many of them have more than one chronic disease: Medicare calculates that 87 percent of enrollees over age sixty-five have multiple chronic conditions, and among hospitalized older people, the rate is even higher.[8]

Hospitals were forced to change in light of the new demographic reality. It was a matter of survival. No acute care facility could expect to fill half its beds with obstetric patients, as had been the norm in 1965, now that women of childbearing age made up a smaller percentage of the population—not to mention that the new standard was for women to stay in the hospital two days after delivery, not ten, and family size had fallen as well. In the emergency department, most of the stretchers were occupied by septuagenarians waiting to move to an inpatient unit, often a CCU or an ICU: 43 percent of the ICU admissions at one major Boston teaching hospital in 2008 were for patients over age sixty-five, and the mean age of these older patients was seventy-eight.[9]

Ironically, some of the regrettable aspects of the older patient's hospital experience today, such as the propensity to develop delirium and the high rate of functional decline, are due to the failure of the hospital to adequately adapt to its graying population. While the hospital of 2015 looks very different from its counterpart of fifty years ago due to the sophisticated technological equipment and the omnipresent women doctors, its basic structure remains unchanged. Doctors make rounds, they order tests and treatments— some of the tests and treatments are different and they are ordered electronically instead of manually, but the process is essentially the same—and nurses and technicians deliver much of the hands-on care. Patients go wherever they are sent and swallow whatever pills the nurse doles out to them. The hospital today is still very much a total institution, organized for the convenience of its medical staff.[10] Efforts to modify the basic organizational principles, for example by introducing specialized acute care units for older people, have run up against the hospital's drive for efficiency. The laser-sharp focus on creating a well-oiled machine geared to the interests of a healthy bottom line is derived from the trend toward consolidation and growth throughout corporate America.

Consolidation and Growth in Corporate America

Talk today about big business getting bigger, about companies becoming "too big to fail," and most people immediately think of the banking industry. But well before the meltdown of 2008, mergers and acquisitions had been transforming America's financial institutions. In 1990, the largest banks held 20 percent of the country's financial assets; twenty years later, the figure had more than doubled. During the same period, the number of financial institutions had decreased from 12,500 to 8,000.[11]

Banks were hardly the only institutions to see the rise of near monopolies. One headline in *USA Today* in 2015 lamented the "incredible consolidating travel industry" as web-based services such as Travelocity and Expedia gradually drove personalized travel agents out of business. Mergers and acquisitions in the airline industry, as well as bankruptcies, have reduced the number of major United States carriers from ten in 2005 to four in 2015.[12]

In health care, consolidations have occurred in multiple arenas. The health insurance industry, for instance, has been contracting for decades. Other than during a brief period during the 1980s and 1990s when health insurance companies proliferated in response to the transient proliferation of health maintenance organizations (HMOs), the private health insurance market has been steadily becoming an oligopoly. By the early 2000s, it was dominated by five giant companies. Given the substantial regional variation, the industry was actually even more consolidated: in every state, over half of all enrollees were insured through just three firms. In fourteen states, the largest three firms jointly controlled at least two-thirds of the market.[13] Facing a stiff challenge from large health care systems that demanded high reimbursements, Aetna made a bid for Humana in the summer of 2015, offering $34 billion for the smaller company, and Anthem set its sights on Cigna, offering $54 billion. These deals, if they survive scrutiny by the Department of Justice, which is investigating their antitrust consequences, would make Aetna and Anthem the largest private insurers, with UnitedHealthcare, having 85 million members, a close third.[14]

The sector that has seen some of the largest mergers and acquisitions is the pharmaceutical industry. Here, too, the phenomenon began as early as the 1980s as companies sought to stamp out competition and improve their bottom line. Some of the mega-mergers took place between foreign drug companies, demonstrating just how international the field is. But when Ciba-Geigy and Sandoz, both Swiss pharmaceutical powerhouses, merged in 1996 to form Novartis, the new company would have important administrative offices in the United States as well as an American sales force and American research labs. The same was true for the acquisition by Britain's Glaxo Wellcome (itself the product of a merger) of SmithKline (the result of still another merger) to form the less than euphonious GlaxoSmithKline for a mere $76 billion. This conjoining, like many others of its time, was between rivals. It would allow diversification—Glaxo brought the anti-ulcer drug Zantac (ranitidine) as well as AIDS-fighting drugs and asthma medication to the marriage, while SmithKline contributed the anti-depressant Paxil (parox-etine) and the successful antibiotic Augmentin (a combination of two drugs, amoxicillin and clavulanate). In addition to creating what at the time was the world's largest drug maker, the new company hoped to save money through economies of scale.[15]

The 2000s brought renewed enthusiasm for mega-mergers as companies found their future profitability threatened by the loss of patent protection, cheaper generics, and a paucity of good drugs in their research and develop-ment pipeline. Attempting to reverse its decline, the world's largest drug company, Pfizer, announced in January 2009 that it would take over Wyeth for a cool $68 billion.[16] The company had a prior history of acquisitions, hav-ing purchased Warner-Lambert in 1999. The new joint company hoped to save money by eliminating duplication, in the process shrinking its R&D ef-fort along with the number of its pharmaceutical representatives and the size of its administrative staff. Many analysts saw the purchase as a desperate move by Pfizer's new CEO, Jeff Kindler, to compensate for his company's im-minent loss of its main cash cow, Lipitor. Sales of this cholesterol-lowering drug accounted for one-fourth of Pfizer's $48 billion revenues in 2007, but the drug would soon lose patent protection and the company didn't have any promising drugs in its pipeline with which to replace it.

The Wyeth acquisition wasn't the end of Pfizer's shopping spree. In July 2010, Pfizer announced it was buying Pharmacia, a move that would so-lidify its global leadership position. Like other pharmaceutical companies, it was under pressure from politicians and hospital chains to limit price increases at the same time that it was under pressure from its investors to increase its earnings. This merger would allow the company to move into several new areas, including cancer and ophthalmology, and potentially improve its bot-tom line.[17]

Not to be left behind, Merck acquired Schering-Plough (already a merged company) for $41 billion. Merck was similarly suffering from lost revenue after its leading blockbuster, the osteoporosis drug Fosamax (alendronate), became available as a generic, and from the imminent loss of one of its other mainstays, the asthma drug Singulair (montelukast). It hoped that its new partner would live up to its reputation as a "juggernaut of drug innovation." (It wouldn't.) And so the churning continued.[18]

Hospitals were likewise infected with the drive toward bigness. The result was the appearance of hospital chains, a surge in mergers and acquisitions, and the creation of entire hospital systems—formal and informal arrangements among hospitals, physician practices, ambulatory surgery centers, and even skilled nursing facilities to share resources in order to take advantage of economies of scale, and above all to gain clout with the insurers by virtue of their large market share. One way to get big was to go from not-for-profit status—the structure of all but 6 percent of American hospitals in 1975—to becoming a for-profit corporation.[19] That proved to be a popular step, first in the 1980s, in response to the enormous increase in demand for medical services generated by the Medicare and Medicaid programs, and then again in the 1990s, in response to the emergence of HMOs. By 1999, 15 percent of American hospitals were for-profit.[20]

Yet another surge in hospital growth came with the realization that the deep pockets of private equity firms constituted an attractive source of capital with which to facilitate growth. Areas of the country such as New England, which had been almost exclusively nonprofit territory, suddenly found themselves with a new kind of hospital in their midst: in eastern Massachusetts, the Steward Health Care System bought up multiple struggling hospitals to build its own empire, financed by Cerberus Capital Management, a large private equity firm.

The job of the hospital CEO has grown in proportion to the increase in size, power, and importance of hospitals. As a result, CEO pay has soared— even at nonprofits. The CEOs at the not-for-profit Boston teaching hospitals all made over $1 million in salary, benefits, and other compensation in 2013. Dr. Elizabeth Nabel, president of Brigham and Women's Hospital, made $2.5 million, and her counterpart at Massachusetts General Hospital made $2.3 million.[21] Moreover, in a national study, there was no discernible correlation between executive pay and mission-driven objectives such as the quality of care and community benefit. Rather, what influenced compensation, aside from hospital size, urban location, and teaching status, was patient satisfaction levels as well as high levels of technology.[22]

The growth imperative among hospitals has been manifest in ways other than ownership. The most dramatic development, and one that makes today's hospitals very different from their earlier selves, is the formation of hospital systems. And while the for-profit HCA is the largest health care system of them all, there are plenty of not-for-profits in the club. Sutter (California) and Partners HealthCare (Massachusetts) are two of the biggest. The CEOs of hospital systems are paid even more than the CEOs of discrete hospitals. For example, the president and CEO of St. Louis-based Ascension earned $7.1 million in 2013, more than double what he made the year before. And the value of his total compensation, including not just his base pay and bonus, but also nontaxable benefits and deferred compensation, was reportedly $8.5 million. He wasn't unique.[23]

Institutions vary in the way they combine to form a system: several of the major New York hospitals, including North Shore-Long Island Jewish, Montefiore Medical Center, and Mount Sinai Hospital, have favored horizontal integration and merged with other hospital systems. A few of their fellow New York institutions, including NY-Presbyterian and NYU Langone, have pursued vertical integration, preferring to tighten their hold on the entire health care chain, from outpatient clinic to hospital to skilled nursing facility.[24] Across the country, hospitals are getting larger and forming chains as they buy up community hospitals or other, smaller chains in their quest for leverage in negotiating with insurers and vendors. The number of community hospitals has stayed constant for the last two decades, hovering around 5,000, but the proportion of hospitals that are part of a system has gone from 45 percent in 1999 to 63 percent in 2014.[25] For patients, this near monopoly growth has meant higher prices and lower quality of care.[26] It has also meant a focus on efficiency as systems seek to streamline their operations.

Alongside corporatization, other engines have been powering the drive to achieve efficiency. One of the most potent has been federal legislation, chiefly in the form of the initial Medicare program and its subsequent amendments.

Legislative Landmarks

The modern transformation of the American hospital dates to the enactment of Medicare and Medicaid by Congress. The passage of Medicare had the immediate result of increasing hospitalization rates for older people. In the early 1960s, only 61 percent of people between the ages of sixty-five and seventy-four had hospital insurance, and an even more paltry 41 percent of those aged seventy-five or older, who were in greatest need, had coverage. As soon as *all* older people had health insurance, they began going to the hospital for the elective surgery they had put off and the nagging symptoms they had ignored. The pent-up demand resulted in a 10 percent increase in hospitalization between 1965, just before the introduction of Medicare, and 1967.[27] The rise in utilization continued as use of the hospital became increasingly acceptable to older people: between 1970 and 1975, admissions for those over age sixty-five increased 30 percent; between 1975 and 1980, they jumped another 29 percent, well beyond the modest growth of the older population.[28]

Medicare was so successful in filling hospital beds with older patients that the program's costs quickly spiraled out of control, leading to the first major legislative change in the way Medicare paid for hospital services. In the beginning, hospitals submitted bills and Medicare paid. Hospitals itemized their bills: every x-ray, every pill, every day of care incurred a charge. The ingenious solution to the problem of unbounded costs introduced in 1982 was payment reform. Instead of paying whatever hospitals charged, the new arrangement reimbursed based on "diagnosis-related groups," essentially providing a fixed fee for each admitting diagnosis at the time of hospitalization. The effect of prospective payment was immediate and profound: all hospitalized older patients, regardless of diagnosis, stayed in the hospital much shorter than previously.[29]

At about the same time that Congress instituted prospective payment, it expanded the Medicare program to include a hospice benefit. Introduced in 1982 as part of the Tax Equity and Fiscal Responsibility Act of 1982 (TEFRA or PL97-248), the initial hospice legislation had a sunset provision—it was set to automatically expire in 1986. Hence, its prognosis was unclear, though as it turned out, the program was reauthorized and has been a feature of health care ever since. The availability of hospice care, most of which is provided at home, has meant a slow but steady change in where older people die. In 1989, just a few years after Medicare hospice first became available, slightly under 50 percent of older patients died in the hospital. By 1997, only 41 percent of the elderly people who died that year spent their last days in the hospital, and by 2009, the figure was 25 percent.[30] To be sure, the site of death for some of the people who no longer died in the hospital was a skilled nursing facility. But a growing number died at home, which is what most people say they would prefer, while enrolled in hospice.

Medicare hospice did not catch on immediately. In 1984, shortly after the first hospices opened their doors, only 200 Medicare beneficiaries enrolled, accounting for less than half a percent of deaths that year. Merely one year later, 6,000 older people enrolled in hospice, and by 1986, the proportion of "Medicare decedents" who were in hospice at the time of death reached 7 percent. That percentage has increased steadily, rising to 19 percent in 1998 and soaring to 47 percent in 2013.[31] Not everyone enrolled in hospice dies at home. Some patients change their minds about concentrating on comfort at the expense of life-prolongation, or they need care that cannot be provided at home and request transfer to the hospital; some patients who live in a nursing home enroll in hospice near the end of life and remain in the institution at the time of death. But what is clear is that the hospital has, to a growing extent, become a place for high-tech, life-prolonging medical treatments and not for the kind of care that most people need when they are dying.

The hospital's rebirth as a palace of technology was furthered by other leg-islation that pushed additional groups of patients out of the hospital. The first to go were those who were only slightly ill, which had the effect of restricting hospital care to the sickest patients. The main stimulus for this development was the introduction of prospective payment, but the increased availability of home care also facilitated getting patients home quickly. Home care, pro-vided by a visiting nurse association, had been included in the original 1965 Medicare legislation, and starting in 1972, Medicare also covered physical therapy and speech therapy (at home or elsewhere). But beginning in 1980, Congress expanded the options for home care by allowing services to be pro-vided by for-profit agencies and by removing the limit on the number of visits allowed for each "episode" of illness. The combination of the greater avail-ability of home care and prospective payment for hospital care resulted in an enormous rise in the use of home health care: between 1988 and 1996, Medicare spending on home health increased an average of 31 percent each year, with the number of beneficiaries using the services increasing by 225 percent, and each beneficiary using more services for a longer time period.[32] Usage in-creased so substantially that Congress felt the need to rein in spending and, as part of the Balanced Budget Act of 1997, it introduced prospective payment for home health services. The result was dramatic: between 1997 and 1999, use of home health care fell by half, but much of the change was the use of less home health aide time and a shorter period of coverage.[33] It was patients with chronic medical problems who lost out; those recovering from an acute illness—the people who were being discharged "quicker and sicker" from the hospital—continued to benefit from enhanced home health care.

Another group of patients who were increasingly excluded from hospital care were those requiring minor surgery or certain procedures. The Omnibus Budget Reconciliation Act of 1980 added a new Medicare benefit: Medicare would cover certain surgical procedures if they were performed in freestand-ing ambulatory surgical centers. To encourage patients to use these centers rather than the hospital, Medicare waived the deductibles and co-pays that patients would otherwise have had to pay for this care. In addition, Medicare instructed physician review organizations, the agencies charged with deter-mining whether a hospitalization was necessary or not, to deny coverage for procedures done in the hospital that could equally well have been performed in an ambulatory surgical center. As a result, inpatient cataract surgery, which once accounted for a large share of inpatient care, fell by two-thirds between 1983 and 1985.[34]

The next legislative landmark to transform the American hospital was the Balanced Budget Act (BBA) of 1997. Designed to contain exploding Medicare costs, the BBA put the screws on hospitals. It lowered reimbursement rates for Medicare patients, who accounted for fully 40 percent of all admissions. It decreased the compensation to attending physicians caring for inpatients, making travel to the hospital to care for patients even less attractive than it already was. And it strongly encouraged hospitals to freeze the size of their residency programs, long a source of cheap labor for them, by limiting Medicare's contribution to the cost of Graduate Medical Education. Faced with an inadequate supply of physicians and a revenue squeeze, hospitals increasingly turned to hospitalists, nurse practitioners, and physician assistants to fill the gap.[35] By 2001, 80 percent of the country's leading hospitals were using hospitalists, fueled in part by the BBA.[36]

The final piece of legislation that has had a major impact on the modern hospital is the Patient Protection and Affordable Care Act (ACA) of 2010. This law does far more than mandate insurance coverage for all Americans, regardless of age. It also has enormous implications for hospitals through multipronged reforms in the way Medicare works in the hospital. Undergirding most of its new programs is the basic principle of "value-based purchasing."[37] In its earliest days, Medicare reimbursed hospitals, along with everyone else who submitted bills, for each item listed on their invoice. Then Medicare reimbursed hospitals a lump sum depending on the patient's diagnosis. Now, Medicare reimburses hospitals based at least in part on the quality of the care provided. That philosophy led to the Hospital Readmissions Reduction Program, one of the many pieces of the ACA legislation, in which hospitals are subject to a monetary penalty if their readmission rates exceed a certain threshold. It led to a similar strategy for hospital-acquired conditions, in which monetary penalties are also imposed when hospital patients develop any of a long list of untoward events. And the commitment to value-based purchasing is at the root of the Medicare Shared Savings Program, which encourages hospitals to collaborate with other health care institutions and to coordinate care across multiple sites.

The ACA is also built on the principle of "patient engagement." Patient participation in their own health care is held to be the key to better health outcomes and lower costs. The idea, deeply engrained in economic thinking about health care, is that patients should be viewed as consumers and informed consumers are savvy purchasers.[38] The ACA translates this ideology into practice by endorsing public reporting of hospital (and physician) performance. The *Hospital Compare* website—allowing potential patients to compare hospitals along a variety of dimensions, from patient satisfaction to safety to timeliness of medical treatment—is the result. All of these programs—the Hospital Readmissions Reduction Program, the hospital-acquired conditions penalties, the Medicare Shared Savings Program, and *Hospital Care*—constitute the main ways that Medicare shapes hospitals today.

Fifty Years of the American Hospital

Superficially, the American hospital of 1965 looked very much like its 2015 counterpart. There were more four-bed rooms than today and some giant twenty-five-bed wards. But the long corridors, the central nursing stations, the general bustle of nurses, orderlies, and doctors, are unchanged. Closer inspection reveals more telling changes: computers are everywhere, with nurses wheeling laptops around on portable stands as they make their rounds; many of the physicians and nearly half of the youngest ones are women; and substantial sections of every building are devoted to radiology and endoscopy suites, to interventional cardiology, or to operating rooms. This metamorphosis reflects developments outside of health care. First and foremost, it reflects scientific progress stemming from fields as disparate as chemistry, physics, and computer science. Computerized tomography scanning, which was conducted 353,000 times in hospitalized patients over age sixty-five in 2007, had its origins in radar and weapons technology. Magnetic resonance imaging, another very popular test, relies on nuclear spectroscopy, used by chemists to reveal the structure of molecules. The treatment of myocardial infarction also changed thanks to developments within biology (a new understanding of the role of blood vessels in the development of disease) as well as epidemiology (the power of a longitudinal, population-based study to uncover lifestyle factors responsible for disease).

Along with dramatic leaps forward in medical science were equally profound social changes. Americans lived longer and developed more chronic diseases. Hospitals, however, were set up to handle episodes of acute illness, not to work with primary care doctors to plan for the aftermath of the acute exacerbation of a chronic condition. In the surrounding society, big was better and corporations had an increasingly free hand in conducting business. The widespread growth and consolidation of industry was echoed in health care, with mergers, acquisitions, and the appearance of hospital chains all affecting the patient's experience of illness.

But even more important to the transformation of the hospital was Medicare, from its original incarnation to the newest version of Medicare ushered in by the Affordable Care Act. The very existence of Medicare forever changed the American hospital, not just by bringing throngs of older patients to its wards, but also by racially integrating hospitals—a prerequisite for accepting federal funds that segregated southern hospitals reluctantly complied with. The institution of prospective payment for Medicare in the early 1980s shortened the average hospital stay for older patients, cramming tests and procedures into a few days, and moving much of what had traditionally been inpatient care out of the hospital altogether. Some types of treatment that were initiated in the acute care hospital, such as hip replacement surgery or antibiotics for pneumonia, were now completed in the skilled nursing facility; other kinds of care, such as colonoscopy screening or cataract surgery, moved to the ambulatory site.

Legislation creating a Medicare hospice program further altered what happened to older patients in the hospital—a growing proportion of older people died at home rather than in the hospital. Restrictions on the number of residency slots funded by Medicare, together with rules limiting the length of a resident's workday, put limits on the hospital's physician workforce, effectively stimulating the use of physician assistants and nurse practitioners to provide hands-on care. And the Affordable Care Act continued the tradition of legislatively reshaping the Medicare program by promoting value-based reimbursement—incentivizing hospitals based on outcomes rather than volume—and by supporting patient engagement in health care—encouraging patients to participate in their treatment through self-management.

In the course of modifying the hospital, Medicare created a new institution entirely, the skilled nursing facility. Built on the model of the long-stay nursing home, where many Americans spent their final months or years, and in many cases taking advantage of the existing nursing home infrastructure, these facilities morphed into something new and different: a short-stay, low-tech facility that was more like an infirmary than either a hospital or a nursing home. A SNF stay would be in the next stop on the health care journey for a growing number of older patients.

Part III
The Skilled Nursing Facility

CHAPTER NINE

Going to Rehab

When I was growing up, I had minimal exposure to older people. I never knew my grandparents: they were all dead, either directly or indirectly at the hands of the Nazis. What few older people I knew lived in their own homes, not in a nursing home. The little I did know about nursing homes was what I learned from two books that were published in the 1970s, Robert Butler's seminal work, *Why Survive? Being Old in America*,[1] and Mary Adelaide Mendelson's consummate exposé, *Tender Loving Greed*.[2] People like me who read these two acerbic critiques of nursing homes decided then and there that we would never, ever live in such a place.

We also thought we would remain healthy and vigorous until, at some very remote date, surely after our 85th birthdays, we would die in our sleep. But, just in case we needed help getting by, we wanted to be sure there would be somewhere to move to other than a nursing home. Assisted living was designed to be that alternative. It offered the privacy that nursing homes lacked and provided the requisite support, or so we believed, without the loss of dignity and independence characteristic of nursing homes. And so, based on the deep-seated conviction that assisted living is the answer to the aging conundrum, it became one of the leading growth industries of the 1990s.[3] We baby boomers breathed a collective sigh of relief: we were safe, we would have plenty of possibilities other than nursing homes waiting for us if the time came. Never did we imagine that we actually would go to nursing homes, and in droves, to nursing homes that had been retooled as short-term, post-acute "skilled nursing facilities." Today, 1.7 million older people each year spend time in such a skilled nursing facility, not for the long haul, but short term, for rehabilitation after a hospital stay.[4]

A brief stay in a nursing home is, of course, different from a far longer stay: a month might be tolerable even if a year would not be. But, to a large extent, these are the same facilities, the same institutions, that provide short-term and long-term care. Older people are once again relying on nursing homes for care at a very significant time in their lives, and the people who make use of SNFs tend to be the frailest, oldest, and sickest of the elderly population. Their experience matters—for their well-being, their dignity, and their future.

The SNF Experience

When Taylor Bryan II was first admitted to the hospital, he didn't think about being discharged. If he thought about the future at all, he imagined that the hospital would fix whatever had made him slump to the ground, unconscious, and then he would return to the house where he had lived with his wife for the previous fifty years. He liked his home and he liked the neighborhood. It was where he had brought up his children—Taylor Bryan III, who was now a well-known physician in the community, and Elizabeth Jane Bryan, who was an attorney in Seattle.

Mr. Bryan was taken aback when he was diagnosed as having blockages in three coronary arteries and a poorly functioning heart valve, and then was told he needed open-heart surgery. He hadn't been sick a day in his life, and the only surgeries he'd had were a hernia repair and an appendectomy. But he was adaptable, and once he'd processed that this time he had a serious medical problem, he focused all his attention on getting better.

Taylor Bryan would get a lot worse before he got better. Surgeons at the hospital gave him a new heart valve and bypassed his blocked coronary arteries, but then the trouble began. As with so many older patients, the operation itself was uneventful, but it was followed by a slew of complications. First, he developed a massive, life-threatening infection. His family was summoned to the hospital late at night and told to say their goodbyes—his blood pressure was plummeting, he was barely conscious, and the on-call physician didn't think he'd make it until morning. Bryan did make it, only to start vomiting blood as soon as his infection was under control. With one violent paroxysm after another, his body ejected blood in volcanic streams. Exhausted and in pain, he endured an upper endoscopy, which pinpointed a stomach ulcer as the cause of the bleeding. He lost half his blood volume, needed a six-unit transfusion, and then, remarkably, the bleeding stopped. But along the way, he developed acute renal failure. Once again his family was called to the ICU for a meeting, this time to discuss whether he should start dialysis. While his son, daughter, and wife were deliberating, his kidney function gradually improved. Taylor Bryan looked as though he might survive after all.

He survived, but not without developing a series of comparatively minor problems—problems that nonetheless took their toll. Even after his renal function was almost back to baseline, he wasn't urinating very much. The problem turned out not to be his kidneys, but rather his enlarged prostate, which made it hard for him to pass his urine. The fix was a bladder catheter, a constant companion that inhibited what little ability he had to get around. While he'd been bleeding, Bryan hadn't been allowed to take anything by mouth, and after he stopped bleeding, he didn't have much of an appetite. Alarmed that he had lost ten pounds since arriving at the hospital, the staff inserted a feeding tube through which they delivered artificial nutrition. That meant yet another tube, along with the bladder catheter and a couple of IVs. If that wasn't enough, Taylor Bryan developed a rapid and irregular heartbeat, which won him a new cardiac medication. Regrettably, either the arrhythmia or the medication used to treat it made him confused. The doctors weren't convinced that the confusion was related to his heart problems, so they ordered an MRI (to rule out a stroke) and an electroencephalogram (to rule out a seizure), even though there wasn't any good evidence to suggest either.

After seven weeks in the ICU, his doctors finally pronounced Taylor Bryan ready for discharge. His family balked. He was far too weak to go home. No problem, the doctors assured the family. He wouldn't be going home, he'd be going to rehab.

Mr. Bryan's family was familiar with rehab. His son, Taylor Bryan III, was an orthopedist who specialized in knees. His patients routinely went to a rehabilitation facility for a week or two so they could literally get back on their feet after surgery. Ditto for the patients of his orthopedic colleagues who specialized in hips. But at this point, Dr. Bryan's father was no longer a surgical patient, he was a medical patient. And his medical problems had all been addressed. Before he could be rehabilitated, he needed to recuperate.

Taylor Bryan II—known all his life as Junior, even after his son was born— had no opinion on the subject of discharge. His heart, his stomach, and his kidneys might be functioning well, but his brain was not. He was still confused, delirious, and couldn't weigh in one way or another.

It was Mrs. Bryan who persuaded her son that the medical team had a point. After all that Junior had been though in the hospital, he was deconditioned. He was weak and disoriented. She certainly couldn't take care of him at home, not without a lot of help. Her son resisted. If his dad wasn't ready to go home, he should stay in the hospital until he was. The resident pointed out that really wasn't possible; Medicare wouldn't allow it. Taylor Bryan II, while clearly a very sick man, wasn't sick enough to warrant hospital care.

Ultimately, Dr. Bryan came around and agreed that his father would benefit from rehab. He spoke to the case manager, a nurse assigned to make sure patients were discharged in a timely fashion and to arrange for what was known in hospitalese as their "disposition." She helpfully printed a list of preferred facilities that were reasonably close to Mrs. Bryan, namely, the institutions with which the hospital had a relationship. That meant the lines of communication between the staff at the hospital and at the nursing home were somewhat better than the usual one-pager that accompanied the patient to the facility, and perhaps the two institutions shared access to electronic medical records. The hospital case manager then indicated which facilities actually had a bed available or would likely have one in the next few days. That narrowed the choices from ten to three, much to Taylor Bryan III's relief as he was encouraged to visit these places and make a decision—preferably in the next twenty-four hours—and he had a full schedule of patients as well as a family of his own to attend to.

How, Dr. Bryan wondered, would he know what to look for if he visited? He knew a great deal about hospitals, but he had to admit that while he had sent plenty of patients to rehab facilities, he had never actually visited one. Would he rely on the sniff test, checking whether the facility smelled more of disinfectant, urine, or air freshener? Wouldn't the facilities simply present him with a sales pitch, a song and dance that was apt to reveal more about the skills of the public relations department and the personality of the tour guide than about the facility's quality?

Nursing Home Compare

Patients and families have two principal ways of picking a SNF. They can go by reputation or they can use the website developed by Medicare called *Nursing Home Compare*. Analogous to *Hospital Compare*, it provides data about safety and clinical care. To simplify the evaluation process, and to help the lay public home in on the essentials, Medicare created a single, overall measure of quality, just as it ultimately did for hospitals.

The Michelin approach to evaluating quality—Medicare again borrowed the idea of awarding between one and five stars for its summary measure— has engendered considerable criticism. Nursing homes, the argument goes, are unlike restaurants or hotels. And like all report cards, the validity of the grade depends on the measurements that go into it. In the case of *Nursing Home Compare*, the specific ingredients are well-defined; there is nothing subjective or mysterious about them. They are not based on hearsay or on expert opinion, components of the controversial *U.S. News and World Report* college rankings. And there's a special list of factors that are used to evaluate post-acute facilities, factors that differ slightly from those used to measure the performance of nursing facilities that provide long-term, residential care. The formula for post-acute facilities has three ingredients: the results of the latest inspection by the local public health department, staffing ratio (formerly based on facility self-report but revised in 2015 to reflect electronically maintained payroll records), and a set of quality indicators.

While patients who are in the throes of an acute illness and need immediate care have little opportunity to use a website to evaluate their options for hospitalization, patients who are already in the hospital and need post-acute care have a little more time. Their family members can even check out the possibilities in person.

In the Beginning

Based on word of mouth, Dr. Bryan dismissed one of the facilities on the list out of hand. It had gotten a lot of bad press recently, something about a disgruntled family member suing the nursing home for neglect, which the local newspaper had picked up on. The reporter documented that the chain of which that facility was a part had a record of negligence suits. Using *Nursing Home Compare*, Dr. Bryan checked on the other two homes on the case manager's list. The results for one of the facilities were impressive: five stars in every category.[5] By comparison, the second facility, that he was embarrassed to say he often used for his own patients, had a rating of three stars on health inspections (average), five on staffing (much above average), and three stars on quality measures (average), for an overall rating (based on a complex weighting of the three ingredients) of four stars (above average). For Taylor Bryan III, it was a no-brainer. His father would go to the German Center for Extended Care in Boston, an unambiguously five-star facility.

Mrs. Bryan drove to the rehab center to meet her husband, who arrived separately via ambulance. She noticed immediately that the place was light and sunny, the rooms clean and spacious. But what impressed her most was how quiet it was compared to the bustle of the acute care hospital. When she first got to the unit, the nursing station was deserted. No receptionist, no staff members reading through patient charts or working at the computer. No one. The halls were wide—and empty. A young woman showed up from the dietary department wheeling a cart with the dinner trays for the residents. A pair of visitors left the unit smiling, seemingly glad to be going. Finally, a nurse emerged from one of the patient rooms and escorted Mrs. Bryan to her husband's room. She sat with her husband, Taylor, made sure he was settled in for the night, and went home.

Mrs. Bryan had been long gone when her husband began complaining of pain. He had a small area of skin breakdown on his heels from being in bed for so many weeks, all the while getting less than optimal nutrition. In the hospital, he'd had a special mattress to keep the friction between the bed and his heels to a minimum, and he'd worn special sheepskin "booties" to further protect his heels. But no one at the hospital had mentioned any of that to the staff at the German Center, so they didn't have the necessary equipment on hand. Mr. Bryan generally got a pill at bedtime to ease the pain and help him sleep. The order for the pain medication had followed him to the German Center, but the medicine hadn't yet arrived.

The rough sheets chafed against his heels. He moaned and was restless. The night nurse tried to soothe him with Tylenol, to no avail. Eventually, she paged the covering physician, who made a few more calls, ultimately authorizing the nurse to open the facility's "emergency kit" and take out one narcotic pill for Mr. Bryan. It was midnight by the time he dozed off, sleeping fitfully.

Medications in the SNF

Skilled nursing facilities, unlike hospitals, do not usually have an in-house pharmacy. They do not allow a patient's medicines to accompany him from the hospital, pre-filled by the hospital's pharmacy, nor do they use neighborhood drugstores as suppliers. Rather, they contract their business to a pharmacy chain that provides medications to many long-term care facilities. The German Center, like many other Boston area SNFs, uses a pharmacy that is part of the Omnicare chain, the single largest supplier of medications to nursing homes in the country.

The lack of an on-site pharmacy means that newly admitted residents do not take any medications beyond Tylenol until their prescriptions are delivered by the outside pharmacy. The pharmacy has a well-honed system in place for handling its SNF customers: as soon as the facility nurse has "confirmed the orders" sent over by the hospital, which she does by reading them on the telephone to the physician who is assuming responsibility for the new patient, she faxes the prescription to the outside pharmacy, which is staffed 24/7. The pharmacy, in turn, fills the prescriptions, typically a several-day supply, and sends them to the SNF by car. All very efficient, except that the pharmacy is unlikely to be in the immediate vicinity of the SNF. And, since the distributing pharmacies make deliveries to multiple area SNFs, it is typically hours before new patients get any of their medications.

A Course of Rehab

By the time Mrs. Bryan returned to the SNF the following morning to see her husband, his medications had arrived from the pharmacy. They'd been ordered shortly after Mr. Bryan arrived, but it was only the next day that they finally came, neatly packaged in bubble wrap containers—all nineteen of them. In addition to four heart medicines (he had, after all, entered the hospital because of heart problems), he was on an antibiotic for a urinary tract infection he'd developed, probably related to the catheter he'd had in his bladder for weeks, an anti-ulcer medication, started when he developed the gastrointestinal bleed, pain medication because of his heel ulcers, a medicated salve to treat the pressure ulcers, a pill to help him pass his urine, two vitamins, and one calcium tablet. Then there were the medicines he had been on before his hospitalization: a thyroid pill for an underactive thyroid gland, a statin for elevated cholesterol, a hypoglycemic to treat his diabetes, and eyedrops for glaucoma. He was also on four as-needed medications, including insulin for diabetes, which he didn't need, but he'd had a few very elevated blood sugars when he'd been extremely ill, resulting in an order to check his blood sugar four times a day and to give him a shot of insulin if necessary.

Later that day, the nurse practitioner, Donna Nicholls, arrived to perform an admission history and physical. "He's a fighter," Taylor Bryan III told her after she finished her exam and telephoned his son to review his code status. "The doctors at the hospital tried to prepare us for the worst," he continued. "They told us it was risky for an eighty-five-year-old man to have an AVR and a four-vessel CABG," he elaborated, using medical jargon for aortic valve replacement and coronary artery bypass graft to make sure that the nurse practitioner knew he was *Doctor* Taylor Bryan. "But they didn't know my father. He just rolled with the punches. First, they couldn't get him off the vent—he had to stay attached to that breathing machine for a week. Then he got septic. He had a gastrointestinal bleed and acute renal failure. He was in the ICU for seven weeks. But he made it through and," he finished ominously, "we're not going to lose him now."

Donna Nicholls listened impassively. She tried her best to see in Taylor Bryan III a devoted son, worried his father was going to die. But she couldn't miss the threat that *they* knew what they were doing at the hospital (even if they'd been wrong about the prognosis); don't *you* mess up. "Dr. Barnes will see your dad tomorrow," she reassured Dr. Bryan. "I'll go over my findings with him." Her voice softened slightly. "It is amazing your father made it this far. But you know, he's a very sick man and he's not out of the woods yet." She chose not to mention that Taylor Bryan II was only able to answer very simple questions, and when he did reply, it was with two- or three-word phrases. Not, she imagined, anything like the way he answered questions when he had been a litigator in a prestigious law firm. He was totally dependent on nursing assistants for his most basic daily activities such as dressing or walking to the bathroom. He had a feeding tube for nutrition. All his major organ systems— his brain, his heart, his lungs, his kidneys—remained severely compromised after the beating they had taken while he was in the hospital. And thanks to chronic diet-controlled diabetes, elevated cholesterol, high blood pressure, an enlarged prostate, and an underactive thyroid, he had not been the most vigorous eighty-five-year-old even before his heart problems became evident.

Once Mr. Bryan had settled in at the German Center, his medications were ready for him, and his medical care had been reviewed by the nurse practitioner and her supervising physician, the business of rehabilitation could begin. A physical therapist worked with him each day to get him walking again. A speech therapist spent time with him to improve his language skills; she strongly suspected he had had a small stroke or two along the way, though nothing of the sort was documented in his chart. In general, the hospital doctors had not made any comments about Bryan's mental functioning. An occupational therapist helped him relearn how to comb his hair and brush his teeth. Over the next few weeks, Taylor Bryan made slow but discernible progress—he could take a few steps to the bathroom on his own and he could wash up at the sink. But then he stopped improving. The therapists concluded that Mr. Bryan was no longer benefiting from rehab and they didn't think he was likely to start benefiting anytime soon.

The Bryan family was in for another shock. They were told that since their father wasn't getting better, he would need to be discharged. Mrs. Bryan was in a tizzy—she was no better equipped to care for her husband at home than she had been three weeks earlier. Dr. Bryan was furious—his father had Medicare, and Medicare paid for one hundred days in a skilled nursing facility, he asserted on the phone with the facility. The family was going to appeal the decision.

Medicare SNF Coverage

What many families misunderstand—just as many families erroneously think that Medicare pays for nursing home care—is that Medicare pays for *up to* one hundred days of short-term rehabilitative care (actually, only in full for twenty days; from day twenty-one on, there is a sizable co-pay—$157.50 a day in 2015). Moreover, payment is contingent on medical necessity, which is determined in large measure by whether the patient is "progressing," as assessed by the facility staff.

Skilled nursing facilities are not unique in defining eligibility for reimbursement based on medical necessity. *All* medical goods and services that older patients use are paid for by Medicare, provided they meet the standard of medical necessity. The original 1965 legislation establishing the Medicare program states that Medicare may only pay for "items and services that are reasonable and necessary for the diagnosis or treatment of illness or injury or to improve the functioning of a malformed body member."[6] The list of exclusions has changed somewhat over time: physical therapy, hospice care, influenza vaccination and, since the passage of the Medicare Modernization Act of 2003, prescription medications, are now in, but hearing aids, glasses, and dental care are not (and never were). And despite repeated attempts to define "medical necessity," Congress has been unwilling to get specific. In general, whether a particular procedure will be covered is determined by "Medicare Administrative Contractors," affectionately known as MACs, which are regional, private health care insurers that process claims for Medicare beneficiaries. (Previously, there were numerous local "Medicare intermediaries"; these have been replaced by the regional MACs. As of February 2014, there were twelve MACs, with the number expected to fall to ten in the next few years.) These companies typically make their own decisions about what to cover, and they sometimes disagree with one another, resulting in some procedures being paid for in one part of the United States but not in another. Only rarely is there a centralized decision about payment, a "National Coverage Determination" that is binding on all the MACs. In one representative year, Medicare issued a total of thirteen National Coverage Determinations, most of which were revisions of previous NCDs. For example, Medicare revised its guidelines about ventricular assist devices, a kind of partial artificial heart, and also its guideline for the reimbursement of pacemakers.

Consistent with the standard of medical necessity, Medicare pays for as much as one hundred days of skilled nursing facility care—*provided* the patient meets certain criteria. And the criterion of medical necessity on which SNFs have traditionally relied is progress. As long as the patient shows measurable improvement, SNFs are confident that Medicare will pay. Once a patient is no longer getting better, it's more difficult to argue that SNF care is necessary and coverage typically comes to an end.[7] And after three weeks of rehabilitative treatment, Taylor Bryan II stopped getting better.

In the Middle

While the appeal was under review, Mr. Bryan seemingly took matters into his own hands. He became acutely ill.

The nurse on duty discovered there was a problem when she made her early morning rounds and could barely awaken Mr. Bryan. His speech was slurred and he was even more confused than usual. She took his vital signs and found his heart was racing and he had a fever. She called the nurse practitioner to evaluate him.

Mr. Bryan almost certainly had an infection, either pneumonia or a urinary tract infection, the NP guessed. She planned to do some blood tests, check a urine sample, and order a chest radiogram—a mobile x-ray van would come to the rehab center. She would start antibiotics while awaiting the results. But first she called Mr. Bryan's son.

He didn't mince words. "I want you to send my father to the hospital. Don't mess around. He's full code." And so Taylor Bryan returned to the acute care hospital.

Hospital vs. SNF

The SNFs in general—and the German Center is no exception—are not designed to provide the same level of care as a hospital. They don't have the staff and they don't have the technology. All they have is the basics: a lab technician who comes around every day, sometimes more than once, to draw blood (the samples then go by courier to an outside lab and the results are faxed back or, if the test was ordered "stat" or if the result is very abnormal, called in); an x-ray technician on-call who arrives rolling portable x-ray equipment to take images of bones (looking for fractures), chests (in search of pneumonia or fluid in the lungs), or abdomens (looking for bowel distension, indicating possible blockage); staff nurses who can insert intravenous catheters and use them to administer fluids and medications; oxygen, pumped from a special wall unit; and an NP or physician off-site but available to perform an assessment.

The German Center was lacking bustle but it was also lacking physicians. For seven weeks, Mr. Bryan had been in the ICU with a ratio of one nurse to every two patients and where one physician was almost always around—a pulmonologist (many ICUs are staffed by ICU specialists who are usually pulmonologists), an anesthesiologist, a cardiologist, or the lowly ICU intern. It had been quite a shock to move from the ICU to a regular medical floor, with its staffing ratio of one nurse to every four or five patients and once-a-day physician rounds. At the German Center, a single physician rounded once or twice a week. Between physician visits, patients were evaluated by a nurse practitioner, if they were examined at all. The orders governing the medications and treatments they were to receive were written at the hospital, faxed over to the facility, and confirmed on the telephone by a facility nurse speaking with the SNF attending physician. The German Center might technically qualify as a medical facility, but it was decidedly not a hospital.

Dr. Bryan's suspiciousness of the quality of care was not entirely unfounded. A recent study by the Department of Health and Human Services' Office of the Inspector General found that 22 percent of patients at short-term SNFs suffer a significant adverse event during their stay, and another 11 percent experience some kind of temporary harm. Fully 59 percent of these events are "clearly" or "likely" preventable. The report attributes much of the preventable harm to substandard treatments, inadequate patient monitoring, and delays in initiating care.[8]

If Dr. Bryan's suspicions about the adequacy of SNF medical care were not entirely baseless, neither was his father's readmission to the acute hospital a rare event for SNF patients. Nearly 25 percent of all patients are readmitted to the acute hospital within thirty days of their arrival at the SNF.[9] The cost of this revolving door is substantial, both to Medicare, which pays an estimated $4.3 billion each year for these readmissions, and to the patients themselves, who are at risk of falls, adverse drug reactions, delirium, and other problems associated with acute hospital care in frail elders.[10] Moreover, careful analysis suggests that as many as two-thirds of readmissions from a SNF are either definitely or probably avoidable.[11] Strategies such as prevention (by identifying and assessing problems early on), management in the nursing home (for certain common conditions), and advance care planning (to determine if patients might prefer a more palliative approach to care) can decrease the rate of readmissions, in some studies by as much as 50 percent. But Taylor Bryan's family wanted him back in the hospital, so back he went.

SNF Care, Round Two

At the acute care hospital, the attending physician ordered blood tests, a urine specimen, and a chest x-ray, exactly the same tests that the NP at the SNF had wanted to obtain. Mr. Bryan proved to have both pneumonia and dehydration, so he was started on intravenous fluids and antibiotics. After a week, he returned to the rehab. He hadn't been out of bed during the entire week. He hadn't seen a physical or occupational therapist. He had lost all his earlier gains in function.

The rehab staff reinstituted their previous plan, but this time Mr. Bryan failed to improve at all. He was too weak and too tired to participate in therapy. The physical therapist modified her approach, coming in the mornings instead of the afternoons; she coaxed Taylor to work with her for a mere fifteen minutes, and then for five minutes. She considered instituting a reward system. She asked the nurse practitioner to check his blood chemistries—everything was in order. She asked the social worker to spend time with him to encourage him. Nothing worked.

The NP and nursing home physician arranged a family meeting to review the situation with Mr. Bryan's family: the therapists reported on his physical status—he was totally dependent on help—the social worker reported on his mood—fatalistic—and the physician gave an update on his medical condition—failure to thrive. Donna Nicholls, the NP, suggested, very tentatively, that perhaps it was time to reconsider the goals of care. Maybe it was time to focus more on comfort than on extending life.

Dr. Bryan responded brusquely. "We want what we've always wanted. We want everything done so that my father can recover."

Dr. Barnes, the rehab physician, didn't miss a beat. "We don't think it likely that your father will recover. We wish it were otherwise. But sometimes the body just can't take any more."

Mr. Bryan's son bristled. "The hospital never said anything like that. They said my father should have rehab. That with rehab he would get better. It was just a matter of time."

The German Center's NP deftly sidestepped the issue of what the acute care hospital had or had not said. "What do you think Mr. Bryan would want, if he could see himself in his current condition? Would he want intravenous fluids and antibiotics and the feeding tube and further trips to the hospital?"

This time, Mrs. Bryan piped up. She was a petite woman of eighty-four, dressed in a well-tailored tweed suit. She had been married to Taylor Bryan for sixty years. "I think he's tired. He's had enough. He just wants to be comfortable." Her son scowled, but she continued, almost inaudibly. "I don't want to lose him. But it would be selfish to keep on doing all these things that he doesn't want."

Her son challenged her. "How do you know he doesn't want the treatment? Dad has always wanted the best treatment."

His mother remained calm. "I know your father. He was angry when the nurse came to start another IV the other day. He's been pulling at the feeding tube in his stomach. He told me all he wants is some coffee ice cream." Dr. Bryan was speechless. He was a surgeon and used to fixing problems. He wasn't used to problems that could not be fixed and he didn't like them, especially not where his father was concerned.

By the end of the family meeting, Mrs. Bryan had agreed to a "do not resuscitate" (DNR) order for her husband along with a "do not hospitalize" order, consistent with the goal of focusing exclusively on his comfort. She suggested offering him ice cream and other soft foods by mouth instead of hooking up the feeding tube to a bag of liquid artificial nutrition. He might choke, but better to have a chance to taste food once more.

Donna Nicholls gave Mrs. Bryan a hug as the meeting broke up. She wished she could arrange to have hospice come in to help support both the patient and his family through the days ahead, but as a short-term SNF patient, he was not simultaneously eligible for hospice services. The facility staff did their best, given their limited resources, to keep Mr. Bryan clean and neat and comfortable. Over the following week he became less and less communicative, but his eyelids fluttered open when his wife kissed him and told him she loved him. Mrs. Bryan did not want to leave him alone. The staff begged her to go home and get some rest. She refused. The staff urged her to go to the cafeteria for a bite to eat. She declined. She left her husband's side only to go to the bathroom or to take calls on her cell phone. After ten days with little food and only sips to drink, Taylor Bryan II passed away while his wife had stepped out of the room.

Dying in the SNF

The hospital medical record showed no indication that Mr. Bryan's physicians ever had a discussion about prognosis. They clearly referred their patient for rehabilitation and not for hospice, a course that hospitals pursue all the time. Sometimes the reason is that the hospital physician is not comfortable talking about end-of-life care. Sometimes it's that hospital physicians are intent on identifying a facility that can provide round-the-clock care, but not because they genuinely believe the patient will recover. And the best way to get twenty-four-hour care paid for after a hospitalization is to go to a skilled nursing facility for post-acute care.

Medicare pays full freight for SNF care after three nights in an acute care hospital—and Taylor Bryan had just spent another week in the hospital, resetting the SNF coverage clock. But Medicare doesn't generally cover inpatient hospice care. Most hospices are home-based, and most hospice care within nursing facilities is supplementary to long-term residential care. The rationale is that Medicare is responsible only for the medical piece; the residential component is paid for by someone else—either the patient, in the case of those paying privately for nursing home care, or Medicaid, in the case of those who qualify based on their low income. The reason that Medicare won't pay for both post-acute care and hospice care at the same time is that they are both Medicare Part A benefits. The presumption is that, at any given moment, patients can get one or the other, but not both. There are rare exceptions: for example, a patient is in the SNF to recover from one medical problem, say a hip fracture, and then enrolls in hospice for a totally separate medical problem, say metastatic cancer. This situation is decidedly uncommon because patients who qualify for hospice based on one diagnosis seldom have a second diagnosis from which they are expected to recover with rehabilitative care. Moreover, the two ostensibly distinct problems typically turn out, on careful analysis, to be related. A fracture, for instance, could well have been caused by a metastasis to the bone, weakening the bone and predisposing to breaks.

Many dying patients need more care than can be provided by their families at home, even with a nurse coming in for half an hour a few times a week and a home health aide providing assistance for a few hours several days a week. The way they can get the round-the-clock help they need—at least until it becomes evident that they are not getting better—is through a SNF admission.

When Taylor Bryan II showed up at the acute care hospital just weeks after discharge, the physicians taking care of him at the hospital may well have realized that he had begun the downhill spiral that would culminate in his death. They might have simply preferred not to discuss prognosis. They might have sent him back to rehab, giving him and his family the message that he would get better, because it was the best way to assure he got the intensity of nursing care he needed. Or they might simply have found it easier to avoid breaking bad news.

Most patients admitted to a skilled nursing facility do not die there. Only 9.2 percent of deaths among older people take place in a short-stay SNF. But fully 30.5 percent of older people who die had been in a SNF at some point during their last six months of life. For people eighty-five or older, the percentage jumps to over 40 percent.[12] Such high death rates indicate that, even though a patient might survive a given SNF stay and be able to return home, his chance of dying in the near future is considerable. The bottom line is that SNF patients are among the oldest, sickest, and most vulnerable people on the planet.

The New Normal

A SNF stay after hospitalization is becoming the norm for older people, especially the frailest and the oldest patients, and particularly after a long, complex hospital stay or an admission for joint replacement. Today's SNF is a
curious hybrid between modern acute care and traditional nursing home
care; at its best, the patient experiences the advantages of both with none of
the drawbacks: round-the-clock nursing care and easy access to physical
therapy without overexposure to invasive and hazardous technology. At its
worst, the patient is subject to the downside of both with few of the benefits:
a sterile, unfamiliar, and alienating environment with little physician contact
and only the most rudimentary technology.

A SNF could look and feel very different for older patients. Instead of lan-
guishing for hours without their medications after arriving at the facility,
sometimes in pain or suffering from a cardiac arrhythmia, their medications
could be pre-ordered. Patients are not sent to the SNF if no bed is available;
why should patients arrive without their medicines ready and waiting for
them? Alternatively, the hospital could arrange to send a one-day, transitional
supply of medications with any patient at the time of discharge, regardless of
whether the patient was going home or to a SNF.

Rather than confining advance care planning to the designation of a health
care surrogate and to discussion of a possible DNR status, every facility could
mandate a family meeting to discuss the goals of care within forty-eight hours
of admission. Today, family meetings typically occur much later in the patient's
course, if they take place at all, usually as discharge looms or in the event of a
conflict over care. Why not clarify up front what is realistic to expect from the
SNF stay and elicit a patient's preferences for treatment, within the constraints of the possible? Surely such an approach would go a long way toward
preventing both unnecessary readmissions to the hospital and inappropriate
treatment in the SNF. The skilled nursing facility also provides an unparalleled opportunity for an interdisciplinary team of clinicians—typically including a physician, nurse, physical therapist, and social worker, but sometimes
a nutritionist, occupational therapist, and others—to work with older people
and their families to assess their function, their needs, and their preferences
for care immediately prior to discharge, once they are as good as they are
going to get. Why not use one of the SNF's regularly scheduled interdisciplinary team meetings to review a patient's progress, to synthesize the results of
their comprehensive evaluation, and to discuss the goals of future care? For
patients who are going home, they could integrate the testing and information

gathering conducted by each member of the interdisciplinary team into a coherent view of the patient that takes into account the home situation, community resources, and personal values.

Finally, the current practice of admitting dying patients to the SNF rather than arranging for hospice care is regrettable, a waste of resources—and unnecessary. Stimulated by the well-meaning desire to push Medicare to pay for much needed twenty-four-hour care, it leads to patients getting more aggressive treatment than they want because physicians and families alike operate on the myth that the patient is there for rehabilitation and will improve enough to go home. Why not allow Medicare to pay for inpatient hospice care at the SNF for those patients who are too needy to be able to remain at home?

The experience of Taylor Bryan II in many ways paralleled the kind of care received by patients across the country in SNFs. But the German Center for Extended Care in Boston is one nursing home in one place. It is average sized (133 beds) and, like most SNFs, it's dually certified for Medicare and Medicaid patients, which means it has a mixture of long-term and short-term residents. Like the majority of nursing facilities, it's in an urban area and doesn't hire its own physician or nurse practitioner. But it is one of only 25 percent of American SNFs that are not-for-profit. It had its origins in 1914 when the German Ladies Aid Society of Boston opened a residence for elderly German-American women needing supportive care. The clientele is no longer predominantly German, although the name out front is "Deutsches Altenheim" and there are "Wilkommen" signs inside, but the organization remains dedicated to service, not profit. To figure out how much the structure and the mission affect the patient's experience, we need to compare places like the German Center to SNFs that are organized along different lines.

CHAPTER TEN

Different SNFs, Different Miffs

During my four years as a medical student and three years as a medical resident, I never once set foot in a skilled nursing facility. I knew that such places existed, and during residency we had numerous patients who lingered in the hospital until they could be "placed," until a bed could be found for them in a nursing home—as though all that mattered was where they would sleep. Still today, when patients go directly into long-term care after hospitalization, it's usually because they were living in a nursing home before their admission. Far more frequently, patients go to a SNF for short-term, post-acute care and few medical residents, and even fewer surgical residents, spend any time seeing a SNF in action. Those young physicians who do have a day allocated for visiting a SNF during the course of their residency don't actually take care of patients in the facility—they are merely tourists, there for a visit. They have little idea of what the SNF can provide, or not provide, for its residents, and what services are available, what technical capabilities the SNF has, let alone how much time is actually required to get an x-ray or a blood test—even a "stat" blood test.

On the rare occasion that a medical student or resident does spend time at a SNF, it will usually be at a single site, affording little awareness of the variety of SNF experience. At Hebrew Rehabilitation Center in Boston, where I worked as a physician for eleven years, the environment was substantially different from what I would later encounter at the German Center. We had a dedicated physician staff, which meant a physician was available to see patients 24/7. Not only that, but physicians were on-site daily, rounding on patients much like at a hospital. Unlike at the hospital, not every patient was seen each day, only those whom the unit nurse felt needed to be evaluated by a doctor, but the threshold for physician visits was far lower than at typical SNFs in light of how easy it was to request one. On the weekends, a member of the medical staff came in for half a day to see those patients scattered throughout the 725-bed facility who had an acute medical problem. And at night, a geriatrics fellow was on call—and expected to come in if the situation warranted immediate evaluation. The medical care was quantitatively and qualitatively different from what was available at more conventional SNFs, where attending physicians gave nurses orders over the phone, seldom first seeing their patient, and routinely arranged for patients to be transferred to the local hospital emergency room if further assessment was deemed necessary. Surely other aspects of the patient's experience were likewise affected by the structure and organization of the SNF? But, perhaps Leo Tolstoy's famous comment about all happy families being alike and each unhappy family being unhappy in its own way applies equally to skilled nursing facilities. Maybe the good ones are all alike in what they do right and the poor ones differ in what they do wrong.

For-Profit Nursing Homes

Post-acute care is a big business and a lucrative business. Because Medicare reimbursement for short-stay patients is so good—Medicare pays on average 84 percent more for short-stay residents than Medicaid pays for long-stay residents—investors are eager to buy facilities that care for them. They're willing to pay a lot for them, forking out $76,500 per bed in 2014. To attract customers, they invest even more money, but often on amenities such as waterfalls or a piano in the lobby. But quality often lags behind the décor.[1]

For-profit nursing homes are nothing new. As long as the United States has had nursing homes, it has had for-profit ones. From the beginning, most have been for-profit and the percentage is growing: it's now at 70 percent.[2] The vast majority of SNFs have both Medicare- and Medicaid-certified beds, which for all practical purposes is another way of saying that they accept both short-term (Medicare eligible) and long-stay (Medicaid eligible) residents. Disentangling these two populations is hard because the data sources tend to mix them, even though they differ in both their needs and their characteristics. Figuring out how to define or measure their respective experiences is harder still. But CMS tries: its *Nursing Home Compare* program uses separate quality indices for short- and long-stay residents, although it also provides a single composite rating of the facility as a whole, ranging from one to five stars. What the star rating system suggests, to the extent that it is a valid proxy for the patient's experience, is that not-for-profit facilities are superior to their for-profit cousins.

Only 18 percent of for-profit SNFs won a five-star rating in 2015, compared to fully 33 percent of nonprofits. Part of the discrepancy is due to size rather than ownership—the smallest facilities are nearly three times more likely than the largest homes to win a five-star rating, and for-profit SNFs are disproportionately large. But ownership status does matter to some extent: among small, for-profit facilities, 33 percent earned five stars, whereas among small nonprofits, the rate was 48 percent. At the opposite extreme, among large for-profits, 24 percent rated only a single star, compared to 11 percent among large nonprofits.[3]

Another way to measure quality is through the state inspections that SNFs regularly undergo. Using this metric, for-profit facilities are more likely than their nonprofit counterparts to have health care deficiencies, including deficiencies that result in actual harm or immediate jeopardy to residents, and are more likely to receive a citation for substandard care. Residents at for-profit facilities are also more likely to be physically restrained and to develop new or worsening pressure ulcers.[4]

Other more comprehensive comparisons of nursing homes by ownership status confirm that nonprofit homes tend to be higher quality, although they lump the short- and long-stay units together. In light of the tendency of for-profit facilities to decrease costs and improve their bottom line by using a low nurse-to-patient ratio, the observation is not surprising: staffing ratios are taken by many as a marker for quality.[5] But what seems to matter more than the for-profit/not-for-profit distinction is whether a SNF belongs to a corporate chain.

The Chains

Finding a for-profit nursing home that *isn't* part of a chain is increasingly difficult. When I searched on-line for SNFs in Cleveland, for example, I found thirty-one homes, of which two are government owned and nine are not-for-profits. The remaining twenty are for-profit facilities and of these, fourteen, or 70 percent, form part of a proprietary chain.[6]

Nursing home chains have been around for some time. In the 1970s, changes in reimbursement and regulatory policies, easier access for chains to capital for expansion, and generous tax policies that reimbursed nursing homes for their mortgage interest and depreciation made nursing homes a popular investment. As a result, between 1972 and 1980, a merger and acquisitions spree led to substantial consolidation within the industry. The largest of these chains, Beverly Enterprises, increased the number of facilities in its empire by 600 percent. To take advantage of the intricacies of the Medicare reimbursement system and the tax code, armies of accountants at the largest firms came up with clever schemes for their corporate bosses to save money, some involving real estate development and others diversifying into the medical equipment business, laundry, and management services.[7]

A second wave of mergers further transformed the nursing home landscape in the 1990s. Existing small nursing home chains were gobbled up by the larger chains. Soon, the eight largest players operated one-fifth of all nursing home beds.[8] Nursing home chains undergo a good deal of shape-shifting, buying and selling pieces of their enterprises ranging from management services to home care agencies so as to maximize their tax advantage—some would say to avoid transparency and minimize their risk of litigation. The net effect is that the list of the largest chains varies from year to year.

As of 2015, the largest by far is Genesis HealthCare, with 49,000 beds in thirty states.[9] Headquartered in Pennsylvania, it has a complicated organizational history: for a time it was publicly traded, then it was bought by a private equity firm, and most recently it acquired another nursing home company, only to go public once again. Because it was privately held for much of its existence, data on its finances are scant. What is clear is that Genesis has long had an uneasy relationship with unions. As a result, when in 2012 Genesis acquired a small Massachusetts chain, Sun Healthcare Group, the nurses working at Sun facilities were not pleased. They protested the company's "poverty wages" and "unaffordable health care" that they said were introduced after the acquisition.[10]

Next on the list of the ten largest nursing home chains is HCR ManorCare which, like Genesis, has a complex history of being privately held, then going public, and then being taken private again, with the private equity firm Carlyle Group its major investor. It seems HCR ManorCare stumbled into the nursing home business. It started out as a manufacturer of glass containers, the Owens-Illinois Company, and got into health care first by making scientific glassware and then by investing in a hospital management group. But it didn't get serious about health care and wasn't at all involved with long-term care until it acquired a lumber company that built nursing homes. From construction to management was apparently not a major leap, and from then on, especially after a few more acquisitions, the company was firmly entrenched in the SNF business.

The next two largest chains are privately held as well. Golden Living, with revenues of $3 billion, is number 148 on the *Forbes* list of America's largest private companies, and Life Care Centers of America, with revenues of just over $3 billion, is number 149.[11] Private companies tend to be secretive: they disclose as little as legally permissible about their finances and their business practices, so it's not so easy to find out much about them. But we do know something about Life Care, and what we know sheds light on both what is the same about this company and other nursing home chains and what is different.

Life Care Centers of America was founded by Forrest Preston, who at age 83 remains the chairman, CEO, and sole shareholder of the corporation. Born in Massachusetts, the son of a Seventh-day Adventist pastor, Preston attended Walla Walla College in Washington State, where he helped support himself by selling vacuum cleaners. His parents hoped he would go into medicine, but young Preston wasn't happy taking the requisite premed chemistry courses and found himself instead on a path toward becoming an x-ray technician. That didn't suit him either, so he moved to Cleveland, Tennessee, to join his brother running a printing business. It so happened that the printing company catered to hospitals, reviving Preston's interest in medicine.[12]

Business proved to be Preston's forte; he just needed to figure out in what arena to apply his skills. Once he decided his mission was to provide medical services for older people, he lined up two partners and together they opened their first old age home, the Garden Terrace Convalescent Center. Over the next six years, the threesome started five other centers and then, in 1976, Preston made the decision to form a management company to operate the centers, a company he called Life Care. He remained in charge of the company until 2006, when he appointed long-standing Life Care executive Beecher Hunter president while retaining the positions of chairman and CEO.[13]

Forrest Preston continues to live in southeast Tennessee with his wife. Some have called him the Sam Walton of the long-term care industry for his formative role in building a nursing home chain. But unlike other leading companies in the industry such as HCR ManorCare and Genesis HealthCare, Life Care Centers of America has diversified only slightly. Its "convalescent homes" include both long-term nursing homes (including some specialized dementia units) and short-term rehabilitation centers plus a few assisted living facilities, but it has not branched into hospice, and it recently divested itself of many of its home care agencies.[14]

Life Care is unusual in another respect: its mission is strongly imbued with a Christian ethos. There's a long tradition of religiously oriented nursing homes, but they are almost exclusively not-for-profit. Forrest Preston, perhaps inspired by the Calvinist Protestant tradition, evidently sees no conflict between pursuing religious aims and the profit motive. "We believe our work is rooted in the Judeo-Christian ethic," the Life Care website asserts, "and that obedience to God is best measured by our service to others. Only by following this principle will our mission and potential as a corporation be fulfilled."[15] And in the quarterly magazine put out by Life Care Centers of America, *Life Care Leader*, Forrest reminds his readers that "each day offers many opportunities to extend acts of kindness to others—by what we do professionally and personally. Let's approach them with a renewed energy."[16]

Situated just a mile and a half from the area's major hospital, Life Care of Elyria (Ohio) is a typical Life Care facility and a typical American skilled nursing facility. It has 99 "certified beds," beds that can be filled with Medicare (short-stay) or Medicaid (long-stay) patients; the average American SNF is just about the same size, boasting 108 beds. It is a freestanding facility that is not part of a continuing care retirement community, though it does also offer assisted living apartments. The center has been in operation since 1999 and is one of 4 facilities owned and operated in Ohio by Life Care Centers of America, which now has over 200 facilities in 28 states.

Life Care of Elyria looks like most other Life Care skilled nursing facilities. It has the trademark front entrance: a brick patio covered by several small tetrahedron-shaped structures, held up by four pairs of white Doric columns. It's a one-story brick and stucco building, set off from the main road which is just off the principal thoroughfare leading into downtown Elyria, a city of 54,000 people in the heart of Ohio's rustbelt. Situated along the Black River, Elyria experienced an improvement in its fortunes in the 1990s, finding itself in the enviable position of being close enough to Cleveland to serve as a suburban bedroom community for Ohio's second largest city, which itself has experienced something of an economic revival. The 2010 census found that 14.3 percent of Elyria's residents are over sixty-five, exactly the same as in the United States as a whole; and 78 percent are white and 15 percent are black, also almost identical to the national average. The city will turn 200 years old in 2017.[17]

Elyria is the proud home to a well-respected school system and two community colleges. In January 2014, its hospital joined forces with the prestigious Cleveland Clinic. Calling itself University Hospitals Elyria Medical Center, the 387-bed community hospital is just a mile and a half from Life Care of Elyria, making it a ready source of referrals. And like the city of Elyria itself, Life Care is in many ways typically American. When evaluated by Medicare in 2014, the facility received an overall rating of three stars, the national average. In the domain of health inspections, it also received three stars. In staffing, as with many of the facilities owned by Life Care Centers of America, it got only two stars, but in the arena of quality indicators, it won four stars. The measures evaluating the short-stay component of the SNF are the most relevant, and here Life Care of Elyria was better than the national average in four out of five areas: the percent of patients with new or worsening pressure ulcers and the percent started on a new antipsychotic medication (where a low number is good), and the percent getting a pneumonia vaccine as well as the percent appropriately receiving a flu shot (where a high number is good). Only in the domain of patients reporting moderate to severe pain was Life Care significantly worse than the national average.

Life Care of Elyria is the only SNF in Elyria proper, but nearby North Ridgeville has one four-star and one five-star facility, both for-profit facilities like Life Care, but owned by smaller nursing home chains. The not-for-profit center, Kendal at Oberlin, is only twelve miles away and is one of the few facilities in the country to have the distinction of being awarded five stars by *Nursing Home Compare* for overall quality as well as for health inspections, staffing, and its performance on quality indicators.[18]

Life Care is responsible for a number of innovations in the nursing home industry that are usually associated with the not-for-profit sector. It has several times been the winner of the McKnight Excellence in Technology Award, earning a gold medal in 2013 and again in 2014. It received an award for using its data analytic capacity to develop an internal ranking system for its facilities based on patients' clinical conditions; the system allowed management to identify facilities that needed improvement. And it received an award for the use of its electronic medical record to improve coordination with area hospitals and substantially decrease the rate of readmissions from its skilled nursing facilities. Life Care has begun hiring full-time physicians to work on-site at some of its facilities, hoping to improve the quality of medical care and to decrease transfers to the acute care hospital. As of the end of 2013, it had recruited eighty physicians to work at Life Care sites in fifteen states.[19] Finally, Life Care reports that it has sought—and obtained—accreditation by The Joint Commission (formerly the Joint Commission on Accreditation of Healthcare Organizations) in every one of its eligible facilities, a stamp of approval sought by only a minority of SNFs. But, at the same time that Life Care continues to bear the stamp of its idiosyncratic founder, it also follows the path of other corporate chains in its efforts to hold down costs and maximize profits.

One strategy used by many large, for-profit chains to improve their bottom line involves gaming the system: they categorize patients as needing the highest intensity of services, particularly physical therapy, regardless of their actual condition and their ability to tolerate therapy. A *Wall Street Journal* exposé found that in 2002, nursing homes billed for "ultra high" therapy (the highest of Medicare's five billing categories) on 7 percent of post-acute Medicare days, compared to 54 percent of patient days in 2013. Billing was further skewed toward the "ultra high" category in the for-profit nursing home chains such as Genesis HealthCare and Kindred Healthcare, both of which billed 58 percent of patient days at the highest rate.[20] A report by the Office of the Inspector General confirmed widespread over-billing by SNFs, which sometimes assigned dying, bedbound patients to the highest level of therapy. That means charging Medicare as much as $620 a day (for "ultra high" therapy needs) compared to $362 a day (for the lowest category of therapy needs), costing Medicare $1.1 billion between 2012 and 2013.[21] Several chains have already settled fraud claims with the Department of Justice for this practice, including Kindred Healthcare and Extendicare. As of 2016, Life Care remains under investigation.

The findings of federal investigators in the ongoing case against Life Care reveal much about the way that the billing strategy plays out—though the company denies any wrongdoing. According to federal investigators, Life Care pushes its facilities and therapists to bill using the "ultra high" physical therapy classification for as many patients as possible. Moreover, it sets high targets for achieving this goal, regardless of the patients' actual diagnoses and needs. The targets, the investigators maintain, are reinforced at corporate meetings as well as through corporate emails and visits from upper management. Facilities and employees who fail to achieve the targets are punished, and those who succeed are rewarded.[22] After investigating Life Care for four years, federal prosecutors decided to name Forrest Preston in their lawsuit, alleging that he "exercised complete control over the company and its board," even determining what materials could be presented at board meetings. The Department of Justice subsequently dropped Preston's name from the suit, indicating, however, that he might be charged separately in a civil suit.[23]

Fending off litigation is another strategy used by the for-profit chains, an approach that was revealed in a three-part investigation conducted by the California newspaper, the *Sacramento Bee*. Trying to piece together the ownership structure for California's twenty-five largest chains, reporters found "extraordinarily elaborate" company structures. Brius Healthcare Services, for example, the state's largest nursing home owner, has a network of eighty distinct entities to oversee fifty-four homes. Some chains create management companies to provide administrative services. Such convoluted ownership structures, which may include a mix of limited liability companies and partnerships, allow owners to "hide assets and shield themselves from civil and criminal liability when patients are abused or neglected in their care." They also make it difficult for regulators to uncover patterns of malfeasance.[24]

As the saga of the nursing home chains and their strategies to maintain high profit margins continues, a new variant of the for-profit model has appeared on the American scene: the nursing home chain bought out by a private equity firm.

Private Equity Companies and the SNF Industry

Over the span of just a few short years, large investment groups have bought up six out of ten of the largest nursing home chains. Just as when they invest in hospitals, private equity firms infuse capital into their acquisitions while simultaneously introducing efficiency measures. Their plan: boost the operation's profitability and then turn around and sell it within a few years. In nursing homes, the principal path to enhanced efficiency is to cut staff.[25]

An investigation conducted by the *New York Times* found that the majority of the homes bought by private equity firms between 2000 and 2006 decreased the number of registered nurses so dramatically that the average nurse-to-patient ratio fell to well below the national average.[26] The result is a decline in the quality of care, with inspections uncovering more health-related deficiencies in facilities owned by private equity firms than in comparable SNFs with a different type of ownership. For short-stay residents, this means more new pressure ulcers and preventable infections.[27]

Private investment companies also affect nursing home performance in another way: they create formidable barriers against potential litigation by creating multilayered corporate structures that make determining who is actually in charge difficult. One plaintiff's lawyer in Florida stopped taking on nursing home litigation cases, complaining that to litigate the last case he had agreed to try, he had had to sue twenty-two discrete companies.[28]

In some instances, the care provided by for-profit, investor-owned chains is so egregiously bad that it leads to a wrongful death suit, as in the case of a sixty-nine-year-old man admitted to such a facility in California. The patient was hospitalized for a stroke and subsequently transferred to Desert Knolls Convalescent Hospital, which is actually a SNF and not a hospital. Neglect at the facility led to a second hospitalization, where he was found to have severe dehydration, malnutrition, infected bedsores, congestive heart failure, sepsis, and a urinary tract infection. The patient was transferred to the hospital's ICU but died despite vigorous treatment.[29] Similar cases are rare in the 20 percent of nursing homes that are not-for-profit.

Not-for-Profit Nursing Homes

A considerable number of the nation's not-for-profit SNFs are ethnically or religiously affiliated. Many of these are the direct descendants of the early nineteenth-century rest homes established to care for the "deserving poor" members of a particular community. The German Center for Extended Care, described in the last chapter, is one example. So, too, is the Menorah Center for Rehabilitation and Nursing Care, a 420-bed SNF in Brooklyn, New York, founded in 1907 when a group of women established the Brooklyn Ladies Hebrew Home for the Aged to house and care for poor, needy, elderly Jewish women. There's even a not-for-profit chain, the Evangelical Lutheran Good Samaritan Society. Established in 1922 by the Reverend August Hoeger, a pastor in North Dakota, its tag line is "in Christ's love, everyone is someone." With 166 facilities in 24 states, it reports annual revenues of $965 million.[30]

These not-for-profit homes are typically mission-driven. They have an unpaid board of directors who view working toward maintaining the facilities as their personal obligation. When the homes have a budget shortfall, they tend to compensate through a fundraising campaign, not by cutting staff. Their performance, on average, is superior to that of their for-profit cousins, especially that of the for-profit chains.[31] And some of them have adopted innovative models of care as they seek to carry out their mission.

Innovative Models of Care

Wellspring Innovative Solutions is a group of eleven nonprofit nursing homes, but it's not a chain because the homes are not linked by ownership. Rather, they comprise a group of Wisconsin nursing homes that banded together to try to improve the quality of long-term care. The coalition got started in 1994, taking as its premise that radical cultural change would be necessary to make nursing homes good places for older people. Its goal is to make nursing homes better places to live, and it is built on the assumption that the best way to reach that goal is by engaging both residents and staff in the process. Patients need to be involved to avoid the loneliness and loss of meaning that routinely result from institutionalization. Staff need to be involved because so many of the problems in nursing homes, such as poor communication and the lack of dignity and respect, are attributable to the high staff turnover in nursing homes.

The Wellspring project is intent on designing and implementing a model of care that improves nursing home life, without distinguishing between short- and long-stay residents. To this end, it has come up with a series of best practices based on existing research and hired geriatric nurse practitioners as well as an interdisciplinary resource team to teach those practices to nursing home staff. Wellspring also routinely involves nursing assistants and nurses in making decisions that affect both the quality of resident care and their own work environment. It also continuously measures outcomes, providing feedback to the staff so they can improve their care. The results are impressive: a careful evaluation of the program found that it succeeded in modifying nursing home culture to achieve its aims. In particular, it led to substantially less staff turnover than was found in the country as a whole, better performance on state surveys of Wellspring facilities, improved quality of life for residents, and better staff/resident communication.[32] The principles and practices endorsed by the original Wellspring coalition have spread to numerous other facilities at sites as far east as the Augsburg Lutheran Home in Baltimore, Maryland, and as far west as the Wellsprings Post-Acute Center in Lancaster, California.

Wellspring's is not the only innovative model of long-term care. Another variant emerged from the fertile brain of Bill Thomas, an iconoclastic physician who began his career as an emergency room doctor, stumbled into work in skilled nursing facilities and then, disgusted with the dehumanization he routinely witnessed in these settings, started his own brand of nursing homes. Called the Eden Alternative, these nonprofit facilities seek to alleviate loneliness and depression among older residents in nursing facilities by bringing in plants and animals. Ultimately, the movement incorporated the Wellspring principles and became the Pioneer Network, another movement for culture change in nursing homes.[33]

The Pioneer approach goes beyond adding plants and animals to redesigning the structure of nursing facilities. Instead of building nursing homes along the model of acute care hospitals, with their large units and central nursing stations, Pioneer nursing homes are broken down into small households of no more than fifteen people. Instead of life on the unit revolving around the nurses' station, it centers on the country kitchen/dining room, a cheery communal space where residents can socialize and help with household chores as well as eat their meals. The staff on each household is supposed to work as a team, sharing patient care responsibilities and involving residents in decisions about their lives, decisions such as when to get up, when to eat, and what to do with their day. Nursing and medical care, instead of dictating the lives of nursing home residents, is administered in the interstices of the patient's day. While many facilities endorse the Pioneer approach in principle, in practice they often utilize only some of its most fundamental precepts. Application of the model to short-stay residents is even more problematic because they tend to be sicker and to need more nursing and medical care than their long-stay counterparts.

Evaluations of Pioneer facilities show mixed results. Frustrated, but convinced he was on to something, Bill Thomas came up with a revised approach, the Green House model. This also focuses on patient-centered care, staff engagement, and small residential units, but it goes further than Pioneer in its conviction that small is better. The buildings are typically home to only ten people, each of whom has a private room and bathroom. The first Green Houses were built in the small southern city of Tupelo, Mississippi. They have since spread and, as of 2015, they can be found in 180 sites in 28 states.[34] One of them is the Leonard Florence Center for Living in Chelsea, Massachusetts, which would never have been built if Barry Berman's mother had not had a stroke.

Barry Berman's mother did have a stroke, which left her profoundly impaired. If that wasn't enough, she also developed pneumonia while she was in the hospital. When it came time for discharge, Berman arranged for her to go to a post-acute care unit for rehabilitation. He thought he knew all about nursing homes, since he had been in the business for twenty-three years. He was particularly enthusiastic about the SNF to which he sent his mother since he owned it.

When he visited his mother at the nursing home, the woman he found bore little resemblance to the dynamic mother he'd known all his life. The staff believed her apathy and despondence were due to the stroke, but she seemed worse than she had been in the hospital. Berman decided to see if his mother would fare better at home. He was in the fortunate position of having the resources to take his mother home and provide her with twenty-four-hour care. Within days, his mother was transformed. Sobered by his firsthand experience with the realities of SNF care, Berman decided to build a radically new type of facility to care for people such as his mother. The critical feature, he insisted, is that "it would be a home, not a hospital, no matter how sick the residents were, and it would allow them to make their own choices and live their own lives." Berman learned about the Green House project and decided to make it the blueprint for his new facility.[35]

The Leonard Florence Center for Living opened as a one hundred-bed facility in 2010 in the small, gritty industrial city of Chelsea, just across the Mystic River from Boston. Built with the help of philanthropic support and government tax credits, it has a bright, spacious lobby complete with a coffee shop, a deli, and a salon, and two residential units on each of the building's five stories. All the units operate according to the Green House principles of staff autonomy, patient-directed care, and teamwork. Patient, family, and staff satisfaction levels are reportedly high, though the most recent Medicare assessment on *Nursing Home Compare* gives the facility an overall rating of three stars.

As they experiment to improve care, some nonprofit SNFs choose to test whether their methods are any better than conventional approaches, and to teach whatever they learn to the next generation of clinicians. The few SNFs that engage in such activities are designated "teaching nursing homes."

Teaching Nursing Homes

Teaching nursing homes have been around since the early 1980s when first the National Institutes of Health and then the Robert Wood Johnson Foundation decided to fund a total of thirty-five self-identified academic programs that operated in nursing homes. When the programs that remained gathered in 2005 to review their accomplishments, they agreed that their most remarkable success was their sheer survival.[36]

The hope all along had been to educate the next generation of long-term care leaders by showing that the long-term care setting could be rewarding for both clinicians and residents. In addition, the idea was to create and test innovative health care practices. Most of what goes on in the SNF is "tried and true practice," much of which has never been subjected to rigorous study to see if it actually works. And many commonly used practices, when analyzed, turn out to be ineffective. Some are downright harmful. Physical restraints—vests or wrist bands tied to the bed or side rails—are supposed to prevent falls. They don't. And when patients climb over the bedrails to get out of bed, or rise from a seated position chair and all, they are more likely to fall and injure themselves than if there had been no restraints.[37]

The dream of the teaching nursing home was to transform the widespread perception that nursing homes are simply warehouses for people waiting to die into a vision of the nursing home as an exciting model of care for some of the most complex and challenging patients anywhere. An early evaluation of six of the teaching nursing homes showed modest improvement in selected patient outcomes.[38] Another early assessment reported that 90 percent of medical schools claimed to have some sort of affiliation with a nursing home, though in most cases this consisted of an elective course that fewer than 20 percent of students—and often fewer than 5 percent—opted to take.[39]

As with Pioneer, Wellspring, and the Eden Alternative, the teaching nursing home movement arose to transform long-stay nursing facilities, not short-stay post-acute units. While it has the potential to improve the quality of care in SNFs, to develop a research base that explores optimal treatment, and to educate a cadre of SNFists, the teaching nursing home has not as yet risen to the challenge. The experience for the 1.7 million people who spend time in a

SNF after hospitalization must rely on the approaches developed by the non-profit and for-profit owners of these facilities.

Peas in a Pod?

Skilled nursing facilities vary in quality, and some of the variability is related to ownership and affiliation. The for-profit facilities that comprise the majority of SNFs tend to have low nurse-to-patient staffing ratios, a practice that improves the bottom line but at the expense of quality. Even without measurable differences in outcomes—markedly worse rates of pressure ulcers or higher use of sedating medications—the relative paucity of staff almost certainly affects the day-to-day experience of SNF care. Patients have to wait longer for someone to respond to their call for help, whether the assistance they need is in getting to the bathroom or receiving a dose of pain medication. But nursing homes don't just tend to be for-profit, they are also apt to be part of a for-profit chain. The chains, by virtue of their size, find it cost-effective to institute profit-making policies and then enforce those strategies through all layers of management: at corporate meetings, through corporate-wide emails, and through periodic site visits by upper management.

Private equity companies, an increasingly influential player on the SNF scene, affect nursing home practice in yet other ingenious ways. By creating a multilayered corporate structure, they limit transparency and accountability, shielding themselves from litigation. Facilities that cut corners, jeopardizing patient health, safety, and well-being, provide few avenues for redress.

Not-for-profits have been at the forefront of the "culture change" movement that seeks to put the patient at the center of care. They have created or endorsed models such as Pioneer, the Eden Alternative, and the Green House, and several facilities joined to create the Wellspring program. But while acceptance of this new and promising approach has been variable among long-stay facilities, it is rare for it to be incorporated into short-stay SNFs. And only a very small number of not-for-profit homes are teaching nursing homes, sites that are dedicated to generating new knowledge, dissemination of best practices, and educating the next generation of nursing home physicians. All in all, not-for-profit facilities tend to be superior to their for-profit counterparts on quality measures, but this may have as much to do with their smaller size as with their corporate structure.

While poor quality, at least as defined by government standards, may be more common in the for-profit sector, it is endemic among all types of SNFs. A 2014 report by the Office of the Inspector General at DHHS found that

22 percent of short-stay Medicare SNF patients experienced an adverse event during their stay. Another 11 percent experienced some kind of "temporary harm," and *all* these incidents were deemed "clearly or likely preventable" by physician reviewers. Typically, the untoward outcomes resulted from substandard care or inadequate monitoring or a delay in instituting treatment. The episodes were sufficiently serious that half of the patients who incurred one returned to the hospital for care—costing Medicare $2.8 billion and costing the patients incalculable pain and suffering.[40]

Government inspections and rankings can detect the most egregiously bad care, but the regulator's view of what constitutes good care is merely the absence of bad care. *Nursing Home Compare* thus implicitly accepts as good care an approach to medical care that routinely involves over-treatment. It unwittingly endorses over-prescription of antibiotics to patients who almost definitely do not have a bacterial infection (thus promoting the spread of resistant organisms), and indirectly encourages the use of statins in patients who are approaching the end of life (for whom such medications are unnecessary). It regards as legitimate transfers to the hospital for aggressive medical treatment of new, unexpected problems, even if a conversation with the patient and family about the goals of care might have led to a decision to keep the patient at the nursing facility for more limited treatment. And it assumes that quality care is being provided if patients are offered pneumonia and influenza vaccines, but fails to criticize a SNF where dying patients receive care focused on cure—whether or not that's what they explicitly want—and are not offered hospice.

That SNFs are more alike than different is not entirely surprising. After all, why the SNF is what it is and does what it does reflects the concerns, motivations, and involvement of the other actors in the health care system that have a vested interest in SNF care: the hospital, which relies on the SNF as a safety valve, a place to send patients who are often still sick and debilitated, so as to keep their hospital length of stay short; the drug companies, that sell a modest but not inconsequential number of drugs to nursing homes; the device manufacturers, which supply equipment used to test and treat patients; and Medicare, which pays for the vast majority of SNF stays. It is the interests and motivations of these entities that provides the key to understanding why SNFs function the way they do—and what happens to older people when they enter their halls.

CHAPTER ELEVEN

Movers and Shapers

One of the most agonizing decisions families make for their relatives with advanced dementia in the nursing home is whether to insert a feeding tube. "Mom no longer knows how to chew and swallow her food," I tell them, or "Dad pushes the nursing assistant away when she tries to spoon-feed him." But no matter how gently I try to suggest that refusing food or losing the capacity to eat are normal parts of the dementing process, families worry that the person they love will "starve to death," and unless they authorize surgical placement of a percutaneous endoscopic gastrostomy (PEG) tube, they will be complicit in that death.[1]

I explain that dying involves a shutting down of various basic bodily functions and that dementia, in its final stage, is no different from advanced cancer. But accepting the notion that someone they care about and for whom they feel responsible will dwindle away is often too much to bear. There seems, after all, to be a technological fix. We can try to counteract nature: we don't have to sit by and watch the end come. I suggest that simple acts of caring such as wiping the lips to keep them moist, offering an ice chip, and holding hands are far more meaningful than calories in this situation, but family members have trouble believing me. The nurturing instinct is very powerful. And won't Mom experience hunger pangs? Won't she suffer?

What helps this conversation along is the work done by geriatrician Dr. Susan Mitchell, who performed a study that provides compelling if not conclusive evidence that feeding tubes do not prolong life in patients with advanced dementia. When she compared nursing home residents in the state of Washington who had a PEG inserted to a group of nursing home residents who did not, despite a comparable degree and duration of cognitive impairment and after adjusting the data for other concurrent conditions, she found that survival in the two groups was identical. Many were dead within six months, most within one year.[2] Families struggling with whether to use a PEG can rest assured that declining artificial nutrition doesn't make them murderers. But does it make them torturers?

That concern is harder to allay. We do have dramatic evidence from alert people dying of advanced cancer that they don't feel much in the way of hunger or thirst when they can no longer take nutrition by mouth. Some report transient thirst or hunger, easily alleviated by ice chips. I also point out that putting in a feeding tube is traumatic—it involves a surgical procedure—and so is its aftermath. People with dementia often pull on alien tubes protruding from their bodies, whether urinary catheters or IV tubing or gastrostomy tubes, and consequently are tied down, "restrained," to prevent them from removing the tubes. Far more humane, I argue, than taking Dad to the endoscopy suite, inserting a tube down his throat and into his stomach, and passing a small plastic tube through the endoscope and through an incision in his abdominal wall, and then tying Dad to the side rails of his bed to prevent him from removing the tube, is to offer him ice cream or Jell-O or whatever he at one time enjoyed, and letting him eat however much—or little—he wishes.

Some families agree to forgo a feeding tube; others, wracked by guilt or disbelief in my claims that their relative is dying and wouldn't suffer, do not. I assumed that the reason some nursing home patients ended up with PEG tubes and others do not has to do with how well their doctors communicate, with their own psychological state, with perceived religious imperatives, and perhaps with the strength (or weakness) of the evidence on the ineffectiveness of tube feeding. What I did not know until Dr. Mitchell studied the phenomenon was that the deciding factor in some cases has nothing to do with emotions or morality, but rather with Medicare rules and financial incentives.

The proportion of nursing home residents with advanced dementia and feeding tubes varies tremendously by geography and by institution, and at least a substantial part of the variability is attributable to organizational factors. For-profit nursing homes and those with a high patient-staff ratio, for example, are more likely to advocate putting in a feeding tube.[3] It's easier and more efficient to feed a person through a PEG rather than by hand-feeding: the former involves hooking a bottle of a nutrient solution to the tube and allowing it to drip in overnight, and the latter entails sitting with a resident and laboriously coaxing him to take a few mouthfuls. But paradoxically, Medicare pays SNFs more for residents who are tube-fed than for those who are hand-fed—a feeding tube qualifies as sophisticated medical technology and residents in a short-term nursing facility who require such technology command greater reimbursement.[4] Dr. Mitchell's work made it painfully clear to me that what happens to patients in skilled nursing facilities is determined by much more than just the quality of the medical care.

The Perspective of the Nursing Home Administrator

In order of frequency, patients at a SNF see nursing assistants, nurses, and therapists. Occasionally, they may see a nurse practitioner. Even more rarely, they see a physician. They probably never see the nursing home administrator, but that's who's actually in charge.

Nursing home administrators are categorized by the Bureau of Labor Statistics as "medical and health services managers." Their salaries in 2015 ranged between $47,860 and $118,706 per year, depending on their experience and the size of the nursing home.[5] In general, nursing home administrators are required to have a BA degree and to have a license from the National Association of Long Term Care Administrators. The exam questions on their board exam reveal the kinds of things an administrator is supposed to know. The questions span five areas: resident-centered care and quality of life (38 percent), leadership and management (21 percent), environment (15 percent), human resources (13 percent), and finances (13 percent).[6] But what really matters to corporate management (in the case of for-profit SNFs) or to the board (in the case of not-for-profits) emerges in job advertisements and the LinkedIn profiles of job seekers.

Sava Senior Care, one of the largest of the for-profit chains, posted an advertisement for a nursing home administrator for a facility in McKinney, Texas, in March 2016. The number one requirement was what every facility lists: the ability to ensure the quality and appropriateness of patient care while meeting company and regulatory standards. More revealing perhaps were the next batch of requirements, which address compliance with legal and regulatory reimbursement guidelines, the ability to prepare a budget, and both recruitment and retention of staff. Number five on the list was making sure the facility is "safe, clean, comfortable, and appealing" in accordance with company guidelines.[7]

A straight shot from McKinney, Texas, 230 miles due south, is Austin, Texas, where Walter Johnson is a nursing home administrator. His LinkedIn profile reveals which of his accomplishments he believes are most likely to attract others to hire him. His top claims to fame are that he improved the census (from 33 patients to 50, at one site) and boosted the state survey scores at the facilities where he worked. He states that he's a "people person who cares deeply about my residents and their families as well as employees," and then hastens to add that he's very "marketing-oriented."[8] Finally, Johnson, who got a BA from the University of Texas, Arlington, and a long-term care administration certificate from a two-year college in Fort Worth, Texas, says he has boosted revenue and created a pipeline of certified nursing assistants.

All these domains are linked: the census affects revenues, as does staff retention; state surveys indirectly influence the census and, in the extreme case where the facility suffers a financial penalty for failing to comply with regulations, directly impact revenue. And matters are complicated further because profit margins are high for short-term patients (they have been running at 10 percent per year since 2000), but abysmally low for long-stay patients since reimbursement for the former is largely by Medicare, and for the latter by Medicaid. Nursing home administrators, not surprisingly, focus much of their energy on the short-stay side of the business. And revenue, whether the facility is not-for-profit or for-profit, looms large over all their other concerns, much as is true for hospital CEOs.

Reimbursement by Medicare to SNFs is based on prospective payment, similar to hospitals but with a twist. The way prospective payment works in a SNF is that patients are assigned to one of sixty-six "resource utilization groups" (affectionately known as "RUGS," as in small carpets) that are supposed to reflect the amount of nursing and therapy care that they need. This computation, in turn, is determined by the diagnosis (stroke patients often need physical therapy, occupational therapy, and speech therapy, while hip fracture patients typically need primarily physical therapy, and patients recovering from a heart attack often need both nursing care and physical therapy), and adjusted for age and co-morbidities (very old people with multiple medical conditions tend to be very sick). The RUG classification corresponds to a baseline per diem rate. What the SNF is actually paid by Medicare is finally determined by modifying the baseline rate depending on the local cost of living.

The net effect of all this elaborate calculation is that nursing home administrators know exactly what sorts of patients are assigned to the higher intensity RUGs and what types to the lower RUGs—and can selectively admit the ones for which Medicare reimbursement is highest. Patients who are particularly attractive are those in whom there is a mismatch between what Medicare thinks they require and what it actually takes to care for them. This mismatch is the reason that nursing homes have an incentive to favor tube-feeding: tube-feeding commands a higher RUG than does hand-feeding, even though the technological approach is less time-consuming than the labor-intensive approach.[9] Just as hospital administrators are at pains to assure that enough lucrative patients are admitted (for example, liver transplant cases) to make up for all the money-losing patients (such as psychiatric cases), similarly, nursing home administrators are concerned about balancing patients for whom Medicare pays little with those for whom it pays generously.

While the budget for the rehab component of the SNF is dictated primarily by Medicare reimbursement, the budget for the long-term care component is determined largely by Medicaid, the major payer for residential nursing home care. The overall viability of the institution in the 90 percent of facilities that accept both types of patients is therefore affected by both Medicare and Medicaid. And while Medicare is a federal program, funded to a large extent by payroll taxes and subject to the whims of Congress, Medicaid is a combined state/federal program. That means that a substantial chunk of the SNF's revenue stream is intimately affected by the fiscal condition of the state where the SNF is located. Medicaid is a major line item in state budgets; nationwide, Medicaid represents 24 percent of total state spending and surpassed K–12 education as the single largest area of state spending in 2012.[10] As a result, whenever a state experiences a financial shortfall, Medicaid is a prime target for cutbacks. And what better place to cut than nursing homes, where few residents can speak for themselves and the staff consists largely of low paid, poorly educated, nonunionized workers?

Maximizing revenue is a very real issue for nursing home administrators. One of the largest nursing home chains, Genesis HealthCare, closed five SNFs in Massachusetts in 2014, to the dismay of the communities where the facilities were located—and no doubt to the administrators who lost their jobs. The facilities weren't sufficiently profitable, so their owners decided to cut their losses.[11] For patients, that means fewer options in their neighborhood; it might mean going somewhere farther from friends and family, who then are less likely to visit during their rehab stay.

The primary way for SNFs to stay above water is to keep their beds full, and running at full occupancy entails having a good relationship with area hospitals because it's hospitals that send patients. Theoretically, patients and their families can choose a rehab facility and Medicare's star rating system of SNFs is intended to help them choose wisely. But unless a patient is having an elective procedure, say a total hip replacement because of degenerative arthritis or scheduled heart valve surgery, going to rehab may come as a surprise. Many patients, much like Taylor Bryan, the patient described in chapter 9, do not expect to go anywhere other than home after discharge and have no knowledge of their options based on previous rehab stays or on the experience of friends. When rehab is broached as the hospital stay draws to a close, families are typically given a couple of choices and a day or two to decide which one they would prefer. Bed availability may further restrict the possibilities, especially if the patient is on special precautions because of an infectious disease. The real decision maker is the hospital case manager, who makes the SNF referrals.

Increasingly, hospitals establish a network of "preferred facilities," SNFs that they recommend to patients. The German Center for Extended Care is one of a small number of facilities that has a special relationship with the teaching hospital where Taylor Bryan was admitted. The decision to put a SNF on a hospital's recommended list may reflect overlapping medical staff—the nursing home medical director might be affiliated with or perhaps even employed by the hospital. But the patient's experience at rehab is shaped primarily by the rest of the facility staff—the physical therapists, nurses, and aides who provide the bulk of the care. One of the SNF administrator's jobs is to worry about the staff.

There is ample reason to worry about the staff members. Being a nurse in a nursing home is not the most glamorous work—there are no gleaming machines, and none of the stimulation of an academic medical center. It's also not the best paying job around: according to the Bureau of Labor Statistics, the median salary of a nurse in a SNF was $58,830 in 2011, more than $8,000 less than what she could earn in a local hospital.[12] The nursing home must rely on a cadre of dedicated nurses who enjoy working with older patients and appreciate the autonomy that comes from being alone on the front lines. The unfortunate reality is that most SNFs are afflicted by very high turnover rates among their RNs (registered nurses) and LPNs (licensed practical nurses), with rates averaging just under 50 percent per year.[13]

If nurses come and go with alarming frequency, the same is true for certified nursing assistants (CNAs), or aides.[14] They are the least appreciated, worst paid, and most critically important part of the health care team. Aides do not even need a high school diploma. All they need for certification is to take a short course. The specific requirements vary from state to state, but the federally mandated minimum is seventy-five hours of training, including sixteen hours of hands-on, clinical training. Currently, this minimum standard, which was introduced years ago, is all that's required in nineteen states. Only thirteen states and the District of Columbia require more than 120 hours, the minimum recommended by the Institute of Medicine.[15] The state with the highest requirement is Maine, which demands 180 hours of training. Massachusetts is at the bottom of the pile, with seventy-five hours required.[16] The 616,550 aides who work in SNFs earn an average hourly wage of only $12.08 and an average annual salary of $25,160.[17] It's the job of the nursing home administrator to try to keep his staff. In most jobs, that involves designing an attractive benefit package, but in the nursing home industry, wages tend to be low across the board. The administrator can, however, develop a pathway for advancement (for example, by offering training to acquire special skills or incentives to attend nursing school); he can also influence retention by improving working conditions and reshaping the SNF's culture.

The culture of the facility is not just important to its employees; it's also a critically important determinant of quality of life for those who live there. It's also notoriously elusive. And while quality of life is of greatest importance to long-term residents, patients in a SNF for short-term rehab also find their experience colored by their interactions with staff, by the patient-staff ratio, the quality of the food, and more generally, the ambiance. The nursing home administrator is the key to setting the tone. He might, for instance, choose to adopt culture change, the resident-centered approach promoted by the Pioneer Network. For the workforce, the model involves empowerment, the flattening of the traditional hierarchical management structure of skilled nursing facilities, and cross-training. While the success of the Pioneer system in improving residents' quality of life is far from clear,[18] its effect on staff retention is unequivocal: in a group of nursing homes that adopted the Pioneer approach, retention of RNs, LPNs, and CNAs rose 70 percent.[19]

Even without embracing the full Pioneer model, the nursing home administrator can mold the facility's culture. In an ethnographic study comparing two nursing homes in South Carolina, one characterized by the high use (41.8 percent) of feeding tubes in residents with advanced dementia and one by low use (10.7 percent), it was attitudes that seemed to account for the difference. The low use facility featured a homey environment, regarded meals as one of the high points of the day, and employed nursing assistants to hand-feed residents. The high use facility has an institutional feel, was poorly staffed during meals, and emphasized regulatory compliance—which was interpreted to require the use of feeding tubes.[20]

Most nursing home administrators are more concerned with their image as a health care facility than as a home. They focus on boosting the number of stars they earn on Medicare's *Nursing Home Compare* website. Winning a high rating requires doing well on the periodic state department of public health inspection, so for administrators, getting a good grade on the inspectors' survey is like winning the gold medal at the Olympics.

It is one of the first things that families notice when they visit: there's a large sign posted conspicuously at the entryway proudly proclaiming that the facility was "deficiency-free" on its most recent survey. Such accolades seem oddly off-key—like a report card that trumpets "no F's" instead of "all A's." But the inspectors are to be on the lookout for noncompliance with federal regulations, and infractions are to be graded for the type of deficiency they represent, with punishment meted out accordingly, from a slap on the wrist to civil or even criminal penalties.

The driver behind the rules are federal regulations, instituted by Medicare both to protect patients and to make sure that Medicare is getting its money's worth. Medicare simply delegates the responsibility for enforcement to state and local authorities. The job of the nursing home administrator is therefore to satisfy Medicare, along with his corporate boss; as a result, Medicare has an outsized influence on the patient's SNF experience.

Medicare and Post-Acute Care

Post-acute care matters to Medicare, which foots most of the bill. In 2012, SNF care accounted for 5 percent of all Medicare expenditures, or $28.7 billion. Medicare pays 100 percent of SNF care for the first twenty days, assuming it is medically justified; after that, patients have a $152 per day co-pay.[21] With so much on the line, the Centers for Medicare and Medicaid Services (CMS) worries about fraud and abuse.

The agency has reason to be concerned. The most recent reimbursement scandal involves over-billing for physical therapy services. Medicare pays more for patients who receive extensive physical therapy than for patients who get just a little therapy, but the amount SNFs have been billing for the highest therapy category has been steadily rising, without any discernible difference in illness type or severity among patients over time. The result was excess billing of over $1 billion in 2012 and 2013.[22]

Actually, CMS is not just worried about cost; it's also concerned about the quality of what it's paying for. And the way it goes about assuring quality is by coming up with regulations that set standards for SNF behavior and then delegating enforcement of those regulations to the individual states. The agencies that actually go into nursing homes to perform inspections are typically part of the state department of public health, and the inspections they perform are referred to as "surveys." In the event of noncompliance with federal regulations, the facility has to submit a remediation plan; if it does not correct the problem, CMS can impose a civil fine and withhold payment for new Medicare admissions. In fact, CMS also imposes staff training regulations and requires nursing homes to establish a Quality Assurance and Assessment Committee to identify and address any quality or safety problems. And CMS uses "quality indicators" to measure performance. The results of the survey, in addition to providing advertising copy for the nursing facility if they are positive, form one component of the rating system used by CMS on *Nursing Home Compare*.

The five-star rating system to measure and publicly report quality is another way that Medicare influences nursing home care. For short-stay residents, the system has three parts: the results of health inspections (carried out by local boards of health), staffing ratios (traditionally self-reported by the facilities, but as of 2015 to be determined using nursing facility payroll data), and quality measures (determined from the Minimum Data Set, a validated, detailed questionnaire filled out by SNF staff or outsourced, describing each patient's diseases, medications, mood, level of function, and other data submitted routinely to CMS).

What the system of quality indicators means for patients is that SNFs make a concerted effort to avoid the problems that comprise the quality measures and pay less attention to most everything else. For years, the three quality measures used by Medicare to evaluate short-stay patients were the percentage of patients reporting moderate or severe pain, the percentage with new or worsening pressure ulcers (bed sores), and the percentage with delirium (acute confusion). As with standardized tests that encourage teachers to teach to the test, this small number of very specific quality indicators shaped staff behavior. At some point, delirium was dropped as a quality indicator and the percentage of patients receiving a new antipsychotic medication was introduced, presumably leading to a shift in emphasis by doctors, nurses, and administrators within SNFs. And effective in January 2017, Medicare is adding four new quality measures to the mix, reflecting its more recently defined concerns. In addition to concerns with pain, pressure ulcers, and antipsychotic medication, Medicare will track the percentage of patients whose physical function improves from the time of admission to discharge, the percentage of patients who are rehospitalized, the percentage with an emergency room visit, and the percentage who are discharged to the community (as opposed to dying or transferred to a long-stay nursing facility).[23]

Despite Medicare's efforts to promote quality, a report by the Office of the Inspector General revealed a distressingly high rate of adverse events in nursing homes: 22 percent of residents experienced an adverse event, of which 59 percent were "clearly or likely" preventable. Over half of those who experienced harm were sent to the hospital at a yearly cost of $2.8 billion to Medicare and incalculable cost to the patients.[24]

Transfers to the acute care hospital from the SNF don't occur solely because of errors or neglect by staff; they also occur because the patients at the SNF tend to have multiple chronic diseases, putting them at risk of acute exacerbations. But whether they have to be hospitalized for treatment of those flares is another question, and Medicare is very concerned about *all* readmissions to the hospital, just as it is concerned about the revolving door from home to hospital. One way CMS tries to prevent such readmissions is to incentivize hospitals to work closely with SNFs. And that, in turn, brings another player into the mix of parties that affect SNF care: the hospital.

Hospitals and Post-Acute Care

It's not just patients and Medicare that are concerned about post-acute care; it's also hospitals. If patients stay in the hospital for a given condition longer than average, the hospital loses money since it is paid a fixed amount based on the reason the patient was admitted in the first place. And on the flip side, if the patient's stay in the hospital is shorter than average, hospitals are still paid as if they stayed the expected period of time—which means they make a profit. Not surprisingly, hospitals are eager to discharge elderly patients as quickly as possible. For them, having a health care facility to which they can send patients, a SNF that can handle some very sick patients, is like getting a bonus check.

But hospitals increasingly are held accountable for readmissions, for patients coming back to the hospital and being readmitted within thirty days after discharge—often, though not always, for the same problem they had the first time around. Medicare has come up with a system for punishing hospitals for this sort of readmission, on the assumption that if patients had been properly taken care of initially, including making the necessary arrangements for follow-up care and explaining how to take their medications, they wouldn't have gotten so sick so soon. The most draconian way to address the problem is for Medicare to simply say they will consider a readmission within a particular timeframe to represent a continuation of the first hospitalization. That is to say, Medicare won't pay all over again for another hospitalization. Even when hospitals do get paid for the repeat admission, their overall readmission rate, when it's greater than what Medicare deems acceptable, triggers penalties for the hospital. Since nearly 25 percent of patients transferred from the hospital to the SNF are readmitted within thirty days, hospitals have suddenly become much more interested in what happens in the SNF.[25] Just as they have designed transitional care programs to smooth the move from hospital to home, they have created similar programs for patients discharged to rehab.

Typically, these strategies include better communication between hospitals and nursing homes, and perhaps a shared medical record. Some of the more innovative approaches assure continuity of care by having the same hospitalist who was responsible in the hospital also assume responsibility in the nursing home. The nursing home chain, Kindred Healthcare, for example, has decided both to use "transitional care" nurses to act as navigators throughout the post-acute care period and physicians from the acute care hospital to provide direct care.[26] This sort of arrangement, in which the same physician directs the medical care in the hospital and the SNF, is particularly attractive under the new CMS "Bundled Payment for Care Improvement" model. In this system, Medicare essentially pays a single fee for hospital and post-acute care, which the two institutions have to share. This means both the hospital and the SNF stand to gain financially if they can provide care that costs less than the standard reimbursement—and to lose if their costs are higher.

One of the principal reasons that SNF patients are readmitted to the hospital—and therefore one of the main problems that these nurses and doctors hope to prevent—is an adverse drug reaction. But hospitals aren't the only ones concerned about what medications patients take in the SNF; an equally interested party is the pharmaceutical industry.

Big Pharma and the SNF

Most SNF patients take a great many medications. Indeed, CMS has been so concerned about polypharmacy in nursing facilities that one of the very first quality indicators it introduced was the use of nine or more medications, where exceeding the threshold indicated poor quality care. By that measure, 40 percent of nursing home patients were in the danger zone in 2004 (lumping long-stay and short-stay residents). More up-to-date data is surprisingly difficult to come by, but one study of hospitalized older patients found that 41 percent were on between five and eight medications at the time of discharge, and 37 percent were on more than nine medications; patients transferred to a SNF rather than home are on average sicker and probably take even more medicines.[27]

Once patients arrive at the SNF, it's the facility that dispenses their medications. Patients don't bring their medications from home or from the hospital. They don't fill their own prescriptions at the SNF. Their medications are prescribed by the physician and/or nurse practitioner assigned by the SNF to care for them during their stay, typically someone they've never met before and won't meet again unless they are readmitted to the same facility. Those clinicians turn out to be the targets of a major push by drug companies.

One strategy used by a major drug company to influence the prescribing behavior of physicians in nursing homes was to deploy a special group of sales reps. According to a whistle-blower suit filed by former pharmacists from Janssen, a division of the mega-pharmaceutical company Johnson & Johnson (J&J), the parent company created a group called ElderForce that was charged with one very specific task: to promote the drug Risperdal (risperidone) for use in nursing home patients with dementia. The only problem was that Risperdal is not FDA-approved for this use as it has never been shown to be helpful in controlling the behavioral problems associated with dementia. And while off-label use of medications is perfectly legal, advertising non-approved usage is not legal, and compensation for the J&J sales reps was directly dependent on the number of prescriptions doctors wrote for Risperdal.

Johnson & Johnson found an even more efficient way of targeting nursing home physicians. The company used an ingenious strategy that derives from a 1987 law requiring nursing homes to use pharmacists to review patient medication lists at SNFs. The requirement is based on studies showing that when pharmacists go over a patient's medicines, they often discover drug incompatibilities or raise questions about whether certain drugs are necessary, leading to enhanced prescribing. The problem with this system in nursing homes is that the pharmacists are typically consultants provided by the distributor supplying the drugs.

The regional distributors used by most SNFs, companies such as Omnicare, offer a package of services including delivery, dispensing of pills in "blister packages," and "drug regimen consulting" by their pharmacists. Those pharmacists advise SNF physicians how to modify their prescribing for particular patients, ostensibly to optimize care, but sometimes to optimize drug company revenues. In a lawsuit settled with the Department of Justice in 2013, J&J paid $2.2 billion for having paid Omnicare pharmacists to supply SNF doctors with *disinformation*: they were instructed to push the J&J drug Risperdal for use in patients with dementia.[28]

Johnson & Johnson is not the only pharmaceutical company to take advantage of pharmacy consultants to influence nursing home prescribing. In 2015, the United States government joined a pair of whistle-blower suits against Omnicare, alleging it had received millions of dollars in kickbacks from the drug company Abbott Laboratories in exchange for pushing Depakote (divalproex) on nursing home patients with dementia. Depakote is an anti-seizure medication that is not FDA-approved for treating dementia. But Omnicare pharmacists gave nursing home physicians kickbacks for prescribing the drug, money that was disguised as "educational funding."[29] Just a few years earlier, Eli Lilly had been found peddling its antipsychotic Zyprexa (olanzapine) for use in patients with dementia in much the same way, and had been fined $1.42 billion.[30] And Omnicare paid $124 million in 2013 to settle a False Claims allegation that it had engaged in a process known as "swapping," in which nursing homes were given deeply discounted drugs for some of their patients in exchange for persuading others to switch to a different Medicare Part D policy—which in turn reimbursed the drug company at a higher rate.[31]

As the nation's largest middleman to SNFs, Omnicare derives three-fourths of its $4.42 billion annual revenues from providing drugs to nursing homes. It is such a lucrative business that it was bought by CVS in 2015 for $10.4 billion.[32] But although it is the drug companies and the distributors that have been penalized for their schemes to modify the drug regimens of nursing home patients, ultimately it's the physician who is responsible for prescribing medications in the SNF, as for other aspects of medical care.

Physicians and the SNF

From the patient's perspective, the main way that physicians influence the rehab experience for patients is by their absence. Taylor Bryan's family noticed right away that there weren't any doctors around when he was admitted in the early evening. Very few doctors actually care for patients either at home or in the SNF, though there is shockingly little data on how many physicians provide this kind of care. An oft-cited AMA survey indicates that over 75 percent of doctors never see patients in nursing homes and those that do spend on average less than two hours per week. But these data are from 1997 and much has changed since then. Today, there is a new breed of physicians who specialize in care of the post-acute, nursing home patient just as there are hospitalists that specialize in the care of hospitalized patients. The actual number of such SNFists (pronounced "sniffists") is unknown.[33]

Traditionally, practice in the nursing home environment has been decidedly unattractive, beset by extensive regulations, lots of paperwork, high professional liability, and inadequate nursing support. But this is changing as the population using nursing home care is growing, both in size and in the complexity of their medical problems. Every SNF is required to have a medical director who bears overall responsibility for the facility's medical care—for assuring that standards are met, guidelines followed, and that the physicians who see patients in the facility adhere to all the relevant regulations. Those medical directors are encouraged to seek formal accreditation, to become a "Certified Medical Director" by meeting clinical requirements and passing an exam administered by the American Board of Post-Acute and Long-Term Care Medicine. They are paid by the SNF for their administrative functions, they are awarded the title of director, and they have their own professional organization, AMDA.

Though AMDA used to stand for "American Medical Directors Association," it has been renamed the Society for Post-Acute and Long-Term Care Medicine but retains its original acronym. It is the only professional society that seeks to represent the 50,000 physicians, nurse practitioners, and physician assistants who work in nursing homes. It has 5,500 members, an annual national conference, and a journal, *JAMDA*, which, mirroring its parent organization, used to stand for the *Journal of the American Medical Directors Association* but now is the *Journal of Post-Acute and Long-Term Care Medicine*. The journal comes out monthly and features articles on such topics as dementia and cognitive impairment, frailty, medication management, fall prevention, and guidelines for nursing home administrators. By awarding medical directors a certificate, giving them a title and a salary, and providing the other accoutrements of a specialty such as a journal and a conference, the Society goes a long way to elevating the prestige of the SNFist.

Whatever regulatory, supervisory, or administrative tasks SNF physicians undertake, their primary responsibility is to provide medical treatment to the patients in their care. That means diagnosing and treating disease, ordering and responding to laboratory tests, referring to specialists, and communicating with families and primary care physicians. It also means prescribing medications—and using medical devices.

Device Manufacturers and the SNF Experience

When Taylor Bryan's nurse couldn't wake him up one morning and then observed that his heart rate was elevated along with his temperature, his son didn't hesitate: he wanted his father to go to the hospital. Not only did the rehab have little on-site medical care, it also lacked technology. There was no radiology department, though a portable x-ray machine could be sent over to take basic films like a chest x-ray, and no on-site laboratory, though a phlebotomist made rounds daily and brought samples over to the lab for processing. By definition, SNFs offer low-tech medicine. They focus on nursing care and on therapy (physical therapy, speech therapy, and occupational therapy); their primary mission is to implement orders instituted elsewhere (typically in the hospital), rather than to diagnose disease and initiate treatment.

Certain kinds of technology are available to rehab patients, ranging from intravenous infusion pumps to special negative pressure wound healing systems, but SNFs are not allowed to charge extra for supplying any of these devices.[34] Their per diem reimbursement is a "bundled" rate that is supposed to include any equipment the patient might need. Nursing homes thus have a disincentive to use elaborate machines, equipment that they would have to purchase for the institution and for which they would not be able to charge patients. If nursing homes don't want to buy expensive devices, then device manufacturers aren't particularly interested in what happens in SNFs. The net effect is that when a facility does obtain access to a particular technology for a given patient, for example, a special bed to avoid pressure ulcers, it generally rents what it needs for the short period of time it is required. As a result, it is medical supply companies—the firms that buy inventory from the manufacturers, rather than from the device-makers themselves—that have a stake in what happens in the SNF.

The medical supply industry is a big business in the United States, and a number of companies have large divisions devoted exclusively to long-term care, whether such care is delivered at home, in the assisted living facility, or in a nursing home. The largest distributor is the privately held company Medline, ranked number 49 on the *Forbes* list of the largest private companies in the United States, with $7 billion in revenue in 2014.[35] The kinds of supplies that Medline and other similar firms provide to nursing homes range from durable medical equipment (such as wheelchairs, walkers, and hospital beds) to wound care and incontinence products. It's generally the job of the nursing home administrator to contract with suppliers. But sometimes the responsibility for contracting is outsourced, and suddenly there are new opportunities for cost-saving—and for corruption.

Hospitals, which have to purchase many of the same kinds of supplies and equipment as skilled nursing facilities, long ago figured out that they would have more bargaining power over prices if they banded together and, as a result, the Group Purchasing Organization (GPO) was born. This organization works as an intermediary between vendors (the device manufacturers) and the health care facilities. The GPO takes on the burden of negotiating a contract. It is funded through a fee charged to vendors, a form of kickback that Congress specifically allowed, making an exception to its Anti-Kickback Statute. The fee is required to be less than 3 percent of the purchase price. But through complex maneuvering, the five largest GPOs managed to collect $2.3 billion in administrative fees in 2012, and those GPOs increasingly include SNFs.[36] And the Government Accounting Agency is increasingly concerned that, far from keeping costs down, as was the original intent of both the congressional exemption and the GPO movement, the arrangement is raising costs; GPOs collect up-front payments from suppliers in return for awarding them sales contracts, even when they don't offer the lowest price.[37]

Nursing home chains sometimes deal with medical supply companies in another way—they buy them. Instead of dealing with an established firm, the chain creates spinoff companies to perform a variety of functions ranging from bookkeeping to physical therapy to supplying medical products. In these arrangements, the amounts charged are above market price, allowing the supplier to enrich the chain's owners while leaving the SNF under-funded.[38] For patients, that typically means poor quality food and inadequate staffing.

All the Actors

Older people who find themselves in a SNF have one overriding goal: to get better. Whatever brought them to the SNF in the first place—a joint replacement, complex medical illness, a stroke, sepsis, or some other condition—is a problem from which they haven't fully recovered. If they are to return home, whether home is the house they've lived in for fifty years, their daughter's house, or an assisted living facility, they have to regain their mobility, get rid of the excess fluid in their legs, relearn how to speak, or complete their course of intravenous antibiotics. To succeed, they need competent medical care, excellent nursing care, and top-notch physical therapy. What they may not appreciate is that the people and the institutions that shape their care—physicians, nurses, and therapists, but also nursing home administrators, drug and device manufacturing companies, hospitals, and insurance companies—share their goals but also have their own agendas. Nursing home administrators selectively accept patients who are complex enough to warrant high levels of Medicare reimbursement but simple enough that they don't require huge amounts of care, which may exclude certain patients in favor of others. At the same time, they try to retain staff by providing in-service training, which has the potential to both enhance employee satisfaction and benefit patients. Medicare tries to maximize quality by requiring states to conduct surveys that check for compliance with federal regulations and rates nursing homes using standard quality indicators, efforts that at best lead to improvement in the domains measured, and at worst lead to neglect of other areas of equal importance to patients. Hospitals have an incentive to avoid readmission to their facilities, and if that means developing more robust channels of communication with nursing home clinicians or even providing that their own doctors spend time working in the SNF, then patients benefit. The pharmaceutical industry deploys consultants to advise SNF physicians regarding their choice of medications, potentially influencing what patients will take for months or years to come. Physicians have historically disdained nursing homes and, even with current Medicare regulations, typically play only a modest role in the SNF, resulting in more transfers back to the hospital for patients.

Patients are probably even less aware of how much more the SNF could do for them—and how disinterested, or even opposed, all those forces are to the SNF playing this potentially crucial role. What the SNF, in principle, can offer older patients is a kind of *intermediate care*, more comprehensive than home care but less sophisticated than hospital care. This is the sort of care that makes sense for patients who are more interested in medical treatment that maximizes their ability to function in the world—to walk and hear and see and think—than they are in living as long as possible.

The less hectic pace of the SNF (compared to the hospital) and the less acute nature of its patients' medical problems are also conducive to providing patients with a comprehensive geriatric assessment. That assessment could serve as the basis for a family meeting which, in turn, would be a forum for discussing the patient's goals of care. The result of such a conversation would be a care plan tailored to the needs, preferences, and abilities of the individual patient, a plan that would immediately translate into treatment in the SNF and that would go with the patient upon discharge, serving as the foundation for all future medical care.

The stars are not aligned for either intermediate care or the assessment and planning process to occur. The physicians who care for SNF patients are often not trained in geriatrics; they may not have the expertise or the interest in either geriatric assessment or advance care planning. Nursing home administrators are more concerned with performing well when the state surveyors visit than they are with evaluating the patient's home situation or eliciting his goals of care, neither of which will earn them high marks and improve their ranking in *Nursing Home Compare*. Pharmaceutical companies would be happy to see a greater emphasis on the development of a care plan if it assured that a patient would take the newest, most expensive medications for the rest of his life. But more likely, the care plan would eliminate expensive medications in an effort to simplify the patient's regimen and decrease his out-of-pocket expenses. Similarly, device manufacturers would be pleased to promote care planning if the plan were apt to include extensive diagnostic workups of any abnormalities found in the hospital that the hospital had been too busy to follow up on. And while occasionally care planning would result in patients pursuing further testing, keeping the hospital's technological gears turning, more often than not, the SNF's interdisciplinary team would explain to the patient why PSA screening is not warranted in an eighty-five-year-old, and why an abnormal test should not prompt a biopsy. Hospitals would not be thrilled if the outcome of the family meeting were the decision to sign a "do not hospitalize" order; over the short run such a step might avoid a readmission within thirty days of discharge, but over the long run it would be counter to the hospital's interest in filling its beds. Medicare, which as of 2016 does pay for this kind of planning meeting and would in principle be supportive, is more concerned with flu shots and pressure ulcers in SNFs than with determining the patient's goals of care.[39]

As it plays out in the contemporary United States, SNF care is a pale shadow of what it could be. It fails to fulfill its potential because it is in the best interests of hospitals, physicians, device manufacturers, and others for nursing homes to operate exactly as they do. But while those same players were already part of the health care system fifty years ago, the nursing home of 1965 looked and functioned very differently from the SNF of today. If the same players, with the same interests, shaped the nursing home then and now, what explains the change? The answer must lie in external forces that shaped the way that the institutions of health care have evolved over time—and how they relate to each other.

CHAPTER TWELVE

Now and Then

Five years after completing fellowship training in geriatrics, I took care of nursing home patients for the first time. Not very many patients, but a few at each of several different Boston area nursing homes. The idea was that, together with my partner (also a fellowship-trained geriatrician), I would provide a modicum of continuity for patients cared for at the hospital where we were on the medical staff. Primary care physicians at our institution, like physicians everywhere, did not continue to care for their patients once they entered a nursing home. Along with giving up their home and their independence, most older people who moved into a nursing home also had to give up their doctor. With our approach, my partner and I would pick up where our colleagues left off. We would take over the records. We would (sometimes) get a handoff from the patients' long-standing physicians. And the patients would at least retain a relationship with the hospital where they had previously received care.

The contours of my role were defined by government regulations and by allowable Medicare reimbursement. I was expected to visit a new admission to the nursing home within three days of her arrival—even if she was transferred from a hospital and had been seen by a physician as recently as the day of transfer. Then I was to make a return visit every thirty days for three months, after which I was to reduce the frequency of my visits to one every ninety days. If, in the interim, my patient was hospitalized, the clock was reset and the process started all over again. And if, between scheduled visits, my patient got sick, I wasn't expected to examine her. In fact, I was strongly discouraged from doing anything other than either telephoning in an order, say for an antibiotic, or requesting that she go to our hospital's emergency room. It wasn't cost-effective for me to travel to the nursing home to see one patient, and I couldn't do very much in the way of diagnosis without access to a good deal more technology than was available in the nursing home, so I might as well just ship the patient out. Or so I was told by hospital management.

I learned a good deal about nursing homes in my first few months as a nursing home physician. I discovered that the facilities that looked the nicest, the ones with the grand piano and the coffee shop in the lobby, tended to provide mediocre care: nobody ever played the piano, the only people who went to the coffee shop were visitors, and what really mattered to the residents was the caliber of the nursing staff, both the nurses and the nursing assistants. I found that the printed forms I was expected to use to document my examinations asked all the wrong questions: they were concerned with heart murmurs and bowel sounds, when it was skin breakdown and mental status that were typically of paramount interest. Few of the standard forms provided space for functional assessment—determination of how well the patient could walk or use the bathroom or feed himself—and none of them had a section for advance care planning, for discussion of the goals of care, and for documenting any potential treatment limitations. But what impressed me most was that even though the nursing home was profoundly limited in the type and amount of medical care it actually offered, it was nonetheless very much a medical institution. The residents were *patients.* Nurses were constantly checking vital signs; often, they weren't allowed to give a patient his daily blood pressure pills without first verifying that the blood pressure was above a particular cutoff. That's the rational approach in an acute situation, when a patient has just started a new medication. But once it's clear that the drug is working and is well-tolerated, there's no more justification for such intensive blood pressure monitoring than there would be in the home setting. Relentless monitoring isn't necessary and isn't entirely benign either—it makes leaving the "unit" for more than a brief period difficult and can make day trips impossible. It medicalizes the person's *life.*

Something was profoundly wrong with nursing homes: they weren't homey. As Robert Butler, the founding father of modern geriatrics, wrote: "A long-term care institution should be homelike—not sterile, antiseptic or reminiscent of a motel. It should be a lively place with many ties to the larger community."[1] What I wanted to know was why, why were nursing homes medical institutions, even though they didn't provide a whole lot in the way of medical treatment? Why were they run by nurses?

The answer, it turned out, is that they hadn't always been like that. Their direct antecedents were "rest homes," small, culturally homogenous residences established in the late nineteenth and early twentieth century by ethnic or religious groups that sought to provide for the "worthy poor." They catered to widows left with no means of support, despite always having led a respectable life, to those who, in the pre-social security and retirement pension era, were on their own with no family and no skills allowing them to get by. The Winchester Home for Aged Women in Charlestown, Massachusetts, for example, admitted thirty-one women between 1911 and 1914. Of those whose backgrounds were documented in the facility's records, seven were housewives, eleven had been housekeepers, and eight were dressmakers or nurses.[2]

In addition to the homes set up by private philanthropists for the poor in their own communities, acute care hospitals also established nursing facilities, usually a special floor of the hospital for chronic cases. Nonprofit hospitals were finding themselves increasingly saddled with "old chronics," patients who were admitted for an acute problem but then were too debilitated to return home. As a result, at institutions such as the Massachusetts General Hospital, the average length of stay in the mid-nineteenth century was eighty-one days. They wanted to free up beds for patients whose illnesses were amenable to the "brave new weapons of medical science." The availability of more suitable accommodations for the chronically ill allowed MGH to lower its length of stay to twenty days by 1900.[3]

In the 1930s, whatever almshouses were still around in the United States emptied their beds, sending their chronic cases to rest homes. They transferred their residents and shuttered their doors in large measure because the Old Age Assistance program established under the Social Security Act of 1935 prohibited old age assistance to residents of public institutions. A quick sleight of hand moved residents of the almshouses, which were public, to rest homes, which were not, allowing them to receive government subsidies. The net effect was a growth in the size and number of rest homes, in the process making them more institutional and less homey.

The full transformation to a medical model, however, would come in the 1950s when, for the first time, government regulations were drawn up to end the most egregious of the many abuses commonplace in rest homes of that era, including fire hazards, inadequate diets, and other safety risks. Further impetus arrived in the form of the Hill-Burton amendments of 1954, which granted public money to build nursing homes (in addition to hospitals, the original authorization). With public money came federal regulations. The federal government designated the Public Health Service as the agency responsible for coming up with rules determining staffing and safety. Public health officials, not surprisingly, recreated the environment with which they were well-acquainted, the general hospital, minus the machines and the medicine. By the time Medicare rolled around in 1965, nursing homes had been thoroughly medicalized. I thought this was a major mistake; older people moved to such facilities in order to live despite their disabilities, not to get better and move on. To focus exclusively on what was wrong with them, rather than to support and encourage whatever was right with them, struck me as profoundly misguided. But while the culture change movement would take this critique to heart and advocate a radical reconceptualization of nursing homes, modestly improving the experience of long-term residents, other forces would conspire to make nursing homes more medical than ever. The emergence and development of the skilled nursing facility as a site for short-term, post-acute care was an indirect result of the Medicare program.

On the Cusp of the Medicare Era

On the eve of the Medicare era, the Public Health Service, the agency also responsible for assuring the quality of American nursing homes, carried out a survey of the institutions that fell under its jurisdiction. The surveyors were interested in discovering who lived in nursing homes, what kinds of problems they had, what kind of care they got, and who provided it. The Public Health Service found a total of 17,098 institutions for "the aged and chronically ill" in the United States as of the spring of 1963. Of these, 728 were hospitals or geriatric units within hospitals. Among the remainder, 46 percent were called nursing homes and were home to the most disabled and oldest residents. Another 21 percent were personal care homes and offered no nursing care whatsoever. These were the direct descendants of the board and care homes of the late nineteenth and early twentieth centuries. Another 29 percent were labeled "personal care with some nursing care," reflecting their status as somewhere between the hospital-like nursing home and the far homier personal care facility.[4]

Nursing homes in the 1960s were small: a typical home had only 39 beds, with fully two-thirds boasting fewer than 30 beds and only 6 percent had over 100. Fewer than half had a full-time nurse on staff. Most of those lacking a nurse were personal care homes, residences that provided a modicum of help, perhaps conjugal meals and a little housekeeping, but not much more. The overwhelming majority of the facilities were privately owned.[5]

The survey reveals a great deal about who lived in the nursing home: the average age of the residents was 77.6, with only 12 percent of the residents under age 65. The majority were women and almost all were white. They could expect to live in the facility for about three years. As to what these residents were able to do for themselves, just over half were "out of bed most of the day" and were able to walk independently or using a cane—which implies that the rest of them stayed in bed almost all day. Three-fourths were continent and half were "aware of their surroundings," suggesting that half were either demented, sedated with medication, or both.[6]

After distilling all the information they had gathered, the staff of the Public Health Service realized they didn't really know what medical conditions were common among nursing home residents, so they returned to collect more data. The 554,000 residents of nursing homes in 1964 had an average of 3.1 chronic conditions. Like their counterparts outside the institution, they suffered from cancer, diabetes, and arthritis. But their rates of heart disease, stroke, and mental conditions (including "advanced senility") far exceeded what was found in the surrounding population.[7]

However many illnesses they suffered from, they didn't receive much attention from physicians.[8] It turned out that, while four-fifths of the 17,000 homes had some kind of arrangement for visits by physicians, half of these visits were on an "as needed" basis only and not regularly scheduled. Only 4 percent of facilities employed a full-time physician and 10 percent had no arrangement for medical care of any kind. How likely a resident was to have seen a doctor in the previous six months varied depending on the type of facility: in nursing homes, including geriatric hospitals, all but 7 percent had had a physician visit; in personal care homes that provided nursing care, 15 percent had had no medical attention; and in purely personal care homes, 18 percent had had no physician evaluation.[9] Little had changed since the U.S. Senate's pronouncement three years earlier that the principal problem in the nursing home field was the "lack of medical care and restorative services in the great majority of the homes."[10] The facilities did have to meet licensing requirements, so they had to conform to standards dealing with sanitation, fire prevention, building and other safety measures, and diet. But not a single facility had a short-term, rehabilitative unit intended for patients discharged from the hospital who needed more time to recuperate from their acute illness. Nursing homes were the last stop, a place for poor, "unbefriended," chronically ill older people to live out their lives, not a place to gain the necessary strength to return home after suffering an acute illness.

Skilled Nursing Facilities, circa 2015

The skilled nursing facility of the early twenty-first century is decidedly a medical institution. Its clientele is typically very old, dependent in many of the basic functions of daily life, and afflicted with multiple chronic illnesses. And today's skilled nursing facility has evolved to care for a distinct subpopulation, patients transferred after an acute hospitalization to complete their recovery before they return home.

On any given day, 14 percent of the beds in a typical skilled nursing facility are occupied by short-stay patients, their care generally paid for by Medicare. These individuals stay in the facility an average of twenty-seven days, compared to the long-term care residents, whose average stay exceeds a year. Because the turnover is so great among post-acute residents, a SNF will serve more than twice as many acute patients as chronic patients over the course of a year.[11] The group of short-stay patients also accounts for a disproportionate share of the facility's revenue.[12]

The patients receiving post-acute care are similar to those receiving residential care, but older and frailer. They are almost entirely over age seventy-five, and the majority are over eighty-five. They have a high degree of disability, with the majority demonstrating limitations in at least four of the most basic activities of daily living. Just about half have cognitive impairment, evenly divided between moderate impairment and severe impairment. They come to the SNF after a joint replacement, after hospitalization for an infection (typically a urinary tract infection, pneumonia, or a blood infection), after treatment for an exacerbation of chronic heart failure, or for any of a host of other less common ailments.[13]

Physicians play a role in SNF care, though they don't have nearly as much of a presence as in the acute care hospital. Just what the physician's responsibilities are varies state by state. In Massachusetts, for example, a physician must document "a medical care plan" including a physical examination and some sort of functional assessment within forty-eight hours of admission. Patients are to be reexamined and reevaluated by the attending physician—or nurse practitioner working under the doctor's supervision—as needed. Other aspects of medical care are also constrained by state regulations. While facilities are typically required to make arrangements for the "prompt" performance of regular and emergency diagnostic tests, they are not allowed to perform lab tests on-site. They are required to have nursing personnel present 24/7, including a full-time director of nursing, a "charge nurse," and to provide a minimum of 2.6 hours of nursing care for each patient each day (a mix of licensed nurse time and care by aides). There are regulations for ordering medication and regulations for what goes into nursing notes, rules about residents' personal care, from how often to bathe or shower the residents to how often to shampoo their hair. There are rules governing shaving, oral hygiene, and foot care—and the list goes on.[14]

The skilled nursing facility is a critical part of the landscape for older people in the United States today. In 2013, 1.7 million fee-for-service Medicare beneficiaries spent time in one of America's 15,000 SNFs and, the older the patient, the more likely that hospitalization will be followed by a SNF stay.[15] Most SNF patients return home, though some die and a few remain as long-stay residents. How nursing homes went from strictly residential facilities housing those who could no longer take care of themselves and could not afford to go elsewhere to medical institutions that provide step-down care for acute hospitals is a function of social, medical, and health policy factors.

Social Factors

The decade following the passage of Medicare and Medicaid saw a huge increase in the number of people living in skilled nursing homes. The number of beds jumped from about 570,000 in 1963 (excluding personal care homes and chronic disease hospitals), to nearly 880,000 in 1969 and reached 1.5 million in 1982.[16] At the time, the experts predicted that by 2000, the United States would need an additional 1.5 million beds for long-term residential care for frail older adults. But then something surprising happened: despite major reforms that improved the quality of care in America's nursing homes, older people decided they didn't want to spend their final days in a nursing home. They didn't want to live in an institutional environment with minimal privacy. They didn't want to spend their time lined up in wheelchairs along the corridor of a nursing home, gazing into space, their medications administered by a nurse. They didn't want to be infantilized, marginalized, and medicalized. They wanted something other than a nursing home life and, when alternatives began appearing, they responded with enthusiasm. The most attractive alternative was assisted living.

The Demand for Autonomy: Assisted Living

Assisted living is an amorphous concept. Facilities that provide assisted living range from large Victorian mansions that have been carved into a small number of private rooms with communal living and dining areas to multistory apartment complexes featuring studios and one-bedroom apartments. What they have in common, according to the industry's trade organization, is that they provide "a special combination of housing, supportive services, personalized assistance, and healthcare designed to respond to the individual needs of those who require help with activities of daily living."[17]

Assisted living took off quickly: between 1991 and 1999, the number of facilities increased by 49 percent, and between 1998 and 2003, by another 48 percent.[18] *Forbes Magazine* predicted that assisted living would be one of just three likely growth industries. Companies building assisted living facilities started to go public as "Wall Street investors, eyeing the impending retirement of millions of baby boomers, fell all over themselves trying to catch a piece of the boom."[19]

The net effect was that, instead of growing in response to the burgeoning population of older Americans, nursing homes found themselves with excess capacity. At the same time, government reimbursement for long-term care—Medicaid is the major payer for long-term nursing home care—was not keeping pace with costs. Skilled nursing facilities desperately needed both a way to fill their beds and a more robust source of revenue. As a result, when Medicare switched to prospective payment for hospitals in 1983, putting pressure on the acute care sector to discharge patients quickly, those excess nursing home beds suddenly seemed like a godsend. Patients who were ready for discharge from a medical perspective but still needed help taking care of themselves could go home with "services" (a visiting nurse and a home health aide), or they could be transferred to a SNF. Short-term, post-acute care was born, rescuing both the hospital and the nursing home.

The Changing Structure of the American Family

Not only did more and more older people opt to move to an assisted living facility, freeing up beds for conversion to short-term, post-acute beds, but those same older people also found themselves increasingly on their own when they got sick. The feminist revolution of the 1970s sent women into the workforce in growing numbers: in 1970, 38 percent of women ages eighteen to thirty-three were employed; today, 63 percent work.[20] It's difficult to serve as a caregiver for an aging parent if you have a full-time job. Moreover, family size has been declining for decades: in 1936, parents claimed that the "ideal" number of children was 3.6, by 1971 they preferred 2.9, and in 2013 they favored 2.6.[21] The fewer children a couple had, the less likely that one of them would be available to help out after an acute illness.

At the same time that family size was shrinking and women were joining the workforce, geographic mobility increased in many parts of the United States. A Pew survey in 2008 found that 63 percent of adults had moved to a new community at least once in their lives.[22] In particular, multigenerational family households have been declining for most of the twentieth century. In 1900, 57 percent of adults over the age of sixty-five lived in a multigenerational household. By 1980, only 17 percent lived with a member of at least one other generation and, in 2012, 22 percent of adults older than eighty-five lived in a multigenerational household; put differently, 78 percent did not.[23] That trend has recently reversed itself, but the change is due principally to adult children transiently living with their parents after graduating from college. Not only aren't older people living *with* their adult children, they are often not even living *near* their adult children. That means they typically don't have their children to help them out after a hospitalization. Short-term SNF care was the perfect solution—for hospitals, for nursing homes, and for families.

The Triumph of the Corporation

If the growth of short-term SNF care was stimulated by the abandonment of residential long-term care by all but the frailest or most demented older individuals, and if the need for such care was magnified by women joining the workforce and by the mobility of the American family, the post-acute experience was also influenced by the consolidation and strengthening of the corporation. Beginning in the 1950s, accelerating in the 1980s, and continuing to the present, American businesses have morphed from moderate-sized firms competing with other moderate-sized firms in quality, customer satisfaction, and profit, to large companies with near monopolistic control of their markets and a single-minded interest in "shareholder value."[24]

Fostered by a pro-business climate that weakened government antitrust and regulatory policies and led to the waning of union power, the United States has been witnessing the era of the corporate giant. Consolidation in industry has affected areas as disparate as banking and agriculture; in health care, it has affected hospitals (see chapter 4), the pharmaceutical industry, and the health insurance industry. And it has had a profound influence on the nursing home industry, shaping the experience of the 1.5 million people who receive institutional short-term rehabilitative care each year.

The nursing home industry, in contrast to the hospital world, has had a long history of for-profit ownership. Already in 1969, 65 percent of nursing home beds were located in proprietary facilities. But the nursing home chain, a national corporation that owns numerous facilities, is a more recent development. In 1966, there were only a handful of such chains, but businessmen recognized that bigger was better because it meant easier access to capital, allowing for the construction of new facilities. The growth rate of the chains in the 1970s and 1980s was, according to an Institute of Medicine report, "spectacular." In 1973, the three largest chains owned 2.2 percent of all nursing home beds; by 1980, their share would nearly triple.[25] But the biggest growth spurt of all was in the 1990s, ushered in by the pro-business Reagan era. Growth was mediated principally by mergers and acquisitions, not by the construction of new facilities. In 1997, the United States had 4,770 nursing home chains, but fully 89 percent of those chains owned between two and ten homes and only 2.6 percent owned over fifty homes. By 2001, the eight largest chains operated nearly 20 percent of all nursing home beds, with each chain owning upwards of 250 facilities.[26]

As of the end of 2014, the list of large chains had shrunk to six. Each of these chains owned at least 200 facilities (a mixture of residential nursing home, short-term skilled nursing facility, and assisted living), which put each of them in control of over 20,000 beds.[27] The management style of the chains is straightforward: control labor costs by keeping nursing staff ratios low, grow rapidly through debt-financed mergers, and accept government sanctions for poor quality care as a normal cost of doing business.[28] Sun Healthcare Group embodied this strategy. Established in 1989 as a small chain with seven facilities operating 954 beds in two states, Sun financed its growth with debt-financed mergers and, by 1998, it owned 397 facilities in twenty-six states. It also purchased ancillary service firms such as pharmacies and home health care agencies to support its business. Its CEO stated publicly he wished to "cut redundancy and fat in the system," which he did by firing direct care staff.

Some of the cost-cutting maneuvers appeared to cross the line into illegality, and Sun was investigated for fraud and abuse by the Office of the Inspector General (OIG). The company was forced to enter into a "corporate compliance program" in 1996. Nonetheless, life continued as usual and the OIG again found Sun guilty of quality problems in 2001. In response to ongoing legal woes as well as financial troubles that led to filing for Chapter 11 bankruptcy protection, Sun restructured itself. But it continued to pursue its goal of "shareholder value," triggering a lawsuit litigated in the California Superior Court. A report by the California attorney general for 2004–05 revealed patient neglect, falsified medical records, inadequate treatment of pressure ulcers, high rates of dehydration, malnutrition, and weight loss among residents, and inadequacies in training and numbers among staff.[29]

Sun Health was not the only chain to be sanctioned for poor performance. In the late 1990s, Kindred paid a $1.3 billion settlement for fraud. The story was much the same when the Synergy nursing home chain moved into Massachusetts in 2013, acquiring ten facilities in the next two years. After the takeovers, several of the homes won a rating of "much below average" from state inspectors, the lowest possible grade. And when Genesis HealthCare, the largest of today's chains with a market capitalization of $675 million,[30] bought competitor Sun Healthcare Group in 2012 (the same Sun Healthcare that had gotten into trouble with the feds and the state of California a decade earlier), acquiring another dozen Massachusetts nursing homes, the local union protested the company's "poverty wages" and unaffordable health insurance. At one facility, state department of public health inspectors found that several quality indicators had slipped noticeably, including the percent of patients with pressure ulcers, the rate of urinary tract infection, and the number of residents on antipsychotic medications.[31] Another chain, Extendicare, agreed in 2014 to pay $38 million to resolve federal claims that it billed inappropriately for physical therapy and provided poor quality care, leading to excess falls and pressure ulcers.[32]

The nursing home chains, in their relentless pursuit of shareholder value, have been moving deeper and deeper into post-acute care, converting long-term Medicaid beds to short-term Medicare beds and, in some cases, eliminating the long-term beds entirely to take advantage of Medicare's higher reimbursement rates. Competition for Medicare patients has heightened. But rather than leading to improved quality of care, competition has led to cosmetic improvements such as attractive lobbies and a snack bar, what some geriatricians have dubbed the "chandelier effect."[33] The approach to care is a direct effect of the growth of chains in the nursing home business, reflecting the broader societal trend toward corporate consolidation. At the same time, who goes to a SNF and what medical problems they have has also been shaped by advances in medicine.

Advances in Science and Medicine

Joint Replacement

Today, one out of two people will develop symptomatic osteoarthritis (wear and tear arthritis) of the knee by age eighty-five; one out of four will suffer from symptomatic hip osteoarthritis.[34] In 1965, the rate was somewhat lower as fewer adults were obese—one of the risk factors for arthritis—but it was still high. And affected older adults then, as now, found they had trouble walking and suffered considerable pain as a result. The difference is that today there is a fix: joint replacement surgery. Patients report such dramatic improvements in their quality of life after they receive a new knee or hip that in 2010, nearly a quarter of a million Medicare enrollees got a new knee and another 210,000 got a new hip.[35] Both procedures are considered "high value," as cost-effective as the widely used benchmark of kidney dialysis and as worthwhile as a pacemaker. Hip replacement surgery has been called the "operation of the century."[36]

As experience with the surgery increased, the age of the joint recipients crept upwards and the duration of the hospitalization shrank. Many of those older patients were in no condition to return home after just a few days in the hospital; instead, they were discharged to an SNF. Between 1991 and 2010, the mean length of stay after a total knee replacement, for example, fell from 7.9 days to 3.5 days and the percent of patients discharged to rehab jumped from 14.6 to 29.4.[37] With time, joint replacement surgery became one of the principal reasons for having a SNF stay. The design of the SNF, which emphasized physical therapy and nursing care, reflected the needs of one of its chief constituent groups, the patient recovering from hip or knee surgery.

This metamorphosis of the nursing home from a site for chronic care to a facility specializing in acute rehabilitation would not have happened if Dr. John Charnley had not designed a hip prosthesis that worked. Born in England in 1911, Charnley became a surgeon, but during World War II he was posted to Cairo, Egypt, where he was put in charge of the orthopedics laboratory. The time spent tinkering with the equipment kindled an interest in both orthopedics and engineering. He also came to appreciate how debilitated older patients could be by their aging hips and knees. At the same time, he recognized that the moment had come to actually make a functional hip prosthesis. The major obstacle had been the inability to control infection: with the availability of antibiotics, plus a special vacuum technique that Charnley designed to keep the operative field sterile, the bacterial foe could be subdued. He also recognized that the second major obstacle to replacing a hip had been the lack of a good material with which to craft the artificial joint. He knew that normal joints, in addition to requiring durability, also needed lubrication, so he sought a way to replicate the slippery surface. By reaching out to specialists in the field of plastics, he ultimately found a type of polyethylene that did the job. In the early 1960s, total hip replacement became a reality.[38] Charnley would be knighted for his work and receive the Lasker Clinical Medical Research prize in 1974.

Total knee replacement would follow. First introduced in the 1970s, it became even more popular than hip replacement, reflecting the higher incidence of osteoarthritis of the knee compared to the hip. In many cases, older patients had both knees operated on at once—clearly requiring rehabilitation afterwards. The development of protocols for starting and monitoring anticoagulation prevented one of the major postoperative complications of joint replacement surgery, a blood clot in the veins of the leg that sometimes broke off and traveled to the lung. Instituting treatment early meant that patients could be discharged even sooner. And over time, the population undergoing knee replacement became older and sicker: they were more likely to have diabetes, kidney disease, and obesity, making transfer to an SNF ever more desirable.[39]

Multimorbidity

Some older patients are admitted to the SNF because they are recovering from a single problem such as joint replacement surgery or pneumonia, but often they have multiple problems, a condition increasingly referred to as "multimorbidity." And many patients start out with one reason for entering the hospital but then develop complications and end up with a cascade of problems, as happened with Barbara Ellis. She was admitted because of a flare of congestive heart failure but was also felt to have depression, for which she was given medication that precipitated delirium. Along the way, she was incorrectly diagnosed with a urinary tract infection, for which she received antibiotics that caused the profuse diarrhea of a *Clostridium difficile* infection. She became dehydrated from all the diarrhea, becoming dizzy, and was then treated with intravenous fluids to cure her dehydration—only to go into congestive heart failure, which is what precipitated the cycle in the first place.

This scenario, or one like it, is all too common in today's hospitals. Nearly half the beds of a typical American ICU, the site of care for the nation's sickest and most complicated patients, are occupied by people over age sixty-five. The most frequent reason for admission to the ICU is cardiovascular disease, with gastrointestinal problems second, and infections third, though often patients will have all three conditions. And as with hip surgery and valve replacement surgery, the past decade has witnessed more and more elderly patients being admitted to an ICU, with the rate rising 5.6 percent each year from 2001 to 2008.[40] A number of these very, very sick patients do not survive the hospitalization. Those who make it to discharge often have developed difficulty walking, dressing, and bathing—more than half of the survivors of critical illness experience functional decline. They frequently require ongoing monitoring of their weight and their blood counts or further medical treatment, sometimes with upwards of ten medications. Not surprisingly, "complex medical illness" is a third reason for transfer to the SNF.[41]

Multiple medical advances have made the path to the hospital and then the SNF possible. Progress in anesthesia has made surgery in octogenarians and nonagenarians far safer than it was fifty years ago. Preoperative evaluation and intraoperative monitoring have helped considerably by ensuring that before a patient is put to sleep for an operation, his hemodynamic condition has been optimized—he is neither dehydrated nor fluid overloaded, which could result in kidney failure or heart failure, respectively, when the stimulus of surgery is added to the already unstable mix. Unless the patient's heart rate and rhythm are well-controlled and the amount of oxygen in his blood satisfactory, he will not go to the operating room: an elective procedure will be delayed until the heart rate has been restored to normal with cardioversion (an electric shock), and the circulation to the heart improved with a cardiac stent. Once the patient is pronounced good to go, continuous monitoring during the procedure allows the anesthesiologist to intervene at the first hint of trouble. Better understanding of geriatric physiology, such as the changes in drug metabolism and excretion that occur with age, have led to smoother recovery in the immediate postoperative period. Intensive study has identified many of the factors that trigger delirium, allowing physicians to prevent and to treat the acute confusion that was previously even more common in hospitalized older individuals than it is today. The net effect is that older patients are more often deemed eligible for procedures than ever before and they have a better chance of surviving their treatments. But they are also desperate for a safe, monitored, well-staffed place to recuperate. Fortunately, the Medicare program offers them just such a place.

The Role of Medicare

Even before Medicare was implemented in 1966, hospitals recognized the value of nursing homes as a safety valve for patients who couldn't be discharged home. Some older patients who entered the hospital with an acute illness were simply too impaired to be able to return home after their treatment. Maybe they had had a stroke and could no longer walk or dress themselves. Maybe they suffered iatrogenic complications in the hospital and had developed incapacities unrelated to the problem for which they were admitted. Or maybe they had been leading a tenuous existence before they got sick and their debilitating pneumonia or their heart attack or their appendectomy tipped them over the edge to dependence. All these patients lingered in the hospital, occupying a bed that could otherwise have been used for a new patient with an acute problem.

Hospitals such as Massachusetts General Hospital, which in 1965 was a 1,000-bed private, nonprofit hospital with a very high occupancy rate, were eager to discharge patients as quickly as possible so as to make space for new admissions. To address the pressing need to free up beds, the hospital established a "Transfer Office" in February of 1965, facilitating what would now be called discharge planning. In its first full month of operation, the Transfer Office dealt with 375 requests for expedited discharge; in response, it referred patients to the Visiting Nurse Association for home care, to nursing homes for long-term placement, and to chronic disease hospitals for ongoing medical care.[42] But it was only with the introduction of Medicare that nursing homes realized they could serve as a bridge to home, not just as an alternative to home for those too debilitated ever to return to their previous abode.

The legislators who crafted Medicare were worried about the cost of hospital care, and in the days of per diem reimbursement, they were especially concerned about patients with lengthy hospital stays. A small number of those patients were very sick and required active and intense treatment by physicians and nurses for an extended period of time. Others needed modest medical care for a protracted period, such as heart attack patients for whom conventional treatment involved two to three weeks of strict bed rest, followed by another three to four weeks of treatment with oxygen and medications to dilate the blood vessels.[43] But while many of these long-stay patients needed to go somewhere other than home, they didn't need the facilities and services of a hospital. Medicare legislation provided for up to one hundred days of care in an "extended care facility" for just such patients after they had spent at least three nights in the hospital.

The legislation opened the door to the creation of short-term institutional care for patients within existing nursing homes. But when Massachusetts General Hospital sent a team of clinicians to evaluate the nursing homes to which its patients had been referred, what they found was not very reassuring. "About one-fourth of the homes visited were found to provide reasonably adequate care, another fourth displayed promise of development, and the shortcomings of the remainder seemed irremediably disappointing," they explained. In particular, although most of the homes were "clean, attractive, safe, and free from odors," they offered no special diets, they did not maintain medical records, staffing was insufficient, and medical supervision was almost absent. Nursing homes would need to provide these services if they were to take advantage of Medicare's extended care provision.[44]

Very gradually, nursing homes added the kinds of care that would be necessary if they were to serve as transitional care facilities. The creation of accrediting bodies for nursing homes facilitated the transformation, as did the setting of standards by professional organizations. And a major step toward recreating the nursing home in the image of the hospital was the passage of the 1972 Social Security amendments (PL 92-608), which added therapy—physical therapy, occupational therapy, and speech therapy—to the menu of services covered by Medicare. Suddenly, the SNF became an appropriate site for all kinds of patients, including patients debilitated after several weeks of bed rest in the hospital and the growing number who had had a total hip replacement.

Diagnosis-Related Groups

An even more potent stimulus to the transformation of the nursing home came with the Social Security amendments of 1983 (PL 98-21), which introduced prospective payment to hospitals. Hospitals, which had previously been interested in emptying their beds for humanitarian reasons—so they could admit other patients who needed their services—were now interested for economic reasons. No longer could they charge Medicare for every day that a patient stayed in the hospital, however many days that amounted to; instead, they could bill only based on the "diagnosis-related group" (DRG), a fixed amount determined by the average length of stay for a given medical problem. Long-stay patients not only deprived other individuals of hospital care; they also cost the hospital money.

As hospitals adjusted to the realities of prospective payment, the length of stay of Medicare patients began to fall and, gradually, increasing numbers of patients were funneled into SNFs on discharge. Determining the exact contribution of prospective payment to the change is difficult since length of stay had been declining *before* DRGs became a reality. In 1970, a few short years after the introduction of Medicare, the average amount of time that individuals ages sixty-five to seventy-four spent in the hospital was twelve days; five years later it had fallen to eleven, and another five years later it was down to ten days. After Medicare started paying hospitals based on DRGs, the duration of hospitalization fell to previously unimaginable levels, down to 8 days in 1990, 6.5 days in 1995, and 5.7 days in 2000.[45]

What is clear is that after the introduction of prospective payment, the amount of money Medicare paid for SNF care began to rise, and starting in 1990 that rise was exponential, especially for patients age seventy-five or older.[46] An ever-increasing proportion of older hospitalized patients made a stop at a SNF before going home, reaching 20 percent in 2013.[47]

Nursing Home Reform

The problem with post-acute nursing home care in the 1970s and 1980s was that the services provided were not much different from those conventionally available in long-stay homes. But traditional nursing home care was intended for people with stable chronic diseases. The new SNF patients, by contrast, were recovering from an acute illness and often needed ongoing medical management. As long as the demand was there but the facilities were not up to the task, growth remained slow. What accelerated growth of the SNF for sub-acute care was another major revision of Medicare, the Omnibus Budget Reconciliation Act of 1987 (PL 100-203), popularly known as the Nursing Home Reform Act or OBRA '87.

In direct response to the recommendations of the Institute of Medicine, whose 1986 report, *Improving the Quality of Care in Nursing Homes*, was in turn an answer to efforts by the Reagan administration to weaken the already minimal regulation of nursing homes, OBRA sought to transform nursing home quality. The law authorized the creation of new, higher standards, it introduced a strong enforcement system, and it subjected both Medicaid and Medicare nursing homes (long-term residential care and short-term rehabilitative care) to a single unified certification system.[48] Each of those three innovations transformed the way nursing homes were operated and significantly affected the daily experience of patients.

The higher standards that were introduced thanks to OBRA '87 changed the SNF world in a new way: they focused on outcomes rather than on the structure and processes of care. Nursing homes were prohibited from using physical restraints, except when specific, narrowly defined conditions were met. They were not allowed to use antipsychotic medication as a form of chemical restraint: only when patients exhibited selected symptoms such as paranoia or hallucinations were these strong medications advised, as these drugs were known to be effective in schizophrenia but not in dementia. Residents were to be treated with respect and their participation in nursing home activities and in decision making was encouraged. To promote quality, a whole host of services, including social work, pharmacy, dental, rehabilitative, and medical were to be made available. Specific staffing requirements were introduced as well, including a registered nurse to serve as director of nursing, the presence of a licensed practical nurse 24/7, and the presence of a registered nurse at least eight hours a day. Certified nursing assistants (aides), who provide as much as 90 percent of the hands-on care, were required to have at least seventy-five hours of training. And all medical care was to be supervised by a physician. Finally, each patient was to undergo a comprehensive evaluation on admission, an assessment that was to serve as the basis for an individualized "care plan."

Whether nursing homes liked the new standards or not, they had no choice but to comply if they wanted Medicare or Medicaid funding. Certification hinged on compliance, and compliance was enforced through the survey mechanism. The federal government dictated the terms and then relied on the states to perform inspections. At least once every fifteen months, according to the regulations, a team was required to show up unannounced at each nursing home receiving Medicare or Medicaid reimbursement and conduct a "survey." These evaluations didn't just involve looking at the written protocols and procedures that nursing homes use; they included speaking with residents and family members, and they entailed looking at outcomes such as the number of patients with a new pressure ulcer or a fall and the fraction of patients prescribed antipsychotic medication. While the specific measures that the surveyors use in compiling their reports have changed somewhat over time, the basic process that was instituted because of OBRA '87 remains in effect today.

The legislation didn't just threaten to decertify nursing homes that were particularly egregious in their failure to adhere to the new requirements; it authorized the Department of Health, Education, and Welfare to come up with a menu of sanctions, ranging from withholding reimbursement for new Medicare patients to withholding reimbursement for all Medicare patients. The net effect of the new regulations, along with the sanctions that gave them teeth, was to substantially improve the quality of institutional post-acute care. In response, more and more older patients were discharged from the acute care hospital to a SNF.

Prospective Payment Comes to the SNF

Nursing homes, especially the large, for-profit chains, had a strong incentive to convert long-stay (Medicaid) beds to short-stay (Medicare) beds. The reimbursement rates for Medicare beds were much higher, allowing them to generate a substantial profit. With a cost-based reimbursement system, the facility could provide unlimited expensive services such as physical and occupational therapy and Medicare would pay whatever it was billed. That policy came to an end with the Balanced Budget Act of 1997, which brought a form of prospective payment to post-acute care, including skilled nursing facilities. The new approach to reimbursement would significantly affect the experience of patients. The Balanced Budget Act mandated that nursing facilities determine in advance the intensity of services that a patient required in order to get better. They stratified patients into "Resource Utilization Groups" (RUGs) depending on their projected need for nursing, therapy, and other services. In 1998, when the law first went into effect, there were forty-four RUG classes; as of 2015, there are sixty-six. Nursing homes charge Medicare by the day, but how much they get paid for each day depends on the RUG classification. And the amount corresponding to the lowest RUG class is dramatically less than the amount corresponding to the highest RUG class. The result is a complex system in which Medicare pays a base amount each day for nursing care, therapy, and room and board, adjusts that amount depending on the geographic area, and then weights the amount depending on the RUG classification. Nursing homes, particularly the large, for-profit chains, have gamed the system by selecting patients who fit into the highest intensity categories. This is achieved in part by categorizing patients as "needing" the highest intensity of services, regardless of their actual condition.[49]

A recent report by the Office of the Inspector General confirmed the widespread overuse of the highest paying RUGs—principally physical therapy, but also intravenous medications and other therapies. Either patients received treatment that they did not need just to boost SNF revenue or the patients did not actually receive treatment for which the SNF nonetheless billed Medicare. The RUG system also means that SNFs have an interest in accepting patients for whom they can bill at high rates (such as those who are tube-fed), and excluding patients for whom reimbursement tends to be lower (such as those with behavioral problems).[50]

Nursing Home Compare

Medicare has gone further still in reshaping the SNF experience. Hoping to pressure nursing facilities to improve their care by making information about quality publicly available, Medicare launched its *Nursing Home Compare* website in 1989. Concerned that its report cards were not sufficiently clear, CMS instituted a five-star rating system at the end of 2008. And CMS now gives each SNF three separate ratings, one to indicate how good its health inspections are, one reflecting its staffing ratios, and a third based on its performance on "quality measures." For short-stay patients, only a handful of quality measures are used. What this means in practice is that the overriding medical concerns by the staff at today's SNFs are on whatever CMS defines as a marker of quality, whether it's the three indicators that were initially considered or the four other indicators added in 2017.[51]

The Affordable Care Act of 2010

The Affordable Care Act (ACA), which dealt principally with private insurance for those under sixty-five, also included a number of provisions affecting Medicare in general and short-term SNF care in particular. In an effort to control costs and to promote physician accountability for medical care, the ACA introduced the concept of "bundling" care. Rather than considering a hospital stay for total hip replacement as unrelated to subsequent care in a SNF, the ACA proposes that Medicare regard both as part of a single "illness episode." Just as it decided back in 1983 to pay hospitals using the prix fixe rather than the à la carte approach, it recommended paying a lump sum for all the medical care involved in replacing a hip joint: the outpatient visit to the orthopedist, hospital care, and rehabilitation in a SNF (or at home). The policy went into effect on a trial basis in 2016. It may well result in longer hospital stays (since the same entity will be responsible for care in the hospital and the SNF). Just how it will change the experience in the SNF remains to be seen, but given that changes in the Medicare program have played a dominant role in transforming SNF care over the past fifty years, it would not be surprising if this change proves key.

The SNF from Infancy to Adulthood

If both the office practice of medicine and the hospital have gone from adulthood to middle age over the last fifty years, the SNF as we know it was born in the 1960s and has progressed through infancy and childhood to emerge into maturity. The specific shape it took was affected by social trends and by developments within medicine. Changes in the family structure, together with an unprecedented degree of geographic mobility, left many older people with no one to take care of them if they went directly home after hospitalization. The concurrent growth of consolidation in industry, together with the free rein given corporations in post-Reagan America, meant there were plenty of companies eager to seize the business opportunity provided by the demand for post-hospital care. And developments in medical science resulted in the SNF evolving as an institution focused largely on physical rehabilitation. The phenomenal success of new orthopedic procedures such as hip and knee replacement, success that was soon achieved in even the oldest of the old, led to an influx of such patients to the SNF. The escalating use of the ICU for medically complex patients, once again including frail older individuals, changed the complexion of the SNF, the institution to which they were sent once the acuity of their symptoms abated. And there are other examples: as heart surgeons became increasingly adept at performing aortic valve replacement, a major operation involving opening the chest and temporarily putting the patient on heart-lung bypass, they offered the potentially life-prolonging surgery to ever more patients. Between 1999 and 2011, the rate of aortic valve replacement surgery increased by 5 percent; in patients over age 85, it increased 47 percent.[52]

But to an even greater extent than the other institutions where older people spend time as they journey through the health care system, the modern SNF is a creature of the Medicare program. It was designed to meet a need for ongoing treatment, recuperation, and rehabilitation that was generated by the spread of high-tech hospital care to older, sicker patients. Making SNF care possible depended on payment, and payment came almost exclusively from Medicare. Not only would Medicare pay for a SNF after hospitalization, but Medicare also encouraged the development of post-acute care, first through instituting prospective payment for hospitals and then by adding physical and occupational therapy to the list of services covered by the program. Medicare also shaped the patient's SNF experience by bringing prospective payment to nursing homes, tying reimbursement to clinical complexity and the anticipated utilization of special services, and thereby favoring certain kinds of patients over others. The regulations introduced as part of the Nursing Home Reform Act, which among other measures included limitations on the use of physical and chemical restraints, further transformed the SNF, as did the publication of survey results based on the inspections undertaken by state authorities in conformity with federal law. Innovations by CMS, including the public five-star system of nursing home evaluation and encouraging Accountable Care Organizations that force SNFs, hospitals, and physician practices to work together, are just the latest in an ongoing series of modifications to Medicare that have affected what happens to patients in the SNF.

Finale

When I first stepped into the hospital as a medical student, I was afraid I'd made a terrible mistake. I went into medicine to take care of people who were sick and suffering, but what I was primarily aware of in the hospital were the machines. Maybe I noticed the equipment because it was so highly visible—from the EKG machine being wheeled down the corridors to a patient's bedside to the beeping monitors and whooshing respirators in the ICU, to the imposing behemoths in the radiology suite. Maybe I was impressed by the technology because I was afraid of it: I couldn't fix a household appliance that stopped working if my life depended on it, I was intimidated by anything that came with the label "assembly required," and I knew nothing about electronics. Moreover, my visual-spatial skills were abysmal: before the GPS era, I invariably got lost whenever I drove to an unfamiliar place.

It would be some time before I came to appreciate that I hadn't made a mistake, and that medicine really was all about guiding people through some of the most vulnerable moments in their lives. It would be awhile before I realized that, while machines could help me carry out my mission, they weren't central to it, and I didn't need to fully understand how they worked to make use of them. But in response to my initial sense of shock and awe, or perhaps to quell my anxiety, my very first research project as a medical student revolved around understanding where the hospital's technology came from. Who invented all those machines? What led companies to make them? What persuaded hospitals to buy them? I decided to focus on a single example and chose the largest, most incomprehensible device I could find: the machines used for radiotherapy, for delivering high-energy radiation to treat cancer.

The radiotherapy machines I studied were linear accelerators; they occupied an entire room and cost between $100,000 and $500,000 in 1977 dollars. And twenty years before I began my study, they had been virtually nonexistent. I spoke to radiotherapists at the fourteen Massachusetts hospitals I visited; I met with a sales representative from Phillips, one of the leading manufacturers, who must have assumed I wanted to become a radiotherapist and that someday I would be in a position to buy his company's products. He agreed to have lunch with me at the top of the Prudential Building—and was taken aback when I insisted on paying my part of the check. I learned about the Certificate of Need process used by Massachusetts, like all other states at the time, to determine whether or not to authorize hospital capital expenditures in excess of $100,000. And I read scholarly works on health policy and sociology, on economics and political science.[1]

What I learned is that there is an entire field devoted to understanding the diffusion of technology. One of the pioneers in the area was Everett Rogers, whose book *The Diffusion of Innovations* was first published in the early 1960s.[2] The earliest models of how technology was developed and spread were linear: a solo inventor has an idea, he develops a machine, a company buys and patents his idea and sells the product, the technology spreads as first early adopters and then late adopters catch on. But by the time I carried out my investigation of radiotherapy, the models had become more complex. There were feedback loops: science influenced the development of technology, but once the technology entered into practice, when it was actually used to diagnose or treat disease in real people, the experiences of those patients affected future development, sometimes even spurring further scientific advances. Similarly, economic incentives stimulated technological development, but technology affected health care expenditures, which precipitated changes in what insurers would pay for, which in turn influenced the creation of new technology.[3] This idea of complex systems with multiple interacting parts went a long way toward explaining where linear accelerators came from and why there were twenty-five of them in the fourteen hospitals I visited. It would also be a powerful tool for understanding the experience of patients as they travel through the health care system. And it's not just that the physicians, hospitals, device manufacturers, drug companies, health insurers, and regulators each affect what happens to the patient in the office, the hospital, and the SNF; they also influence each other, reinforcing some of the tectonic forces that shape today's health care institutions and subtly modifying others. To understand these interactions—what they are and how they work— it's helpful to look at another case history, this time following an older patient's entire journey through the health care system.

The Health Care Journey: The Office

At age eighty-two, Rosa Gottlieb felt she was pretty healthy. She and her husband of sixty years led a very independent life, although her two children, who lived nearby, kept an eye on them. Rosa was an avid reader and regularly frequented her neighborhood public library. The couple went to museums and the symphony. Rosa corresponded with some of the many students for whom she'd served as a surrogate mother during her years as the administrator of the Hematology Department at a major medical school in New York City. And, very grudgingly, she took the pills her primary care doctor prescribed.

Rosa Gottlieb had always been leery of medications. Maybe it was a libertarian streak—she liked to feel she was master of her body and believed that taking medicines meant ceding control to chemicals. Maybe she harbored a deep-seated suspiciousness of doctors, resulting from the death of her closest childhood friend, a victim of Dr. Josef Mengele's twin experiments in the Auschwitz concentration camp. Or maybe, like many of her friends, she'd experienced enough side effects from medications to be appropriately cautious.

Not that Rosa had had many encounters with American medicine before she reached her eighties. She'd had two children—two beautiful, full-term baby girls who had been born the way babies had been born for millennia. Then in middle age, she developed thyroid cancer and had undergone surgery to remove the thyroid gland, an operation that cured her cancer but sentenced her to take thyroid replacement pills the rest of her life. And she'd had high blood pressure for decades, resulting in prescriptions for all kinds of different medications as the medical fashions changed: diuretics and beta-blockers and angiotensin-converting enzyme (ACE) inhibitors. Often the drugs didn't seem to work, so her primary care doctor ordered higher doses or switched to other medications, perhaps unaware that Mrs. Gottlieb wasn't actually taking the medication as directed. Two pills a day seemed like a lot to her, so she compromised by taking only one. And, of course, high blood pressure, known as 'the silent killer,' didn't produce any symptoms until finally, when Rosa was well into her ninth decade, her heart began beating irregularly and she developed congestive heart failure.

High blood pressure wasn't Rosa's only risk factor for heart disease. She also had moderately elevated cholesterol, high enough that her primary care doctor prescribed a statin to lower it. Within weeks of starting the new drug, Rosa began experiencing aches and pains in her legs. Statins cause muscle pain (myalgia) in a very small percentage of patients, somewhere between 1 and 3 percent. In its most severe form, statin toxicity takes the form of myopathy, or weakness of the muscles, along with pain. Her doctor wanted to run tests. He wanted her to consider undergoing electromyography to record the electrical activity in her muscles. Or perhaps, he suggested, she could have an MRI to get a look at the muscles themselves. At the very least, he wanted to measure enzymes in her blood that rose if muscles were being destroyed, as happened with relatively unusual and serious conditions like polymyositis, an inflammation in multiple muscles.

Mrs. Gottlieb was adamant that it was the pills that caused her pain, and when she stopped the medication, the achiness vanished. Then her doctor proposed trying her on a different statin—Lipitor was the most potent statin, but there were others, several of which were available as generics. He acknowledged that if one statin caused muscle aches, the others often did as well, so he suggested as an alternative one of the older cholesterol-lowering drugs. But Rosa vetoed these other less effective medications. She was an exceptional patient, and was perhaps exceptional also in her ability to withstand the many forces buffeting the outpatient practice of medicine.

Rosa's physician was just trying to be a good doctor when he prescribed antihypertensive medications and tried everything in his power to lower her cholesterol level. He was influenced by the Healthcare Effectiveness Data and Information Set (HEDIS) measures that Medicare, along with 90 percent of American health care plans, use to evaluate physician performance. And for older patients, those over age sixty-five, two leading HEDIS measures are high blood pressure and high cholesterol. Her physician's choices about how best to spend the twenty minutes he spent with Rosa Gottlieb during an office visit, not surprisingly, were dictated in large measure by his efforts to comply with the guidelines for effective care.

Drug companies also sought to shape Rosa Gottlieb's experience, though they may have met their match in this strong-willed woman who figured she knew a thing or two about surviving under adversity. A major way that drug companies try to influence care is by marketing medications to patients, the consumers. At the height of its marketing campaign, Lipitor's manufacturer, Pfizer, spent $180 million just on television ads for this one drug.[4] But television commercials, including spots during the popular medical show *ER*, weren't Pfizer's only strategy for reaching consumers. The company also launched the "Know Your Numbers" campaign in which it encouraged patients to have their cholesterol checked and explained what levels warranted treatment.[5]

Device manufacturers also set their sights on the office practice of medicine. Rosa Gottlieb may have declined the opportunity to have blood tests, electromyography, or an MRI to evaluate her muscle aches and pains, but her doctor was eager to prescribe one or another of these tests, each of which involved some form of technology. Despite Rosa's skepticism about procedures, she would have seventy-nine discrete radiologic procedures in the last five years of her life, many done in the hospital but a good number performed in the outpatient setting.

Hospitals would exercise their influence on Rosa's outpatient care later on, after she had spent time as an inpatient. In its quest to avoid a costly readmission, the hospital would make sure that Rosa had a follow-up appointment with her primary care physician within days after discharge. The hospital would do its best to ensure that the medications Rosa took at home were the ones prescribed for her in the hospital, if necessary by sending a nurse to compare the medication list sent home with Rosa and the pill boxes on her kitchen table.

But beyond all these ways in which the various actors in the health care system directly affected Rosa's care were the ways they indirectly affected her care by interacting with each other. In the case of Lipitor, her doctor's prescribing patterns were likely affected by the drug company, which lavished much of its marketing budget on physicians. In 2010, a year before Lipitor lost patent protection, Pfizer spent $660 million advertising the drug, the majority directed at physicians—and achieved worldwide sales of just under $14 billion.[6] But the drug company itself had been affected by the research establishment, which had showed that statins could lower the risk of cardiac events, stimulating Pfizer to come up with its own statin in the first place— even though, at the time, four other statin drugs were already on the market. And the researchers in turn were affected by the availability of NIH funding, which in fiscal year 2015 included just under $3 billion for the National Heart, Lung, and Blood Institute research grants, or nearly 10 percent of the total NIH budget.[7] The cycle doesn't stop there. National Institutes of Health funding priorities are shaped in part by the number of subspecialists in each field—there are more cardiologists, for example, than geriatricians and, correspondingly, far more research in cardiology than in geriatrics. But the number of specialists is dictated in large measure by the number of fellowship slots available for advanced training, and it's Medicare that effectively determines the total number of fellowship positions. Medicare also influences physician behavior by working with the National Committee for Quality Assurance to choose what HEDIS measures to use for the older population. A similar web of relationships affects what happens to older patients when they are admitted to the acute care hospital.

The Health Care Journey: The Hospital

For years, Rosa Gottlieb never had an illness that produced symptoms. But shortly after her eighty-second birthday, she had a nasty fall and was sent to the emergency department. X-rays showed she hadn't broken anything, but the doctors admitted her anyway to investigate why she had fallen in the first place. They quickly discovered that she sometimes had a very rapid and irregular heartbeat. Medication slowed down her racing heart, but the price was a dangerously slow heartbeat. The fix for that was a pacemaker.

Rosa duly had a pacemaker inserted and, because her persistently irregular heart rhythm put her at risk for a stroke, her doctors advised anticoagulation. Her cardiologist recommended the drug warfarin, a tried-and-true blood thinner, but Rosa was skeptical. She didn't like the sound of warfarin (brand name Coumadin): first of all, she observed, it was rat poison; secondly, it was a tricky drug for people. Too much of it caused bleeding, which could be severe, and too little predisposed to a stroke. To navigate the narrow path between hemorrhaging and clotting, patients needed to have their blood checked regularly, every day at first, ultimately every week or two. Rosa didn't like any of that. Fortunately, a new blood thinner had just come on the market that didn't require monitoring at all. A fixed dose worked well for everyone, or so the drug company asserted. It was even supposed to be more effective than warfarin in preventing stroke and less likely to cause bleeding.

And so Rosa Gottlieb was discharged from the hospital on the miracle drug dabigatran (brand name Pradaxa). It cost a small fortune each month, while warfarin, which was available as a generic, was relatively cheap.[8] At first, everything went well. A beta-blocker medication controlled her rapid heart rate, the pacemaker compensated if the beta-blocker overshot and her heart rate slowed too much, and Pradaxa protected her from developing a clot in her fibrillating heart, a clot that could in principle travel to her brain, causing a stroke. But then the trouble started.

It began without warning. Rosa didn't have any abdominal pain or black stools. She just had a sudden urge to go to the bathroom, and then the blood began pouring out of her. She was rushed to the hospital for her second hospitalization as an octogenarian. Tests revealed she was bleeding from an abnormal blood vessel, an arteriovenous malformation in her large intestine. A hotshot young gastroenterologist managed to see the culprit through a colonoscope and was able to make the tangle of abnormal blood vessels stop bleeding, essentially by stapling it shut. So much for Pradaxa being virtually risk-free.[9]

Rosa felt she was treated well in the hospital; her only complaint was that her regular physician was not involved in her care. The hospital used a hospitalist system, which was the way the hospital administrators liked to run things (hospitalists had been shown to be associated with shorter lengths of stay) and the way primary care doctors liked them to be run (allowing them to avoid disrupting their busy office practice with hospital visits).

Big Pharma also influenced what happened to Rosa by persuading her cardiologist that Pradaxa was superior to warfarin in the first place. The data that convinced her doctors was published in the *New England Journal of Medicine* and the results of that initial drug trial were used to extensively promote the drug.[10] In fact, the drug's manufacturer, Boehringer-Ingelheim, would later be found to have concealed data showing that monitoring drug levels and adjusting the dose of Pradaxa, contrary to widely publicized claims, *did* reduce the risk of bleeding. In fact, checking levels and adjusting the dose of Pradaxa, much as was routinely done with warfarin, could reduce the risk of serious bleeding by as much as 30 percent. Moreover, without dose adjustment, the risk of bleeding with standard dose Pradaxa was statistically the same as the risk of bleeding with warfarin.[11]

Years after Rosa Gottlieb was rushed to the hospital with gastrointestinal bleeding, claims were filed in federal court against Boehringer-Ingelheim by 4,000 patients (or their families) who had died or suffered major internal bleeding while on the drug. The drug company disputed the charges but settled for $650 million to avoid "the distraction and uncertainty of protracted litigation."[12]

What happened to Rosa once she entered the hospital was also shaped by the devices that helped diagnose and treat her problems. In fact, she had the two of the most common procedures performed in hospitalized people over age sixty-five, endoscopy and pacemaker insertion. In each case, the procedure probably saved her life and certainly improved her quality of life by halting her internal bleeding, and preventing her from fainting, respectively. She didn't realize that in addition to using a "hemoclip" to stop the offending vessel from bleeding, her gastroenterologist also used an experimental technique, argon plasma coagulation, to cauterize a second blood vessel that wasn't actively bleeding but was at risk of causing problems in the future. Argon plasma coagulation is a sophisticated electrosurgical procedure that has the virtue of delivering high frequency current to tissues without direct contact by a surgical probe, thus avoiding collateral damage to nearby structures. It's relatively simple and safe, but at the time Rosa underwent the procedure, its efficacy had been documented in only a handful of case reports. Not many hospitals have the technology, which requires an electrosurgical generator, argon gas, and a special probe manufactured by only a few medical device companies. But the teaching hospital where Rosa was undergoing treatment, eager to be on the cutting edge of innovation, evidently had both the technology as well as eager young gastroenterologists who were eager to use it.[13]

Rosa was also blissfully unaware that the specific type of pacemaker that was inserted was made by St. Jude Medical, one of the three largest firms in the U.S. market. Medtronic, the world leader, had global sales of $1.9 billion in 2013, St. Jude's was number two with $1 billion in sales, and Boston Scientific was third with $514 million. The Big Three have worked hard to maintain their market dominance, carefully cultivating relationships with major teaching hospitals and thought leaders in the field of cardiology to assure their products would be the pacemakers of choice.[14]

Medicare was another potent force influencing Rosa's hospital stay, particularly through its system of prospective payment, which encouraged early discharge to a SNF. The program also affected how Rosa was treated through its emphasis on the transition between hospital and home. But, in addition to the individual forces converging on Rosa as she lay unsuspecting in her hospital bed are all the interactions among the drivers: Medicare affected what technology was available to doctors by promoting innovation and diffusion in the device industry, which it accomplished through its almost unrestricted reimbursement policy. And the device industry affects physicians in their choice of which devices to use, for example, which pacemaker to insert, by paying them as consultants and advisors, as well as awarding them sizable royalties for their participation in designing new products. St. Jude Medical, the manufacturer of Rosa Gottlieb's pacemaker, made $52.9 million in payments to close to 22,000 physicians in 2015, with $5.8 million related to "electrophysiology products" (such as pacemakers) alone.[15]

The Health Care Journey: The SNF

Rosa recovered from her gastrointestinal bleed and was discharged. Once she was home, her primary care physician asked her if she would be willing to go on warfarin as prophylaxis against a stroke. Rosa wasn't sure, so she consulted with her older daughter, who was a biostatistician. When her daughter learned that the risk of stroke in non-valvular atrial fibrillation, the technical name for Rosa's arrhythmia, was on the order of 4 percent each year, she didn't think the potential benefit was worth the risk. With no guarantee that she wouldn't have further bleeding if she took an anticoagulant, and only a small risk of stroke if she didn't, Rosa stayed away from warfarin.

Two years later, at age eighty-five, Rosa Gottlieb had a stroke. Her right side was paralyzed, she had difficulty expressing herself, and she was confused. After a brief hospitalization, Rosa was discharged, this time to a SNF for rehabilitation.

It was not an experience she would want to repeat.

The medical care, or rather the paucity of medical care, was a major source of frustration for Rosa's daughters. But physicians had little motivation to see patients in the SNF setting, in light of the lack of prestige associated with nursing home care. Their inclination to avoid SNF work was exacerbated by Medicare, which offered them only mediocre levels of reimbursement, scarcely enough to compensate for the time required to travel to and from one or more facilities.

Soon after Rosa arrived at the facility, she became confused and agitated. Her mental function had been affected by her stroke, but it was more than likely the unfamiliar environment of the SNF that pushed her over the edge; as soon as Rosa returned home, her mental status improved dramatically. And it was Medicare's prospective payment policy that prompted the hospital to discharge her to a SNF in the first place rather than remaining an inpatient a little longer and then going home directly. The hospital didn't want patients to linger any longer than the number of days that Medicare paid them for, and that, in turn, was determined by the average length of stay for the patient's admitting diagnosis. Medicare's reimbursement policy fostered the hospital's view of the SNF as a kind of extension of itself, a mini-hospital but devoid of much of the technology and most of the physician care.

One evening Rosa became agitated, crying out and trying to get out of bed without the assistance the nursing staff felt she needed to be safe, and the facility physician prescribed an antipsychotic medication. Her primary care physician, who was a board-certified geriatrician, probably would not have recommended antipsychotic medications, but Rosa was cared for in the facility by someone who didn't know her, who assumed she was far more demented at baseline than was actually the case. Moreover, Medicare regulations mandated the use of consultant pharmacists in the SNF and the consultant pharmacists who, in many instances, were employees of pharmaceutical firms, tended to advocate the use of whatever brand-name antipsychotic their employer manufactured. The facility's consultant pharmacists recommended treating Rosa with antipsychotic medication and the SNF doctor complied, only rescinding the order after her daughters' strenuous opposition.

Other aspects of Rosa's care at the SNF were likewise determined by the behind-the-scenes interactions among hospitals, Medicare, physicians, and supply companies. While Rosa was hospitalized, her physical therapist suggested the use of a particular kind of brace to help her walk in the wake of her stroke, but that model, which she had adapted to while in the hospital, was unavailable in the SNF. Even though the SNF was part of the hospital's network of preferred facilities, ostensibly promoting integration of care across both sites, the two institutions contracted with distinct medical suppliers. The SNF supplier didn't deal with the manufacturer of the brace that Rosa was used to, so she had to start over with a new device.

What mattered most to Rosa Gottlieb and her family was her quality of life. They wanted her to become sufficiently strong and independent so that she could return to the duplex where she lived downstairs with her husband while her daughter lived upstairs. But Medicare, in an attempt to assure decent care, rated facilities based on their adherence to standards for health and safety. The result was an overweening focus on health and safety, sometimes to the detriment of quality of life.

The Health Care Journey: Home Care

Over time, Rosa regained her strength and the ability to walk. She could communicate without difficulty—the speech center of her brain had been unaffected by the stroke. Her personality was unchanged—she was as hypercritical and irritable as ever—but her mind wasn't the same. She had been a writer, publishing several children's books, but she could no longer write. She had been an avid reader, making weekly trips to her local public library, but she no longer had the necessary power of concentration to read books. She had always been fiercely independent, but she could no longer manage on her own and had to move, with her husband, to an assisted living facility.

The staff at the facility made sure Rosa took all her medications: one pill to slow her heart rate, one to control her blood pressure, thyroid replacement medication, something against stomach and intestinal bleeding—and, at long last, warfarin. It was the best of all worlds in that Rosa was no longer responsible for her husband, who also suffered from cognitive impairment, but she could still spend time with him. Her children and her grandchildren lived nearby. But after a year and a half in the assisted living facility, Rosa's husband fell and broke his hip. That proved to be the beginning of the end: he started on a rapid downward spiral. Within months, he enrolled in a hospice program to supplement the care at the assisted living facility and died soon afterwards. A mere nine months later, Rosa herself fell and broke a hip.

This time she went home after her hospitalization, home to the assisted living facility. The problem was that she needed more help with all the basics of life than the assisted living facility was equipped to provide—she couldn't get dressed on her own or make her way to the bathroom, and she certainly couldn't find the dining hall or figure out how to telephone her daughters.

The director of the assisted living facility told Rosa's family that he couldn't in good conscience keep her in her apartment. It was too risky, both for Rosa and for the facility. But for Rosa, it was home. After all her recent losses—her husband, her mental acuity, her independence—not to mention her remote losses, decades earlier—another move would be devastating. It would undermine her increasingly tenuous grasp of reality, throw her into a quasi-psychedelic state of overwhelming stimuli and dizzying novelty. Her children decided that they would do whatever they could to keep her where she was for whatever time she had left. They wanted, above all, to keep her comfortable and to maintain her dignity. They opted to add hospice care and a personal attendant to the basic services provided by the assisted living facility.

For two months Rosa continued her slow but steady decline. She had good days when she could converse with her family, and bad days when she was restless and uncomfortable, often for unclear reasons. But her hospice nurse visited daily and reported her findings to Rosa's primary care doctor. The primary care doctor worked closely with a nurse practitioner who actually made periodic home visits, adding a layer of medical sophistication to Rosa's care. When Rosa developed shortness of breath, the nurse practitioner treated her with additional diuretics and oxygen—though in her confusion, Rosa often ripped off her oxygen mask. When Rosa moaned, the nurse practitioner prescribed very low dose opioid medication, trying to balance the need for pain control with the risk of worsening confusion. Her personal attendant bathed and dressed her and, as the end approached, fed her and changed her diapers. And then suddenly, Rosa took a turn for the worse. She fell asleep and was difficult to awaken. Her breathing became shallow and her pulse erratic. Her daughters were called to her bedside and were with her when, just days before her 88th birthday, she took her last breath.

Rosa was one of the lucky ones. Thanks in large measure to her children's determination and willingness to use every penny of their mother's financial resources, she was able to have the best possible last few months of life, given the constraints of her physical and mental condition. Thanks in part to her having a geriatrician as a primary care physician, a system was put in place that enabled her to get treatment for her medical problems without leaving her home. She was able to escape the more common end-of-life experience in which patients lose all contact with their principal physician once they enroll in hospice and must forgo technology, even technology designed to promote quality of life, once they substitute their Medicare hospice benefit for conventional, fee-for-service Medicare. She was able to remain in the assisted living facility with major involvement of her medical team despite regulatory standards that regarded assisted living as a quintessentially non-medical environment. But she is the exception that proves the rule—the person who circumvents the interacting forces that conspire to excessively medicalize care near the end of life.

Medicare as the Key

As Rosa journeyed through the health care system in the last five years of her life, as she encountered American medicine in the office, the hospital, and the skilled nursing facility, she received many of the benefits of modern medical care. The others whose stories appear here, Saul, Barbara, and Taylor, similarly experienced much that was admirable about American medicine, but however good their medical care at various points along the way, it could have been a great deal better. Geriatricians who designed a set of quality indicators to assess the adequacy of medical care in vulnerable older patients found that patients received optimal treatment of conditions such as falling and incontinence in less than one-third of cases.[16] And in international comparisons, the United States also performs poorly: compared to other economically advanced countries, our nation is ranked 20 out of 34 in life expectancy at age 65 for men and at 25 out of 34 for women. Moreover, the gap between the United States and the healthiest other countries has been growing. Swiss men can expect to live four years longer than their American counterparts and Japanese women five years longer.[17]

For most older patients, what American medicine considers the best care entails a stay in a hospital or SNF that may be confusing and disorienting and lead to a decline in independence and daily functioning. The best care often involves invasive and burdensome tests and diagnostic procedures that confer only a very small chance of benefit and substantial risk, and treatment with medications or devices that are likewise hazardous and seldom helpful.

Understanding why our best medical care often proves highly problematic for patients begins with the recognition that Americans are living long lives, affording them the opportunity to develop multiple chronic conditions. Older people as a group live longer today than in any previous era, even if they do not live as long as in select other countries: in 1900, sixty-five-year-old Americans could look forward to 11.9 years of additional life; by 1960, they could anticipate 14.4 years; and by 2009, they could expect another 19.2 years on this earth. And while those few hardy souls who made it to age eighty-five in the year 1900 could count on an average of another 4 years of life, and their counterparts in 1960 could expect 4.6 years, those reaching eighty-five in 2009 could expect to live an additional 6.7 years.[18]

While older people are surviving longer than ever before, modern medicine was designed to treat diseases one at a time. We know about what medications work and what procedures are beneficial for a given disease based on studies of people who had nothing wrong with them other than that one disease. But older patients typically don't have just one disease; rather, they have multiple chronic conditions, any of which may act up at any given time. Having multiple underlying conditions also means that when they develop some brand new problem, as older people statistically are wont to do, that new problem, whether it's pneumonia or a stroke or cancer, both impacts and is affected by all their other problems. As a result, the approach to care that many older patients need, unlike patients without other chronic conditions, involves much more than treating the particular body part that is out of kilter. It requires considering the effect of any proposed new medications on all the patient's other chronic diseases as well as taking into account their cognitive and physical functioning. The ability to monitor their illness, to get to the pharmacy to buy medications, and to remember to take their pills at the right times are just as critical to successful treatment as a correct diagnosis.

The American health care system also fails many older patients because it focuses single-mindedly on the individual, seldom considering that person's family, home, and community. That approach may suffice for middle-class people who don't depend on anyone else for shopping or transportation, let alone dressing or bathing. It is particularly effective for well-educated patients with the resources, both financial and organizational, to manage their own care. But for frail elders who need assistance to get by, going to the doctor and navigating the hospital and the SNF are a considerable challenge. What they need is medical care that begins by taking an inventory not just of their diseases, but also their level of functioning and their environment. They need their physician to come up with a plan of care that considers their home and their community in its design, along with their emotional, social, and financial resources. This kind of assessment and management is very different from what most primary care physicians and virtually all subspecialists have been trained to do; in fact, it's more than even a well-trained geriatrician can do. It's a job for a multidisciplinary team, a group of clinicians who work together to provide continuity of care to patients as they wend their way through the office, the hospital, the skilled nursing facility, and back home.

Despite all its limitations, the American health care system has accom-plished a great deal for older individuals. It is, after all, responsible for much of the improvement in life expectancy after age sixty-five. A considerable por-tion of that improvement comes from better health, with the death rate from heart disease and stroke each plunging over 50 percent between 1981 and 2009. And while lifestyle factors such as smoking cessation, a low-fat diet, and regu-lar exercise all contributed to the drop in mortality, improved medical treat-ment probably accounted for at least half of the improvement.[19]

Moreover, some older patients don't have multiple chronic diseases, they don't have any limitations in their daily activities, and they have sufficient economic resources to get by when they become sick.[20] They do just fine with the contemporary health care system—although even they might do better with a system that focused more on functioning. Evaluating even the most vigorous older people for their risk of falling or their hearing might identify incipient problems early, before they cause difficulties, and allow prevention of other problems. Other older people fare reasonably well, even without a system that effectively integrates the different pieces of the health care system into a coherent whole, because they have *some* elements of a good system and they have strong family support. Rosa had a generally positive experience—but she had devoted, involved, and well-educated family members who lived nearby and advocated on her behalf, trained geriatricians who actively par-ticipated in her care, and the financial resources to supplement conventional care along the way.

How can we make the system better so that it provides technically compe-tent, compassionate care to *all* older patients, including the frailest and oldest among them, care that is both consistent with what they value most and that is also achievable, given their personal and family circumstances? It's fairly clear what this kind of medical care would look like—it would be interdisci-plinary, coordinated, and accessible—but it would be more than that. It would begin with a comprehensive assessment of the person including his ability to hear and see, to walk and to think, to get dressed and use the bathroom, to shop for food and pay his bills. It would evaluate his emotional state, his de-gree of social engagement, his support system, his medical insurance, and his access to transportation. It would involve the patient and family, caregiver, or health care surrogate to be certain that they all understood the patient's health state and the implications of that state for the immediate future. Next, it would elicit the patient's preferences for care *in light of his overall condition.* Based on both the facts and the preferences, and with the input of the patient and family, the medical team would design a plan of care, a program for what should happen now (what pills to take, what exercises to perform, what health care services, such as physical therapy, nursing, and social work, to utilize), and a rough map of what should happen in the future if the principal foreseeable problems arise (for example, what to do if the person with heart failure has an acute episode of shortness of breath), such as what medications to take, whom to call, when and whether to go to the hospital. Optimal medical care for frail older people would have a large home care component, it would entail strategies for avoiding hospitalization to minimize the perils of iatrogenesis and transitions of care, and it would empower and engage both patients and caregivers in its implementation. How can we get from where we are today to such a radically different approach?

The dominant theme of this book is that medical care for older people looks very different from this ideal because hospitals, physicians, the medical device industry, pharmaceutical companies, and the Medicare program, operating within the larger social context, have made it what it is. Together, they determine where patients receive care, who provides it, and what it consists of. Medical schools, lawyers, scientific researchers, and the FDA, which I touch on only briefly and sporadically in this account, also figure into the mix. With so many interlocking moving parts, changing the system to make it more effective, function-oriented, and safe—and less fragmented, confusing, and alienating—is a formidable task.

Reform is particularly daunting because all the parties purport to be interested in improving health, but they each have their own interests to promote and turf to defend. Pharmaceutical companies want to sell drugs and make a profit. They may from time to time adapt their strategy to achieve this end: for decades, they sought to bring "blockbusters" to market that would generate over a billion dollars in revenue by virtue of a huge volume of sales; as the prospects for identifying high volume candidates declined, they switched their focus to low-volume "specialty drugs," drugs that are taken only by five to ten thousand patients a year, but compensating by charging $1,000 for a one-month supply of medication, or even more. Device manufacturers similarly want to sell equipment, from IV catheters to pacemakers to PET scanners. They are interested in innovation but only if they are reasonably confident the idea will pan out—unlike the pharmaceutical companies that try hundreds of chemical compounds, searching for something with the desired effect, they tend to promote designs that they think have a very good chance of becoming a product, a product that they are certain Medicare will pay for because it pays for just about any device that the FDA approves as "safe and effective."

Even physicians, who usually go into medicine to help people and treat disease—and who, despite losing some of our idealistic enthusiasm over the course of our long, arduous training, remain advocates for their patients—are not entirely selfless and dedicated. As a group, we want to preserve and protect our lifestyle. We want to practice a style of medicine that we find rewarding, both intellectually and financially, and that allows us to maintain our professional autonomy. And we are deeply imbued with a medical culture that values and promotes a highly specialized, technology-intensive approach to care.

Hospitals are businesses and often, when they are part of a network or system, very big businesses. The mission statements of both for-profit and not-for-profit hospitals may emphasize their role as providers of a community service, but the reality is that they are both focused on their bottom line. They would be quite willing to modify their processes and their structure to better accommodate the needs of geriatric patients—if they could do so without adversely affecting their overall profitability and without alienating their powerful constituents, the physicians who care for patients, the device manufacturers who supply them with sophisticated machines, and the drug companies that fill their pharmacies.

That leaves Medicare, the only participant in this drama that is single-mindedly concerned with access to and quality of health care for its members. Despite the political undercurrents that threaten to derail or at least impede change within CMS, Medicare is the best candidate to serve as the lever that can improve the system. In fact, for the fifty years since its inception, Medicare has repeatedly demonstrated that it can radically alter business as usual across multiple sectors of American health care.

The very creation of the Medicare program was transformative: by providing insurance coverage for the 56 percent of older Americans who didn't have a private policy, medical care suddenly became affordable for millions of people.[21] Use their policies they did, in order to have more hospital stays in general and more elective surgeries in particular, and also to see more physicians in the office, with a striking fall in mortality. And because Medicare placed essentially no restrictions on reimbursement of diagnostic and therapeutic procedures, device manufacturers were given an enormous boost, encouraged to produce and sell equipment such as pacemakers, and later CT scanners, to hospitals and doctors who were thrilled to have them and eager to use them on patients.

The introduction of prospective payment for hospitals in 1983 was another game changer. It triggered a ripple effect throughout the health care system, shortening hospital stays, then dramatically changing the kinds of activities that took place in the hospital and diverting them elsewhere. The SNF had scarcely existed as a site for short-term rehabilitative care until diagnosis-related groups created a demand for a bridge between the hospital and the home. The ambulatory surgery center was another offspring of prospective payment, born when hospitals and physicians redefined hospital care.

Even modest reforms to the Medicare program have had major consequences for older patients. The Balanced Budget Act of 1997 is remembered primarily for its introduction of prospective payment to the world of home health care, resulting in shorter periods of time during which a patient recently discharged from the hospital could have a visiting nurse and restricting who was eligible for home health care altogether. But it did far more. The BBA also made it easier to enroll in a Medicare HMO, a private plan that contracted with Medicare and assumed full risk for all elements of a patient's care. While the newly renamed "Medicare + Choice" plans didn't catch on to nearly the extent that legislators had hoped, they were more widely accepted than their predecessors. Later, when further modified to become "Medicare Advantage" plans, they would see dramatic growth in popularity—today they account for 31 percent of Medicare enrollment, compared to 18 percent in 1999—opening the door to more comprehensive and coordinated care for older patients.[22] A final feature of the BBA, which also got relatively little attention and is seldom remembered today but which had a major effect on health care for older people, is that it capped the number of residency slots that Medicare pays for—and Medicare pays for the costs of training most of the country's 110,000 young physicians. By limiting the number of positions, Medicare effectively froze both the supply of new doctors and the allocation between specialists and generalists at 1996 levels. What older patients need is more and better primary care, not more specialists, but the BBA had precisely the opposite effect.[23]

Today, the Affordable Care Act is ushering in a new era of potentially transformative changes to Medicare—with correspondingly significant implications for patient care. Through its web of incentives to bundle care, the ACA is forcing hospitals, physicians, SNFs, and home care agencies to collaborate or lose their shirts. Patients are beginning to experience the kind of more integrated and cohesive care that is essential to address the chronic diseases so common among older people. Mandating use of the electronic medical record, though much maligned and not without its drawbacks, may one day further promote coordination of care. Through its system of penalties for adverse events, including hospital-associated infections and falls, Medicare has embarked on an ambitious program to restructure the modern hospital, making it safer and more patient-centered. With its vendetta against hospital readmissions and its experiments in providing care in alternative sites rather than taking the easy road of hospitalizing patients, Medicare is promoting a style of care that is safer, less alienating, more consistent with patient preferences, and cheaper—and that just may be more effective than the technologically intensive, doctor-centric model that is common today. And with its *Hospital Compare* and *Nursing Home Compare* websites, Medicare is pushing hospitals and SNFs to make changes that enhance patient satisfaction, hoping to shame the institutions into improving quality by publicly reporting patients' opinions about their physicians, their nurses, and other aspects of comparison. How well these initiatives are working is debatable. But Medicare is on the right track in using its leverage to effect change throughout the health care system.

There is still more that Medicare could do. If Medicare negotiated with pharmaceutical companies over how much it would pay for prescription drugs—which it is currently prohibited by law from doing—it could push down the price of drugs. Patients would have fewer out-of-pocket medication expenses and be more likely to be able to afford gym memberships or social activities that have the potential to prevent cardiac disease, mitigate against depression, and perhaps delay the onset of dementia. If Medicare introduced cost-effectiveness as a criterion for determining whether to reimburse medical device manufacturers for a new technology, companies would have less incentive to invest in high-cost, low-benefit technology than they do currently. Right now they are free to work on invasive and risky devices, basking in the knowledge that physicians will be willing to use whatever technology they make available as long as Medicare is willing to pay for it. And Medicare will pay as long as they can show in a controlled study that the technique, on average, is just a smidgeon more effective than available alternatives. The result is a cycle of innovation and expansion that knows no bounds. Once Medicare agrees to pay for a new technology, doctors come to see it as the standard of care, and as soon as doctors have accepted the technology as normal, patients assume it's essential to their health and well-being.[24] But if Medicare didn't routinely pay for everything—right now it interprets the statutory requirement that it pay for devices that are "reasonable and necessary" to imply that it can't take cost into consideration—then companies might not have been so enthusiastic about developing the left ventricular assist device in the first place, a technology that had a cost-effectiveness ratio of between $500,000 and $1.4 million per quality-adjusted-life-year when it was introduced.[25] Hospitals would find their costs falling, allowing them to devote resources to creating a better environment for frail, older patients, if they didn't spend so much on the latest, greatest technology. They might be more willing to develop special units for geriatric patients, the acute care for the elderly (ACE) units that have repeatedly proved to be effective in reducing falls, delirium, polypharmacy, and other hazards of hospitalization.

There's more. Not only does Medicare affect nursing home and hospital care, but it could also take steps to shape the way young people who just got their MD degrees learn to become practicing physicians. The way forward is by introducing requirements into the training programs, the internships and residencies, that Medicare supports.[26] It could, for example, demand far more contact hours devoted to communication with patients and families about goals of care. It could insist that residents in training demonstrate proficiency in comprehensive geriatric assessment. It could mandate time spent on advance care planning.

Public financing pays $15 billion a year for graduate medical education, of which $9.7 billion is from Medicare alone. The money covers 90 percent of the costs of the nation's nearly 118,000 residents, but Medicare has no control over how that money is used. The hospitals to which it doles out support (in the form of direct payments that go to residents' salaries and indirect payments that go to the hospital for the increased costs associated with having a training program) are responsible for the allocation of the funds between primary care and subspecialty training slots and for what goes into the education they provide. A totally separate private body, the Accreditation Council of Graduate Medical Education, determines accreditation standards.[27] When MedPAC, the advisory council that recommends changes to the Medicare program, looked into graduate medical education a few years ago and discovered that Medicare had never linked its generous subsidies to any educational goals, the authors were shocked. Their dismay emerges between the lines of their sober, measured, and generally matter-of-fact report. After marveling that despite Medicare's "enormous financial stake in health care and graduate medical education," it does not now and never has done anything to promote the training of doctors who are well-equipped to take care of our aging population, the report quietly concludes that "Medicare should consider ways to ensure that residents . . . obtain the skills they need to provide efficient, coordinated, high-quality care."[28]

In fact, MedPAC enumerates many of the ways in which the current training system falls short: residents do not learn enough about measuring quality and effective ways of improving the quality of practice; they don't spend enough time working as part of a multidisciplinary team; they know little about the costs of any of the tests they order or the drugs they prescribe; they spend entirely too much time in hospitals even though most care is delivered outside hospitals; and they don't learn much about communicating with patients, especially about their goals and preferences for care. Medicare, if given the green light by Congress to introduce incentives into its support of medical education, could change its reimbursement to allow for residents to spend more time out of the hospital without their program losing money, and could reward programs that do a good job of teaching all those skills that are currently largely ignored.

Medicare could also encourage physicians to spend as much time on functional assessment and advance care planning as they do on optimizing the control of blood pressure and diabetes. Medicare could incentivize hospitals to work with primary care physicians and skilled nursing facilities so as to provide truly integrated and comprehensive health care: it simply needs to hold them collectively responsible for all of a patient's health care. Medicare could channel innovation in the medical device industry by reimbursing for technology based on its cost-effectiveness rather than on a rate set by the manufacturers.

Not every change in the way Medicare works requires new federal legislation; some of Medicare's influence on the health care system arises from the rules and regulations it imposes. When OBRA '87 established a framework within which Medicare could impose controls on skilled nursing facilities, the specific requirements that followed, regulations specifying the temperature of the food served as well as the circumstances under which antipsychotic medications could be used, were the brainchildren of CMS. Similarly, federal legislation mandated the creation of a Hospital Readmissions Reduction Program but left the details of how this plays out to Medicare.

Perhaps the most dramatic change Medicare could make, one that would require legislation, might be to develop a new benefit package designed to meet the needs of the frail elderly. Such a plan would offer a more intensive home care program than is currently available in exchange for decreased coverage of invasive, expensive, and often non-beneficial hospital-based technology such as ICU care and open-heart surgery. The model for this approach is hospice: choosing to enroll in hospice in lieu of conventional Medicare has been an option since 1983 and, after a slow start, it's been a very successful approach—nearly half of all older people are enrolled in hospice at the time of their death. It's also similar to the various other alternatives—HMOs and PPOs (Provider Preferred Organization)—that allow patients to substitute a comprehensive plan for fee-for-service Medicare and, as of 2015, fully 30 percent of Medicare enrollees choose that option. A variant that also relies on a modified funding mechanism, in this case a modified Accountable Care Organization, is "MediCaring." Intended for frail elders and built on a foundation of comprehensive geriatric assessment and individualized care planning, this program would offer transportation, nutrition, and caregiver support, along with geriatrically oriented medical care, using a local service delivery system.[29]

Relying on Medicare as the lever for change in the complex system that comprises modern American health care is not without risk. Medicare, as a government program, is subject to external influences. It has to pay attention to costs, though interestingly, it has never been required to operate within a predetermined budget, making allocation decisions within that total. It is concerned with cost because its expenditures affect how much money will be left for the federal government to spend on schools, roads, and all the other institutions and services that are crucial to a vibrant, prosperous country. And making major changes to Medicare requires an act of Congress, which is problematic in times of an extremely polarized, dysfunctional legislature. It's also been a concern because Senators and Representatives are subject to intense pressure from lobbyists—and the device manufacturing and pharmaceutical industries are among the largest, most effective lobbyists in Washington, DC. And over the past fifty years, during which time Medicare has successfully functioned as one of the prime drivers of change for the growing number of Americans enrolled in the program, Medicare hasn't always gotten things right. There have been unintended consequences of some of its bolder initiatives: the introduction of prospective payment and the mandated use of electronic medical records are two examples that I return to repeatedly in *Old and Sick in America* precisely because they have had such profound and far-reaching effects.

Despite its missteps and its weaknesses, Medicare is the best and most plausible candidate for a beneficent change agent. At its inception, all it was expected to do was to provide short-term acute hospital care for older people. In the eyes of the founders, most of those older people were not going to be alive for many years, and those who exceeded actuarial expectations would surely not want or demand expensive hospital treatment. Very slowly, Medicare has had to adapt to a new reality in which patients routinely live into their eighties, suffer from multiple chronic diseases, and think nothing of undergoing surgical procedures or other aggressive interventions in their ninth decade. And as Medicare has evolved, it has forced change in physi-

cians, hospitals, and SNFs and, to a more limited extent, in device manufacturers and pharmaceutical companies.

For the last five years, Medicare has moved forward in response to its own
research initiatives, conducted through the Center for Medicare and Medicaid Innovation, funded by the Affordable Care Act to the tune of $10 billion
over a ten-year period. The Center's mission is to develop and test innovative
delivery models and payment systems to see if they can decrease costs and
improve quality and, if they are successful, to encourage widespread adoption. Thanks to the demonstration projects sponsored by the Innovation
Center, Medicare has promoted bundled payments, accountable care organizations, and home care. Its "Comprehensive Primary Care Initiative," for
example, paid clinicians substantial case management fees that resulted
in improved care for high-risk patients.[30] And its "Independence at Home
Demonstration" found that providing services in the home saved an average
of just over $1,000 per beneficiary by preventing hospital readmissions, de-
creasing the use of emergency rooms, and adding more extensive advance
care planning.[31]

There's a long way to go before all Americans can expect medical care that
is tailored to their needs and preferences, care that is both effective and cost-
effective, and that takes into consideration their ability to function as well as
their diseases, their family and community supports, as well as their individual resources. The challenge is formidable as many of the linchpins of the
health care system—the physicians, the hospitals, the skilled nursing facility
owners, the drug companies, and the device manufacturers—benefit from
the system as it is today. The task is also daunting because all those players do
not merely stand to lose something precious, whether autonomy, power, or
money; they are all interlinked, and the fortune (or misfortune) of any one
affects the well-being of each of the others. But that interconnectedness is
also the key to successful change, if only we can identify the lever that affects
all the parts of the system. Medicare is that lever. Modifying Medicare, a process that has already begun, can assure that, one day, all older people will be
able to look forward to an auspicious journey as they ail and age.

Acknowledgments

This book is my attempt to understand how the health care system that I have worked in as a geriatric and palliative care physician for over thirty years works, what it's like for older patients to navigate this system when they become ill, and why it functions the way it does. It reflects my understanding of what happens to patients, for better and for worse, as well as what doesn't happen that should. In addition to relying on my experiences taking care of patients, it rests on research in history, politics, economics, sociology, and other areas that don't fit neatly into a single academic discipline. The result is both a very personal book, a synthesis of existing work in multiple fields, and, I hope, a manifesto on how to make the care of older people better in the future.

Old and Sick in America couldn't have been written without my Swarthmore College undergraduate professors who taught me to write seminar papers. Those essays, which during the Honors Program at Swarthmore were cranked out every few weeks, required me to synthesize a host of disparate sources and come up with a way of tying all the strands together. At some level, I've been writing seminar papers ever since: my thought pieces in the *New England Journal of Medicine*, the *Annals of Internal Medicine*, and *Health Affairs* are all modeled on this format, and *Old and Sick in America* is in many ways made up of multiple seminar papers. I'm particularly indebted to Paul Beik in the History Department and Patrick Henry in the Religion Department for their mentorship and encouragement.

Many of the chapters in this book start with a vignette about my earliest reactions to the health care system, either as a medical student or a medical resident, at a time when everything in medicine was new and fresh. For the perspective I developed during this crucial, formative period, I owe a debt of gratitude to my teachers at Harvard Medical School, particularly Charles Hatem and Robert Lawrence. They taught me much of what I know about the essentials of good doctoring. Other physicians I have gotten to know as colleagues, mentors, and role models have also contributed in sometimes subtle but always important ways to my understanding. Bob Buxbaum, a fine internist and pioneer in palliative care, died this past year—his wisdom and joy in doctoring are very much missed.

Thanks as well to those family members who agreed to share their relatives' stories with me, and to editorialize on what the experience of the health care system was like for both patients and families. For reasons of confidentiality, the names and identifying characteristics of these patients have been modified, so I will not mention the names of their family members either, but you know who you are. Thank you, thank you, thank you.

This book is a synthesis of material from medical science, history, political science, and economics, and it rests on the scholarship and investigative journalism of many.

Their names and works are listed in the Bibliography. *Old and Sick in America* is also an interpretation of the experience of older patients as seen through my clinical lens. I am grateful to all those I have cared for over the years because it was my patients, in the office, in the hospital, in the skilled nursing facility, and in their homes, who showed me what it was like to be a patient in the American health care system—and who made me realize how the experience could be improved.

I would particularly like to thank those friends and colleagues who read preliminary versions of several chapters, and whose comments and insights were invaluable in shaping this book, with the usual disclaimer: I alone am responsible for any errors of fact as well as for the judgments that are liberally dispensed throughout the book. My colleague in the Department of Population Medicine of Harvard Medical School, Jim Sabin, made many useful suggestions on the manuscript in addition to serving as a springboard for my thinking over the past ten years. Daniel Callahan, biomedical ethicist par excellence and, in my view, one of the few philosophers who really "gets" the important issues in clinical practice, is still going strong at age 85, was incredibly generous with his time, and read numerous chapters. He is a true mensch and was the gentlest of critics. Sharon Kaufman, a distinguished medical anthropologist, likewise made thoughtful comments on the manuscript and has contributed to my thinking through her complementary perspective over several lunches we shared when I was in California to visit my sons. Finally, my most invaluable critic is my husband Larry, who not only reads and comments on most everything I write, but encourages me whenever I falter in my work.

Notes

Prelude

1. Blesch, "Baptist Health South Florida."
2. Kolata, "Patients in Florida."
3. *Dartmouth Atlas*, 2015.
4. Gillick, "Medicine as Ecoculture."
5. Institute of Medicine, *Conflict of Interest*.
6. In a terrific piece of investigative journalism, Rick Weiss of the *Washington Post* revealed that Michael Phelps, PET's inventor, urged his friend Senator Ted Stevens (R-Alaska), chair of the appropriations committee in charge of the CMS purse strings, to pressure CMS to change its policy on reimbursing for PET scans in the diagnosis of dementia. Phelps paid a lobbyist at a prominent Washington lobbying firm over $500,000 to work for expanded Medicare coverage and also repeatedly donated to Stevens's senate campaigns. The story appeared in "A Tale of Politics" in the *Post* in October 2004.
7. Gillick, "How Medicare Shapes the Way We Die."
8. National Hospice and Palliative Care Organization, *NHPCO Facts and Figures 2015*.
9. National Center for Health Statistics, *Health, United States, 2014*. A man who turned sixty-five in 1960 could have anticipated living for another 12.8 years; in 2013, he could expect to live for 17.9 years.
10. Chay, "Medicare Hospital Utilization."
11. Docteur and Berenson, "How Does the Quality of US Health Care Compare."
12. Kwok et al., "Intensity and Variation of Surgical Care."
13. Earle et al., "Aggressiveness of Cancer Care."
14. Plsek, "Complexity and the Adoption of Innovation."

Chapter One

1. Centers for Disease Control, "National Ambulatory Medical Care Survey: 2012."
2. Cherry, Lucas, and Decker, "Population Aging and the Use of Office-Based Physician Services." The average number of visits made by the elderly to a physician was 6.9. Of these, 45 percent were to primary care doctors, 25 percent to medical specialists, and 30 percent to surgeons.
3. The exception is recent immigrants or someone who neither worked in the United States nor was married to someone who worked.
4. Kane and Peckham, *Medscape Physician Compensation Report, 2014*.

5. Alexander, Kurlander, and Wynia, "Physicians in Retainer ('Concierge') Practices." This study reported that a physician in a concierge practice has on average about 900 patients compared to 2,300 in a conventional practice.

6. Brennan, "Luxury Primary Care."

7. Physicians Foundation, *2014 Survey of America's Physicians*. In this survey of practicing physicians, 7 percent reported they practice some form of concierge medicine and another 13 percent said they were planning to transition, at least in part, to this model.

8. Ibid. The 2000 primary care shortage is 9,000; the projected shortage in 2020 will be 45,000. Starting salary was $185,000 for a family physician and $205,000 for an internist, compared to $300,000 for a neurologist and $424,000 for a urologist.

9. Ibid. Physicians are retiring at the rate of 9 percent per year and are cutting back their hours at a rate of 18 percent per year.

10. West and Dupras, "General Medicine vs Subspecialty Career Plans."

11. Physicians Foundation, *2014 Survey of America's Physicians*.

12. Doyle, Lennox, and Bell, "A Systematic Review of Evidence."

13. Yahoo Finance, "Press Ganey Holdings."

14. Ibid.

15. The Picker Commonwealth Institute and the National Quality Forum, converts to this perspective, designed their own surveys.

16. Kane and Peckham, *Physician Compensation Report*, 2014. Eighteen percent of visits are nine to twelve minutes in length, 29 percent last between thirteen and sixteen minutes, and 25 percent last from seventeen to twenty minutes.

17. Terry et al., "Top 15 Challenges Facing Physicians." Just one year earlier, 58 percent of doctors spent a day or more per week on paperwork.

18. Woolhandler and Himmelstein, "Administrative Work."

19. Centers for Medicare and Medicaid Services, "Chronic Conditions among Medicare Beneficiaries." Among patients over sixty-five enrolled in fee-for-service Medicare, 61 percent have high blood pressure, 48 percent have elevated cholesterol, 34 percent have ischemic heart disease, 31 percent have arthritis, and 28 percent have diabetes. Among patients who are between 75 and 84, 27 percent have four or five chronic disorders and another 18 percent have at least six; in people 85 or older, 29 percent have four or five conditions and 25 percent have six or more.

20. Park, Cherry, and Decker, "Nurse Practitioners in Physician Offices."

21. Northeastern University, Bouvé College, "Physician Assistant Studies."

22. Levinson and Pizzo, "Physician Communications." It shouldn't be surprising that physicians in general, and those who go into procedure-oriented specialties in particular, are not well skilled in communication since they receive little teaching in this area in either medical school or residency programs.

23. Levinson, Hudab, and Tricco, "A Systematic Review of Surgeon-Patient Communication."

24. According to the Association of American Medical Colleges, *2014 Physician Specialty Data Book*. Only 36.9 percent of family doctors and 35.8 percent of internists are

women. Interestingly, 49.3 percent of geriatricians are women. According to Young et al., "A Census of Actively Licensed Physicians," 20 percent of active physicians are between 60 and 69 and 10.9 percent are 70 or older.

25. Cherry, Lucas, and Decker, "Aging and the Use of Office-Based Physicians." Of the 6.9 office visits made to doctors by older people in 2008, only 45 percent were to primary care doctors, down from what it was in 1978, when 62 percent of their office visits were for primary care.

26. John Hartford Foundation, "Brief History of Geriatrics."

27. Institute of Medicine, *Retooling for an Aging America*. In 2007, only about 250 out of 400 available positions were taken.

28. Ibid.

29. PerryUndem Research, "Survey of Adults 65 and Over." Eighty-two percent of older adults report very high levels of satisfaction with their primary care doctors.

30. Osborn et al., "International Survey Finds Shortcomings." In this international comparison, the United States fares poorly compared to other countries in how promptly older patients can see their doctor, in the cost of care—despite universal Medicare coverage—and in coordination of care.

Chapter Two

1. Accenture, "Clinical Transformation."

2. Kane and Emmons, "New Data on Physician Practice."

3. Hargrave et al., "Retainer-Based Physicians."

4. Page, "Rise and Further Rise of Concierge Medicine."

5. Kane, "Updated Data on Physician Practice." Among surgical subspecialists, 71.9 percent are practice owners; among medical subspecialists, the rate is 62 percent. For internists, it's 46 percent, for family practitioners, it's 39.8 percent, and for pediatricians, the rate is lowest at 37 percent.

6. Kirchhoff, "Physician Practices."

7. Ibid.

8. Monegain, "Intermountain, Geisinger Share the Spotlight."

9. Ibid. Overall, only 22.1 percent of doctors work in a multispecialty group. Among internists, the rate is 36 percent.

10. Altman, "Dr. Russell Lee."

11. Palo Alto Medical Foundation, "About Us: History."

12. At the time of the merger, Sutter included thirty-four acute care hospitals, five home care organizations, and five acute rehabilitation facilities.

13. Palo Alto Medical Foundation, "About Us: History."

14. Ibid. The website listed 141 doctors on staff, including 10 general internists and 13 family practitioners as of December 2015.

15. Inouye et al., "Geriatric Syndromes."

16. Boult et al., "A Randomized Controlled Trial of Outpatient Geriatric Evaluation."

17. Beyer et al., "Prevalence and Characteristics of Outpatient Palliative Care."

18. Meyer, "Changing the Conversation in California."

19. May, Norman, and Morrison, "Economic Impact of Hospital Palliative Care Consultation."

20. Temel et al., "Early Palliative Care."

21. American Academy of Family Physicians et al., "Guidelines for Patient-Centered Medical Home Recognition."

22. Fishman et al., "Impact on Seniors of the Patient-Centered Medical Home."

23. Meyer, "Group Health's Move to the Medical Home."

24. Counsell et al., "Geriatric Care Management."

25. Boult and Wieland, "Comprehensive Primary Care for Older Patients."

26. Boult et al., "The Effect of Guided Care Teams," and Boult et al., "A Matched-Pair Cluster-Randomized Trial."

27. National Center for Quality Assurance, "Future of Patient-Centered Medical Homes."

28. Old data is from Meyer and Gibbons, "Housecalls and the Elderly"; new data is from Peterson et al., "Trends in Physician Housecalls."

29. Reisman, "End of a Chapter."

30. De Jonge et al., "Effects of Home-Based Primary Care."

31. Fye, "The Origins and Evolution of the Mayo Clinic."

32. Porter and Kellogg, "Kaiser Permanente."

33. Kaiser Permanente, "Fast Facts about Kaiser Permanente."

Chapter Three

1. Friedberg et al., "Factors Affecting Physician Professional Satisfaction."

2. Association of American Medical Colleges, "Medical Student Education: Debt, Costs, and Loan Repayment."

3. Peckham, "Medscape Compensation Report, 2015."

4. Grayson, Newton, and Thompson, "Payback Time."

5. Friedberg et al., "Factors Affecting Professional Satisfaction."

6. Schulte and Donald, "Cracking the Codes."

7. Terry et al., "Top 15 Challenges Facing Physicians." The percentage of physicians who spend more than one day per week on paperwork increased from 58% in 2013 to 70% in 2014.

8. Hanover, "Business Strategy: Ambulatory EHR Buyer Satisfaction."

9. Woolhandler and Himmelstein, "Administrative Work." This was the conclusion reached based on data collected from a random sample of U.S. doctors in 2008.

10. The Physicians Foundation, *2014 Survey of America's Physicians*. Among the 20,000 physicians who responded to a detailed questionnaire about their views on the state of American medicine, 44 percent said they were planning to cut back services.

11. Centers for Medicare and Medicaid Services, *Chronic Conditions*.

12. Sirovich et al., "Discretionary Decision Making."

13. Physicians are trained on how to bill by specialized "coding experts." The patient's history also has three components: the "history of the present illness"; the "review of

systems"; and a conglomeration of past history, family history, and social history. The physical exam is made up of "elements," where each element is a part of the body that was examined. Finally, medical decision making is rated as low-, medium-, or high-risk, depending on whether what the doctor does is routine (like refilling a prescription or checking the blood pressure), new (such as prescribing a new medication), or a matter of life and death (discussing chemotherapy or advance directives).

14. Medicare does evaluate physicians based on whether they ask patients if they have fallen in the recent past, but it doesn't require them to do anything about it if they have. Similarly, it now pays for advance care planning discussions that don't have to be linked with a physical exam, but the standard Medicare payment is lower than was already available using "time" rather than visit complexity.

15. Rockoff, "Drug Reps Soften Their Sales Pitches."

16. Ibid.

17. Rockoff, "As Doctors Lose Clout, Drug Firms Redirect the Sales Call."

18. Kassirer, *On the Take.*

19. Ventola, "Direct-to-Consumer Pharmaceutical Advertising." Pharma spent $1.6 billion on DTC advertising in 1999, $2.5 billion in 2000, $3.1 billion in 2003, $4.4 billion in 2004, and $5.4 billion in 2006.

20. Silverman, "Drug Makers Are Targeting Patients in Physician Offices."

21. Kirchhoff, "Physician Practices."

22. Ludmerer, *Let Me Heal.*

23. CMS, "Accountable Care Organizations." CMS lists the participants in each of its ACO models, the Pioneer ACO Model, the Advance Payment ACO Model, and the Medicare Shared Savings Programs, on its website.

24. McWilliams et al., "Change in Patients' Experience."

25. CMS, "New Hospitals and Health Care Providers Join Federal Initiative."

26. Loftus and Walker, "Drug and Medical-Device Makers Paid $6.49 Billion." The data was made public by CMS in its Open Payments Report, as required by a provision of the Affordable Care Act that promotes transparency, dubbed the "Sunshine Provision."

27. Carreyrou and McGinty, "Medical Lab Tests Anti-Kickback Law."

28. Ibid.

29. Carreyrou, "Lab Reaches Deal with Government."

30. Carreyrou and Tamm, "A Device to Kill Cancer, Lift Revenue."

31. Smith-Bindman, Miglioretti, and Larson, "Rising Use of Medical Imaging."

Chapter Four

1. Miller and Miller, *Making the Rounds.*

2. Ibid.

3. Balfe, "A Survey of Group Practice, 1965."

4. Kane and Emmons, "New Data on Physician Practice Arrangements."

5. U.S. Department of Health and Human Services, "Characteristics of Office-Based Practices."

6. See Groves, "Changing Demographics of Women in Medicine," for the historical data, and Kaiser Family Foundation, "Distribution of Medical School Graduates by Gender," for the more recent data.

7. Sutter Health, "Find the Doctor Who Is Right for You." As of April 2016, fifteen of the twenty-three adult primary care physicians listed on the PAMF website for the San Carlos practice were women.

8. Kaiser Family Foundation, "Distribution of Medical School Graduates by Race/Ethnicity." The remaining nonwhites were 21 percent Asian, and 5 percent Hispanic.

9. National Center for Health Statistics, "Office Visits by Persons Aged 65 and Over."

10. Hsiao et al., "National Ambulatory Medical Care Survey."

11. U.S. Department of Health, Education, and Welfare, "Volume of Physician Visits. United States—July 1966–June 1967."

12. Peterson, Landers, and Bazemore, "Trends in Physician House Calls." Strikingly, 5.6 percent of physicians billed Medicare for at least one house call in 2006. However, over half of these doctors made only one or two house calls in an entire year. Rural solo practitioners accounted for fully 86 percent of the house calls made to geriatric patients.

13. U.S. HEW, "Volume of Physician Visits. July 1966–June 1967."

14. Bureau of Labor Statistics, *CPI Inflation Calculator*.

15. Centers for Medicare and Medicaid Services, "Medicare Final CY 2015 Physician Fee Schedule."

16. SHEP Cooperative Research Group, "Prevention of Stroke."

17. Staessen et al., "Comparison of Placebo with Active Treatment."

18. Gillespie and Hurvitz, "Prevalence of Hypertension."

19. Centers for Medicare and Medicaid Services, *Chronic Conditions among Medicare Beneficiaries*.

20. Knatterud et al., "Effects of Hypoglycemic Agents on Vascular Complications."

21. Diabetes Control and Complication Trial Research Group, "Effect of Intensive Treatment of Diabetes."

22. UK Prospective Diabetes Study Group, "Intensive Blood-Glucose Control with Sulphonylureas or Insulin." This study would be extensively criticized for suggesting that oral medication might result in worse outcomes than diet alone. But its finding that type 2 diabetes is a serious illness was a major breakthrough.

23. Greene, *Prescribing by the Numbers*.

24. Association of American Medical Colleges, "The Changing Gender Composition of US Medical School Applicants."

25. Gomory and Sylla, "The American Corporation."

26. Relman, "The New Medical-Industrial Complex."

27. Frack and Hong, "Physician Practice Management."

28. American Medical News, "Negotiating Your Productivity Target."

29. Lee, Bothe, and Steele, "How Geisinger Structures Its Physicians' Compensation."

30. The Physicians Foundation, *2014 Survey of America's Physicians*.

31. Gerteis et al., *Through the Patient's Eyes*.

32. Zgierska, Rabago, and Miller, "Impact of Patient Satisfaction Ratings."

33. Ludmerer, *Time to Heal.*

34. The system is actually even more complicated: the dollar amount assigned to a given CPT code is determined not just by the physician's work, but also by practice expenses and malpractice insurance. Each of these three components is weighted depending on the RVU assigned. My abbreviated description refers to the major component, which is the physician's work.

35. Sinsky and Dugdale, "Medicare Payment for Cognitive vs Procedural Care."

36. Kohn, Corrigan, and Donaldson, eds. for Institute of Medicine, *To Err Is Human.*

37. DeVita and Chu, "A History of Cancer Chemotherapy."

38. Association of American Medical Colleges, "Diversity in Medical Education."

Chapter Five

1. Gorina et al., "Hospitalization, Readmission, and Death Experience."

2. Barnett, Hsu, and McWilliams, "Patient Characteristics and Differences in Hospital Readmission Rates."

3. Covinsky, Pierluissi, and Johnston, "Hospitalization-Associated Disability."

4. Russo and Elixhauser, "Hospitalizations in the Elderly." In a sample of older, fee-for-service Medicare beneficiaries from 2003, 839,300 people were hospitalized for CHF, or 6.3 percent of all admissions in the elderly. There were 770,400 hospital pneumonia stays in elderly people (5.8 percent of the total).

5. Hinami et al., "Worklife and Satisfaction of Hospitalists."

6. White and Glazier, "Do Hospitalist Physicians Improve Quality?"

7. Welch et al., "Use of Hospitalists by Medicare Beneficiaries."

8. Yarbrough et al., "Multifaceted Intervention Reduces Inpatient Laboratory Costs."

9. Hall et al., "National Hospital Discharge Survey, 2007."

10. Inouye, "Delirium in Older Persons."

11. Witlox et al., "Delirium in Elderly Patients." In this review of the literature, physicians found that the mortality rate by two years after discharge was 38 percent in older patients who had developed delirium in the hospital, compared to 22.7 percent in those who had not. The risk of nursing home placement after a little over a year of follow-up was 33.4 percent in the delirium sufferer compared to 10.7 percent in controls.

12. Schimmel, "The Hazards of Hospitalization."

13. Gillick, Serrell, and Gillick, "Adverse Consequences of Hospitalization." In this study, we did not consider symptoms to be potentially related to the hospitalization if they were commonly associated with the admitting diagnosis. For example, patients with meningitis, a brain infection, were expected to become confused. Patients admitted with a stroke were clearly at risk of falling, patients with a bladder infection might be expected to be incontinent, and patients with a stomach ulcer often did not eat.

14. Covinsky, Pierluissi, and Johnston, "Hospitalization-Associated Disability."

15. Klevens et al., "Estimating Healthcare-Associated Infection in US Hospitals."

16. Kaye et al., "Effect of Nosocomial Bloodstream Infections on Mortality."

17. Jencks, Williams, and Coleman, "Rehospitalizations among Patients in Medicare."

18. One example of a successful intervention is Coleman et al., "The Care Transitions Intervention."

19. Krumholz, "Post-Hospital Syndrome."

20. National Center for Health Statistics, "Utilization of Short-Stay Hospitals." For people over sixty-five, the average length of stay was 5.5 days in 2010, compared to 14.1 days in 1967.

21. Wier, Pfuntner, and Steiner, "Hospital Utilization among Older Adults."

22. Teno et al., "Change in End-of-Life Care for Medicare Beneficiaries."

23. Flory et al., "Place of Death: US Trends since 1980." These statistics are for all deaths, not just deaths in people over sixty-five, but most deaths occur in older individuals so these numbers are roughly representative of the older group.

24. SUPPORT Principal Investigators, "A Controlled Trial to Improve Care." A total of 38 percent spent between three and ten days in an ICU and 50 percent reported pain.

25. Goodman et al., "Trends in Cancer Care." The percentages are 62 and 29, respectively.

26. Tschirhart, Du, and Kelley, "Factors Influencing the Use of Intensive Procedures." Just under one-fifth of patients got at least one such procedure in the six months before death.

Chapter Six

1. The terminology is confusing. The federal government defines a community hospital as any hospital that's not a psychiatric hospital, not a chronic disease hospital, and not run by the federal government. I will instead use the term "general hospital" for these facilities and will distinguish between large, teaching institutions on the one hand and community hospitals on the other. Dunn and Becker, "50 Things to Know about the Hospital Industry."

2. U.S. Department of Health and Human Services, "NIH Research Portfolio Online Reporting Tools (*RePORT*), NIH Awards." Beth Israel Deaconess Medical Center was number 5 in the country with 237 awards; BWH was number 2 with 535, and MGH was number 1 with 772. https://report.nih.gov/award. Accessed February 22, 2016.

3. Papanikolaou, Christidi, and Ioannidis, "Patient Outcomes with Teaching versus Nonteaching Healthcare."

4. Wennberg et al., "Use of Hospitals during Last Six Months of Life."

5. Ibid.

6. Kaiser Family Foundation, "Hospitals by Ownership Type." This research found that 58.4 percent of hospitals are nonprofit and 21.4 percent are for-profit. The for-profit hospital proportion in Nevada is 51.7 percent, and in Florida it's 51.4 percent.

7. McLaughlin, "Private Equity and Non-Profit Hospitals."

8. Banner Estrella Medical Center, "Mission, Values, Vision and Brand"; Memorial Hospital, "Mission Statement."

9. Horwitz, "Making Profits and Providing Care."

10. Eggleston et al., "Hospital Ownership and Quality of Care."

11. Joynt, Orav, and Jha, "Association between Hospital Conversion to For-Profit Status and Clinical and Economic Outcomes."

12. Auerbach, Weeks, and Brantley, "Health Care Spending and Efficiency in the U.S. Department of Veterans Affairs." It's very difficult to be more precise about how many older vets get their care in the VA system because almost all veterans eligible for VA benefits (and only those with service-related injuries qualify) also have Medicare. Many patients go to VA facilities for some services and to private health care institutions for others. They also cycle in and out of the VA system.

13. Kizer and Dudley, "Extreme Makeover."

14. Rubenstein et al., "Effectiveness of a Geriatric Evaluation Unit."

15. Cohen et al., "A Controlled Trial of Geriatric Evaluation and Management."

16. Jha et al., "Effect of the Transformation of the Veterans Affairs Health Care System on the Quality of Care." In 2000, the VA did better on 12 out of 13 quality indicators, compared to Medicare patients.

17. Healthcare Cost and Utilization Project, "Bedsize of Hospitals."

18. Riley and Lubitz, "Outcomes of Surgery among the Medicare Aged."

19. Goodman et al., "Trends in Cancer Care." A total of 9.4 percent of patients got life-sustaining treatment in the last month of life.

20. Bynum et al., "Our Parents, Ourselves."

21. American Hospital Association. "Fast Facts on US Hospitals, 2016."

22. Goodman et al., "Trends in End-of-Life Care."

23. Ibid.

24. Dafny, "Hospital Industry Consolidation."

25. Carrier, Dowling, and Berenson, "Hospitals' Geographic Expansion."

26. Kowalczyk, "Partners Hospitals, Doctors Top Health-Payment List."

27. Gamble, "15 Things to Know about the Deal."

28. Weisman, "Steward Reshapes Mass. Health Care Business."

29. Barber and Goold, "The Strategic Secret of Private Equity."

30. Donnelly, "Steward Health Care: Layoffs Are Needed."

31. Adams, "Physicians Group Sues Steward over Payments."

32. Fisher et al., "The Implications of Regional Variation."

Chapter Seven

1. Massachusetts passed legislation in 1971 establishing a "Determination of Need" process that was intended to "promote availability and accessibility of cost effective, high quality health services to Massachusetts citizens and to assist in controlling health care costs." Approval was required for capital projects in excess of a certain amount—the cutoff changed yearly, and in 2015 it was $17,826,988 for a project proposed by a

hospital. Massachusetts overhauled the regulations in January, 2017. Bicknell and Walsh, "Certificate-of-Need: the Massachusetts Experience."

2. American Hospital Association, "Economic Contribution of Hospitals Overlooked."

3. Evans, Wood, and Lambert, "Patient Injury and Physical Restraint Devices."

4. Goodman et al., "Trends and Variation in End-of-Life Care."

5. IMS Institute for Healthcare Information, "Medicines Use and Spending Shifts."

6. Hajjar et al., "Unnecessary Drug Use in Frail Older People."

7. Mizokami et al., "Polypharmacy with Common Diseases."

8. Staats, "On the Case: Clues to Hospital Selling."

9. American Society of Health Systems Pharmacists, "ASPH Guidelines."

10. Rockoff, "As Doctors Lose Clout."

11. Kassirer, *On the Take.*

12. Loftus, "For Doctors, Fewer Perks."

13. Kane, "Updated Data."

14. Pfuntner, Wier, and Stocks, "Most Frequent Procedures in US Hospitals."

15. Millman, "Keeping Up with the Joneses, Hospital Edition."

16. Juo et al., "Is Minimally Invasive Colon Resection Better?"

17. Gold, "Proton Beam Therapy Heats Up Hospital Arms Race."

18. Yu et al., "Proton versus Intensity-Modulated Radiotherapy."

19. American College of Healthcare Executives, *Annual Survey, 2014.*

20. Creswell and Abelson, "A Giant Hospital Chain Is Blazing a Profit Trail."

21. Available on the Medicare.gov website.

22. Centers for Medicare and Medicaid Services, *Hospital Compare.*

23. Ackerman, "Disaster of the Day: HCA." To be sure, the fraction of total receipts attributable to the sickest patients went up at all hospitals, but not as dramatically as at HCA, rising from 58 percent in 2000 to 76 percent in 2006.

24. Aiken et al., "Hospital Nurse Staffing."

25. Evans, "Juggling the Lineup."

26. Gorman, "Cedars-Sinai to Cut Most Psychiatric Services."

27. Baghai, Levine, and Sutaria, "Service-Line Strategies for US Hospitals."

28. Rodak, "Structuring Hospital Service Line Management for Success."

29. Brown, *Body of Truth: How Science, History, and Culture Drive Our Obsession with Weight.*

30. Halpern, "The Incredible, Perilous, Money-Making, People-Shrinking Machine."

31. Abelson and Creswell, "Hospital Chain Inquiry."

32. For units designed in the 1990s, see Landefeld et al., "Care in a Hospital Medical Unit Especially Designed to Improve Functional Outcomes." For ACE units today, see Barnes et al., "Acute Care for Elders Units."

33. Clark, "If ACE Units Are So Great."

34. In the "Annual Survey" conducted by the American College of Healthcare Executives, the top three issues in 2014 (as reported in January 2015) were financial concerns, health care reform implementation, and government mandates. In 2015 (as

reported in February 2016), the top three concerns were financial, patient safety and quality, and government mandates.

35. Chaudhry et al., "Systematic Review: Impact of Health Information Technology."

36. Cubanski and Neuman, "The Facts on Medicare Spending and Financing."

37. Weiss and Elixhauser, "Overview of Hospital Stays."

38. Centers for Medicare and Medicaid Services, "Eliminating Serious, Preventable, and Costly Medical Errors."

39. Centers for Medicare and Medicaid Services, "Hospital-Acquired Conditions."

40. Lee et al., "Effect of Nonpayment for Preventable Infections." This study examining the effect of nonpayment for preventable infections concluded that the policy did nothing because rates of health care-associated infections had already been falling *before* the policy was instituted in late 2008, and the rate of decline remained unchanged after 2008.

41. Jencks, Williams, and Coleman, "Rehospitalizations among Patients." By ninety days after discharge, 34 percent have been readmitted.

42. MedPAC Report to the Congress, *Reforming the Delivery System.*

43. Rau, "Medicare Fines 2,610 Hospitals."

44. Goodman, Fisher, and Chang, "After Hospitalization."

45. Eisenberg et al., "A Study of the Impact of Meaningful Use."

46. CMS, *Hospital Compare.*

47. Ibid.

48. Agency for Healthcare Research and Quality, "Public Reporting on a Quality Improvement Strategy."

Chapter Eight

1. Devlin, "Einstein Hospital Opens in Bronx."

2. Nabel and Braunwald, "A Tale of Coronary Artery Disease and Myocardial Infarction."

3. Ibid.

4. Cohen, "Critical Questions Regarding Medical Technology."

5. Damadian, "Tumor Detection by Nuclear Magnetic Resonance."

6. Cohen, "Biomedical Innovation and the Development of Medical Technology."

7. Statista, "Density of Magnetic Resonance Imaging."

8. Steiner et al., "Trends and Projections in Hospital Stays."

9. Fuchs et al., "Trends in Severity of Illness."

10. Goffman, *Asylums.* This classic work described "total institutions," including jails, hospitals, and psychiatric facilities, as places that controlled every aspect of the lives of the "inmates."

11. *Mother Jones*, "How Banks Got Too Big."

12. McGee, "The Incredible Consolidating Travel Industry."

13. Robinson, "Consolidation and the Transformation of Competition."

14. Lam, "Health-Care Mergers."

15. Sorkin and Peterson, "Glaxo and SmithKline Form Largest Drug Maker."

16. Sorkin and Wilson, "Pfizer Agrees to Pay $68 Billion for Rival Drug Maker."

17. Sorkin, "Pfizer to Buy Large Drug Rival."

18. Singer, "Merck to Buy Schering-Plough."

19. Gray, ed., *For-Profit Enterprise in Health Care.*

20. Kaiser Family Foundation, "Hospitals by Ownership Type."

21. McCluskey, "Pay Continues to Rise for CEOs of Major Hospitals."

22. Joynt et al., "Compensation of Chief Executive Officers."

23. Sandler, "CEO Pay Soars at Top Not-for-Profits."

24. Goldberg, "New York's Leading Health Systems."

25. Avalere Health, *Trendwatch Chartbook, 2014.*

26. Gaynor and Town, "The Impact of Hospital Consolidation."

27. National Center for Health Statistics, "Utilization of Short-Stay Hospitals: Summary of Non-Medical Statistics, 1967." In 1965, 26 of every 100 older people were hospitalized; in 1967, 29 out of 100 were hospitalized.

28. National Center for Health Statistics, "National Hospital Discharge Survey, 1965–1998."

29. National Center for Health Statistics, "National Hospital Discharge Survey: 2000." In 1967, the average length of stay for patients sixty-five and older was 14.1 days; by 1985, it was down to 8.7 days. Teasing out what changes resulted from the introduction of prospective payment and what changes were due to other factors is difficult, but most authorities agree that DRGs did have a profound effect on hospitals. See Guterman and Dobson, "Impact of the Medicare Prospective Payment System."

30. For the period 1980–98, see Flory et al., "Place of Death," and for the period since 2000, see Teno et al., "Change in End-of-Life Care."

31. Data from the early years are from Davis, "Medicare Hospice Benefit: Early Program Experiences"; the recent data are from MedPAC Report to the Congress, *Medicare Payment Policy* (2015).

32. McCall et al., "Medicare Home Health Benefit."

33. Ibid.

34. Leader and Moon, "Medicare Trends in Ambulatory Surgery."

35. Punke, "Hiring of Non-Physician Providers on the Rise."

36. Wachter and Goldman, "The Hospitalist Movement Five Years Later."

37. Porter, "What Is Value in Health Care?"

38. Tomes, *Remaking the American Patient.*

Chapter Nine

1. Butler, *Why Survive?*

2. Mendelson, *Tender Loving Greed.*

3. Stevenson and Grabowski, "Sizing Up the Market for Assisted Living."

4. MedPAC Report to the Congress, *Medicare Payment Policy* (2015).

5. The five-star rating was the most recent report listed on *Nursing Home Compare* in January 2015, not the date of the actual admission.

6. Social Security Act, Sec. 1862.

7. Recent court cases have overturned the long-standing assumption by SNFs that progress is Medicare's criterion for ongoing coverage. However, this finding is not widely known, nor is it easy to enforce since "benefit" is difficult to define.

8. Office of Inspector General, *Adverse Events in Skilled Nursing Facilities*.

9. Mor et al., "The Revolving Door of Rehospitalization."

10. Ouslander and Berenson, "Reducing Unnecessary Hospitalizations."

11. Ouslander et al., "Potentially Avoidable Hospitalizations."

12. Aragon et al., "Use of the Medicare Post-Hospitalization Skilled Nursing Benefit."

Chapter Ten

1. Thomas, "In Race for Medicare Dollars, Nursing Home Care May Lag."

2. MedPAC Report to the Congress, *Medicare Payment Policy* (2015).

3. Boccuti, Casillas, and Neuman, "Reading the Stars."

4. Centers for Medicare and Medicaid Services, *Nursing Home Data Compendium* (*2013*). For health deficiencies, the difference is 6.3 percent versus 4.8 percent, for deficiencies that result in actual harm or immediate jeopardy to residents it's 17.1 percent versus 14.8 percent, for receipt of a citation for substandard care it's 3.4 percent versus 2.2 percent, for physical restraints it's 6 percent versus 4.2 percent, and for new or worsening pressure ulcers it's 14.2 percent versus 13.1 percent.

5. Comondore et al., "Quality of Care in For-Profit and Not-for-Profit Nursing Homes."

6. This sort of data fluctuates over time. My search was performed in April 2016.

7. Hawes and Phillips, "The Changing Structure of the Nursing Home Industry."

8. Kitchener et al., "Shareholder Value."

9. *Provider Magazine*, "Top 50 Largest Nursing Facility Companies."

10. Lazar, "Complaints Follow Nursing Home Chain's Expansion."

11. *Forbes*, "America's Largest Private Companies."

12. Green, "How Forrest Preston Built Life Care Centers."

13. Ibid.

14. Alexander, "Life Care Founder Becomes Billionaire on Aging Population."

15. Life Care Centers of America, "Mission and Values."

16. Preston, "Letter from the Chairman."

17. *Elyria Magazine and Community Guide, 2015*.

18. The star ratings for Medicare approved nursing homes can be found at "Nursing Home Compare" on the Medicare.gov website, accessed in 2014, https://www.medicare.gov/nursinghomecompare/search.html. The ratings are revised regularly, and these have been replaced by more recent ratings. To find the most recent data for Life Care Center of Elyria, type "Elyria, Ohio" into the space for location and "Life Care" into the space for the name.

19. Tumlinson, "Physician Relationships Hold Key to SNF Success."

20. Weaver, Mathews, and McGinty, "How Medicare Rewards Copious Nursing Home Therapy."

21. Office of the Inspector General, "The Medicare Payment System Needs to Be Reevaluated."

22. Mongan, "Kindred, RehabCare Settle False Claims Allegation for $125 Million."

23. The progress of the lawsuit was reported by the *Chattanooga Times Free Press*, the local newspaper based closest to Life Care's corporate headquarters in Cleveland, Tennessee. Todd South, "Judge Scolds Prosecutors in Whistle-Blower Medicare Fraud Investigation," reported the addition of Preston's name, and Alex Green, "Feds Drop Motion to Add Preston," reported on its withdrawal.

24. Lundstrom and Reese, "Unmasked: Who Owns California's Nursing Homes?" and "California Falls Short."

25. Harrington et al., "Nurse Staffing and Deficiencies in the Largest For-Profit Nursing Home Chains."

26. Duhigg, "At Many Homes, More Profit and Less Nursing." The *Times* reported that 60 percent of homes reduced their nursing staffs. On average, their staffing ratios were then 35 percent below the national average.

27. Stevenson and Grabowski, "Private Equity Investment and Nursing Home Care."

28. Duhigg, "At Many Homes, More Profit."

29. Johnson, "Nursing Facility Sued for Wrongful Death."

30. The Evangelical Lutheran Good Samaritan Society, "Spiritual Well-Being."

31. Comondore et al., "Quality of Care in Nursing Homes."

32. Stone et al., "Evaluation of the Wellspring Model."

33. Pioneer Network, website.

34. Gustke, "Small Residences for the Elderly Provide Personal Care."

35. Samuels, "Building Better Nursing Homes."

36. Mezey, Mitty, and Burger, "Rethinking Teaching Nursing Homes."

37. Evans, Wood, and Lambert, "Patient Injury and Physical Restraint Devices."

38. Shaughnessy et al., "Quality of Care in Teaching Nursing Homes."

39. Schneider, Ory, and Aung, "Teaching Nursing Homes Revisited."

40. Office of the Inspector General, "Adverse Events in Skilled Nursing Facilities."

Chapter Eleven

1. Mitchell et al., "The Clinical Course of Advanced Dementia." In this prospective study of nursing home residents with advanced dementia, the authors found that 55 percent of the residents died within eighteen months; of those who died, 86 percent developed problems with eating.

2. Mitchell, Kiely, and Lipsitz, "The Risk Factors and Impact on Survival of Feeding Tube Placement."

3. Mitchell et al., "Clinical and Organizational Factors Associated with Feeding Tube Use."

4. Mitchell et al., "Tube-Feeding versus Hand-Feeding."

5. Bureau of Labor Statistics, *Occupational Employment and Wages.*

6. National Association of Long Term Care Administrator Boards, "Exam."

7. Indeed.com, Jobs listing for Nursing Home Administrators.

8. LinkedIn, Profile for Walter Johnson.

9. Mitchell et al., "Tube-Feeding versus Hand-Feeding."

10. State Budget Crisis Task Force, "Report, July 31, 2012."

11. Donnelly, "Genesis Health Care to Close," and Clossey, "Coolidge House Nursing Home in Brookline to Close."

12. Bureau of Labor Statistics, *Occupational Employment.*

13. American Health Care Association, "Report of Findings: Nursing Facility Staffing Survey."

14. Ibid.

15. Institute of Medicine, *Retooling for an Aging America.*

16. Paraprofessional Healthcare Institute (PHI), "Nurse Aide Training Requirements."

17. Bureau of Labor Statistics, *Occupational Employment.*

18. Shier et al., "What Does the Evidence Really Say about Culture Change?"

19. Stone et al., "Evaluation of the Wellspring Model."

20. Lopez et al., "The Influence of Nursing Home Culture."

21. MedPAC Report to the Congress, *Medicare Payment Policy (2015).*

22. Office of Inspector General, "The Medicare Payment System for Skilled Nursing Facilities." There are two RUGs, or resource utilization groups, for patients requiring therapy. The RUGs are further subdivided into five categories, with patients in the highest intensity category, "ultra high," requiring 720 minutes a week, and those in the lowest category requiring 45 minutes per week. As discussed in the previous chapter, the Department of Justice has successfully prosecuted nursing home chains for over-billing, collecting $3.75 million from Kindred Healthcare in 2014 (and another $125 million from Kindred in 2016), and $3.5 million from ArchCare, owned and operated by the Catholic Health Care System, in 2015. Cases against two giant chains, HCR ManorCare and Life Care Centers of America, are ongoing.

23. Centers for Medicare and Medicaid Services, "Design for Nursing Home Compare Five-Star Quality Rating System."

24. Office of Inspector General, "Adverse Events in Skilled Nursing Facilities."

25. Mor et al., "The Revolving Door of Rehospitalization."

26. Johnson, "Kindred Seeks to Shake Up Post-Acute Care Continuum."

27. Maher, Hanlon, and Hajjar, "Clinical Consequences of Polypharmacy."

28. Thomas, "J&J to Pay $2.2 Billion."

29. Schenker, "Suit Alleges Abbott Supplier Omnicare Involved in Illegal Kickback Scheme."

30. *Wall Street Journal* Roundup, "Eli Lilly Agrees to Settle."

31. Lueck, "In Nursing Homes, A Drug Middleman Finds Big Profits." This wasn't the first time that Omnicare got in trouble with federal authorities for manipulating

drug prescribing in nursing homes. In 2006, the company settled with forty-two states and the federal government for illegal activities involving medications and long-stay nursing home residents on Medicaid. Interestingly, Omnicare was formed in 1981 from two chemical companies, one of which, W. R. Grace, is perhaps most famous for dumping toxic chemicals into the water supply, poisoning its workers and town residents, as described in *A Civil Action*.

32. Walker, "CVS to Buy Drug Providers."

33. Katz and Karuza, "Nursing Home Physician Specialists."

34. Negative pressure wound therapy involves covering a wound with a sealed dressing and connecting it to a vacuum pump.

35. *Forbes*, "America's Largest Private Companies."

36. Andrews, "GPOs Gaining Ground."

37. Government Accounting Organization, "Group Purchasing Organizations."

38. Lundstrom and Reese, "Unmasked: Who Owns California's Nursing Homes?"

39. Centers for Medicare and Medicaid Services, "FAQs about Billing the Physician Fee Schedule." Contrary to widespread impression, it was possible for physicians to bill for advance care planning prior to the introduction of the new regulation. However, the patient had to be present at the meeting (after the new regulation was instituted, planning meetings could involve physicians and families without the patient), and the note in the medical record had to include comments about the physical examination.

Chapter Twelve

1. Butler, "Geriatrics and Internal Medicine." Ignatz Leo Nascher is sometimes referred to as the father of geriatrics. An Austrian psychiatrist who coined the word "geriatrics," Nascher is credited with recognizing that normal aging is associated with a variety of physiologic changes that physicians need to understand to diagnose and treat accurately. However, he was also very much a creature of his time (1863–1944). In his groundbreaking geriatrics textbook he wrote that "the appearance of the senile individual is repellent both to the esthetic sense and to the sense of independence, that sense of mental attitude that the human race holds toward the self-reliant and self-dependent . . ." (Nascher, *Geriatrics: The Diseases of Old Age and Their Treatment*). Accordingly, I prefer to regard Robert Butler (1927–2010), also a psychiatrist, as the father of modern geriatrics.

2. Gillick, "Long-Term Care Options for the Frail Elderly."

3. Clark et al., "Patient Care in Nursing Homes." This delightfully revealing paper written by members of the pioneering Social Service Department of Massachusetts General Hospital in Boston details both the problems facing MGH and the adequacy—or inadequacy—of the available solutions.

4. U.S. Department of Health, Education, and Welfare, "Institutions for the Aged and Chronically Ill. United States: April–June 1963."

5. U.S. Department of Health, Education, and Welfare, "Nursing and Personal Care Services Received by Residents of Personal Care Homes (1964)."

6. The results of the survey appeared in several separate reports published by the U.S. Department of Health, Education, and Welfare. Information on residents appeared in "Prevalence of Chronic Conditions and Impairments among Residents of Nursing Homes" and "Characteristics of Residents in Institutions for the Aged and Chronically Ill."

7. U.S. Department of Health, Education, and Welfare, "Chronic Illness among Residents of Nursing and Personal Care Homes (1964.)"

8. U.S. Department of Health, Education, and Welfare, "Arrangements for Physician Services to Residents of Nursing and Personal Care Homes (1964)."

9. Ibid.

10. The United States Senate Subcommittee on Problems of the Aged and the Aging conducted its own survey in 1960. See: Edwards and White, "About Nursing Homes."

11. American Health Care Association, *2013 Quality Report*.

12. MedPAC Report to the Congress, *Medicare Payment Policy (2015)*. In 2014, short-stay residents accounted for 22 percent of the facility's revenues.

13. Centers for Medicare and Medicaid Services, *Nursing Home Data Compendium*, 2013 ed. As CMS reports data by type of facility, that means it lumps together short- and long-stay residents for the 96 percent of all SNF dwellers who are in a facility that admits both types. Since the short- and long-stay residents are demographically and medically different, the data I have included stem from the 2 percent of SNF residents who are in a facility that cares exclusively for Medicare short-stay patients. In this population, 28 percent are between 75 and 84 years of age, 45 percent between 85 and 95, and another 9 percent over 95. In terms of physical function, 47 percent have limitations in four ADLs and another 15 percent have five deficits.

14. Massachusetts Executive Office of Health and Human Services, "Regulations (2015)."

15. The SNF data are from MedPAC, *Medicare Payment Policy (2015)*. The hospital discharge data are from Wier, Pfuntner, and Steiner, "Hospital Utilization among Older Adults." For people aged 65–74, 17 percent will go from the hospital to a SNF, for those 75–84, the rate is 29 percent, and for those over 85, it's 44 percent.

16. Hawes and Phillips, "The Changing Structure of the Nursing Home Industry."

17. Assisted Living Foundation of America, website.

18. Redfoot and Pandya, *Before the Boom*.

19. Goldstein/Eagan, "Better than a Nursing Home?"

20. Patten and Fry, "How Millennials Today Compare."

21. Gao, "American Ideal Family Size."

22. Cohn, Morin, and Wang, "Who Moves?"

23. Fry and Passel, "The Growth in Multi-Generational Family Households."

24. Gomory and Sylla, "The American Corporation."

25. Hawes and Phillips, "Changing Structure."

26. Kitchener et al., "Shareholder Value."

27. Oberst, "Dementia Care."

28. Kitchener et al., "Shareholder Value."

29. Ibid.

30. Yahoo Finance, "Genesis Healthcare."

31. Lazar, "Complaints Follow Nursing Home Chain's Expansion."

32. Thomas, "Chain to Pay $38 Million."

33. Thomas, "In Race for Medicare Dollars."

34. Centers for Disease Control, "Lifetime Risk of Symptomatic Osteoarthritis."

35. Cram et al., "Clinical Characteristics and Outcomes of Medicare Patients Undergoing Total Hip Arthroplasty," and Cram et al., "Total Knee Arthroplasty by Volume, Utilization, and Outcomes among Medicare Beneficiaries."

36. Learmonth, Young, and Rorabeck, "The Operation of the Century."

37. Cram et al., "Total Hip Arthroplasty." For total hip replacement patients, mean length of stay went from 9.1 days in 1991 to 3.7 days in 2008, with the percentage of patients going to SNF rising from 17.8 to 34.3 percent.

38. Jackson, "Father of the Modern Hip Replacement."

39. Cram et al., "Total Knee Arthroplasty."

40. Fuchs et al., "Trends in Severity of Illness."

41. Ferrante et al., "Functional Trajectories among Older Persons." Mortality in the ICU ranges from 11 percent for those aged 65–74 to 14.6 percent for those over 85, and the 28-day mortality goes from 20.4 percent to 34.6 percent.

42. Clark et al., "Patient Care."

43. Braunwald, "The Treatment of Acute Myocardial Infarction."

44. Clark et al., "Patient Care."

45. Kozak, Hall, and Owings, "National Hospital Discharge Survey: 2000."

46. Lubitz et al., "Three Decades of Health Care."

47. MedPAC, *Medicare Payment Policy (2015)*.

48. Weiner, Freiman, and Brown, "Nursing Home Quality."

49. This phenomenon was discussed in chapter 10, describing how the for-profit chains game the system to maximize revenue.

50. Office of Inspector General, "The Medicare Payment System."

51. Centers for Medicare and Medicaid Services, "Design for Nursing Home Compare Five-Star Quality Rating System."

52. Barreto-Filho et al., "Trends in Aortic Valve Replacement for Elderly Patients."

Finale

1. Gillick, "The Criteria of Choice in Medical Policy."

2. Rogers, *Diffusion of Innovations.*

3. Cohen, "Diffusion of New Medical Technology."

4. Rockoff, "Goodbye, Lipitor."

5. Greene, *Prescribing by the Numbers.*

6. Rockoff, "Helping Lipitor Live Longer."

7. U.S. Department of Health and Human Services, "NIH Budget Overview."

8. It's very difficult to find out what drug prices were in the past. As of June 2016, the retail cost for Pradaxa (still brand name only) is $378 for a sixty-day supply. The retail cost of a typical 2 mg dose of warfarin is $50 for a sixty-day supply.

9. The drug's manufacturer would later be sued for concealing data: Thomas, "$650 Million to Settle Blood Thinner Lawsuits."

10. Connolly et al., "Dabigatran versus Warfarin."

11. Cohen, "Concerns over Data in Key Dabigatran Trial."

12. Husten, "Boehringer Ingelheim Settles US Pradaxa Litigation for $650 Million."

13. Cohen, "Argon Plasma Coagulation" in *UpToDate*, 2016. Argon plasma coagulation equipment is sold by small- to medium-sized privately held device manufacturers such as Erbe-USA (headquarters in Marietta, Georgia) and US Medical Innovations (headquartered in Takoma Park, Maryland), as well as by the larger, publicly traded company Bovie Medical Corporation (market capitalization $47.5 million as of June 2016).

14. Hollmer, "The Pacemaker inside Me."

15. Ornstein et al., "Dollars for Docs." Thanks to the Affordable Care Act of 2010, drug and device manufacturers are required to report money they pay to physicians and hospitals. The data are available on the CMS website, OpenPaymentsData.CMS.gov.

16. Wenger et al., "The Quality of Medical Care Provided."

17. OECD, "How Does the United States Compare?"

18. Federal Interagency Forum on Aging-Related Statistics, *Older Americans, 2012.*

19. Costa, "Causes of Improving Health and Longevity."

20. One-third of older Medicare enrollees have no more than a single chronic disease—but 32 percent have 2–3 chronic diseases, 23 percent have 4–5, and 14 percent have 6 or more. For those over eighty-five, only 17 percent have a single chronic disease, with 29 percent suffering from 2–3, another 29 percent from 4–5, and 25 percent with 6 or more. In terms of functional limitations, as of 2009, 41.4 percent of older people had some kind of limitation of their daily activities. As to income, 30.4 percent of older adults are considered middle income and 31.4 percent high income as of 2010, with greater levels of poverty among the oldest old. See CMS, *Chronic Conditions among Medicare Beneficiaries.*

21. Gornick et al., "Thirty Years of Medicare."

22. Kaiser Family Foundation, "Medicare Advantage."

23. Technically, the BBA froze the number of slots but not the allocation among specialties. However, with the total fixed, the only way to increase the number of primary care slots was to decrease the number of some other slots—which subspecialist physicians resisted mightily, effectively holding both the number and the distribution of positions constant.

24. Kaufman, *Ordinary Medicine.*

25. Gillick, "Technological Innovations." There is no established cutoff for what constitutes cost-effective care since Medicare doesn't use cost-effectiveness as a criterion for decision making, but between $50,000 and $100,000 is widely considered to be the benchmark for cost-effective care.

26. Statutory change would be required to modify Medicare's mandate, but once that was accomplished, Medicare could design the actual rules and incentives it imposed to graduate medical education programs.

27. Eden, Berwick, and Wilensky, eds., *Graduate Medical Education.*

28. MedPAC Report to the Congress, "Medical Education in the United States."

29. Lynn, *MediCaring Communities.*

30. Dale et al., "Two-Year Costs and Quality in the Comprehensive Primary Care Initiative."

31. Neergaard, "Doctor House Calls Can Save Money."

Bibliography

AARP. "Prescription Drug Use among Midlife and Older Americans." 2005. Accessed July 13, 2012. http://assets.aarp.org/rgcenter/health/rx_midlife_plus.pdf.

Abelson, Reed, and Julie Creswell. "Hospital Chain Inquiry Cited Unnecessary Cardiac Work." *New York Times*, August 6, 2012.

Accenture. "Clinical Transformation: New Business Models for a New Era in Healthcare." September 2012. Accessed February 9, 2016. http://www.mindsailing .com/uploads/1/3/7/8/13788354/accenture-clinical-transformation-new-business -models-for-a-new-era-in-healthcare.pdf.

Ackerman, Roger. "Disaster of the Day: HCA." *Forbes*, December 15, 2000.

Adams, Dan. "Physicians Group Sues Steward over Payments." *Boston Globe*, September 26, 2014.

Agency for Healthcare Research and Quality (AHRQ). "Public Reporting on a Quality Improvement Strategy. Closing the Quality Gap. Revisiting the State of the Science." Evidence Report/Technology Assessment. AHRQ Publication No. 12-E011-EF. July 2012.

Aiken, Linda, Sean Clarke, Douglas Sloane, Julie Sochalski, and Jeffrey Silber. "Hospital Nurse Staffing and Patient Mortality, Nurse Burnout, and Job Dissatisfaction." *Journal of the American Medical Association* 288, no. 16 (2002): 1987–93.

Alexander, Annelise, "Life Care Founder Becomes Billionaire on Aging Population." *Bloomberg Business*, August 7, 2014.

Alexander, G. Caleb, Jacob Kurlander, and Matthew Wynia. "Physicians in Retainer ('Concierge') Practices." *Journal of General Internal Medicine* 20, no. 12 (2005): 1079–83.

Altarum Institute. Health Sector Economic Indicators, September 2012. Accessed October 11, 2014. http://www.altarum.org/files/imce/CSHS-Spending-Brief _Sept%202012.pdf.

Altman, Lawrence. "Dr. Russell [*sic*] Lee, 86, Physician; a Pioneer in Group Practice." *New York Times*, January 29, 1982.

American Academy of Family Physicians, American Academy of Pediatrics, American College of Physicians, American Osteopathic Association. "Guidelines for Patient-Centered Medical Home (PCMH) Recognition and Accreditation Programs." February 2011.

American College of Healthcare Executives. *Annual Survey, 2014*. March/April 2015. https://www.ache.org/pubs/Releases/2015/top-issues-confronting-hospitals-2014 .cfm.

American Health Care Association. *2013 Quality Report*. Accessed December 10, 2015. http://www.ahcancal.org/qualityreport/documents/ahca_2013qr_online.pdf.

———. "Report of Findings: Nursing Facility Staffing Survey, 2010." October 2011. https://www.ahcancal.org/research_data/staffing/Documents/REPORT%20 OF%20FINDINGS%20NURSING%20FACILITY%20STAFFING%20 SURVEY%202010.pdf.

American Hospital Association. *AHA Fast Facts on US Hospitals, 2016.* Accessed March 23, 2017. http://www.aha.org/research/rc/stat-studies/101207fastfacts2016 .pdf.

———. "Economic Contribution of Hospitals Overlooked." *Issue Brief, 2014.* Accessed February 15, 2015. http://www.aha.org/content/11/11econcontrib.pdf.

———. "Trendwatch: Hospitals Develop Commitment to Quality Improvement." October 2012. Accessed October 12, 2015. http://www.aha.org/research/policy /2015.shtml.

American Medical News. "Negotiating Your Productivity Target: The New Payment Structures." August 2, 2010. Accessed June 16, 2016. http://www .amednews.com.

American Society of Health Systems Pharmacists. "ASPH Guidelines on the Pharmacy and Therapeutics Committee and the Formulary System." *American Journal of Health-System Pharmacy* 65 (2008): 1272–83.

Andrews, John. "GPOs Gaining Ground: Using Group Purchasing Organizations to Your Advantage." *McKnight's,* November 1, 2010.

Aragon, Katherine, Kenneth Covinsky, Yinghui Miao, et al. "Use of the Medicare Post-Hospitalization Skilled Nursing Benefit in the Last 6 Months of Life." *Archives of Internal Medicine* 172, no. 26 (2012): 1573–79.

Argentum. Accessed April 24, 2017. https://www.argentum.org/.

Association of American Medical Colleges. "The Changing Gender Composition of US Medical School Applicants and Matriculants." *Analysis in Brief* 12, no. 1 (March 2012). Accessed March 23, 2017. https://www.aamc.org/download/277026 /data/aibvol12_no1.pdf.

———. "Diversity in Medical Education: Facts & Figures 2012." Accessed March 23, 2017. https://members.aamc.org/eweb/upload/Diversity%20in%20Medical%20 Education_Facts%20and%20Figures%202012.pdf.

———. "Medical Student Education: Debt, Costs, and Loan Repayment Fact Card." October 2015. Accessed March 23, 2017. https://members.aamc.org/eweb/upload /2015%20Debt%20Fact%20Card.pdf.

———. "2014 Physician Specialty Data Book." Accessed March 27, 2017. https://www .aamc.org/download/473260/data/2014physicianspecialtydatabook.pdf.

Auerbach, David, William Weeks, and Ian Brantley. "Health Care Spending and Efficiency in the U.S. Department of Veterans Affairs." Santa Monica, CA: RAND Corporation, 2013. Accessed June 21, 2016. http://www.rand.org/pubs/research _reports/RR285.html.

Avalere Health for the American Hospital Association. *Trendwatch Chartbook, 2014.* Accessed June 24, 2016. http://www.aha.org/research/reports/tw/chartbook /2014/14chartbook.pdf.

Baghai, Ramin, Edward Levine, and Saumya Sutaria. "Service-Line Strategies for US Hospitals." *McKinsey Quarterly*, July 2008, 1–9.

Balfe, Bruce. "A Survey of Group Practice in the United States, 1965." *Public Health Reports*, no. 84 (1969): 597–603.

Banner Estrella Medical Center. "Our Mission, Values, Vision and Brand." Accessed June 21, 2016. https://www.bannerhealth.com/Locations/Arizona /Banner+Estrella+Medical+Center/About+Us/Mission+Vision+Values.htm.

Barber, Felix, and Michael Goold. "The Strategic Secret of Private Equity." *Harvard Business Review*, September 2007.

Barnes, Deborah, Robert Palmer, Denise Kresevic, et al. "Acute Care for Elders Units Produced Shorter Hospital Stays at Lower Cost While Maintaining Patients' Functional Status." *Health Affairs* 31, no. 6 (2012): 1227–36.

Barnett, Michael, John Hsu, and Michael McWilliams. "Patient Characteristics and Differences in Hospital Remission Rates." *JAMA Internal Medicine* 175, no. 11 (2015): 1803–12.

Barnett, Michael, Zirui Song, and Bruce Landon. "Trends in Physician Referrals in the United States, 1999–2009." *Archives of Internal Medicine* 172, no. 2 (2012): 163–70.

Barreto-Filho, José, Yun Wang, John Dodson, et al. "Trends in Aortic Valve Replacement for Elderly Patients in the United States, 1999–2011." *Journal of the American Medical Association* 310, no. 19 (2013): 2078–84.

Beyer, Gabrielle, David O'Riordan, Kathleen Kerr, and Steven Pantilat. "Prevalence and Characteristics of Outpatient Palliative Care Services in California." *Archives of Internal Medicine* 171, no. 22 (2011): 2057–59.

Bicknell, William and Diana Walsh. "Certificate-of-Need: the Massachusetts Experience." *New England Journal of Medicine* 292 (1975): 1054–61.

Blesch, Gregg. "Baptist Health South Florida to Pay $7.8 Million Settlement." *Modern Healthcare*, May 12, 2008.

Boccuti, Cristina, Giselle Casillas, and Tricia Neuman. "Reading the Stars: Nursing Home Quality Star Ratings, Nationally and by State." Kaiser Family Foundation Issue Brief. May 2015.

Boult, Chad, Lisa Boult, Lynne Morishita, et al. "A Randomized Controlled Trial of Outpatient Geriatric Evaluation and Management." *Journal of the American Geriatric Society*, no. 49, no. 4 (2001): 351–59.

Boult, Chad, Bruce Leff, Cynthia Boyd, et al. "A Matched-Pair Cluster-Randomized Trial of Guided Care for High-Risk Older Patients." *Journal of General Internal Medicine* 28, no. 5 (2013): 612–21.

Boult, Chad, Lisa Rieder, Bruce Leff, et al. "The Effect of Guided Care Teams on the Use of Health Services: Results from a Cluster-Randomized Controlled Trial." *Archives of Internal Medicine* 171, no. 5 (2011): 460–66.

Boult, Chad, and G. Darryl Wieland. "Comprehensive Primary Care for Older Patients with Multiple Chronic Conditions." *Journal of the American Medical Association* 304, no. 17 (2010): 1936–40.

Bozic, Kevin, Steven Kurtz, Edmund Lau, et al. "The Epidemiology of Bearing Surface Usage in Total Hip Arthroplasty in the United States." *Journal of Bone and Joint Surgeons of America* 91, no. 7 (2009): 1614–20.

Braunwald, Eugene. "The Treatment of Acute Myocardial Infarction: The Past, the Present, and the Future." *European Heart Journal: Acute Cardiovascular Care* 1, no. 1 (2012): 9–12.

Brennan, Troyen. "Luxury Primary Care: Market Innovation or Threat to Access?" *New England Journal of Medicine* 346, no. 15 (2002): 1165–68.

Brown, Harriet. *Body of Truth: How Science, History, and Culture Drive Our Obsession with Weight and What We Can Do about It.* Boston: Da Capo Press, 2015.

Bureau of Labor Statistics. *CPI Inflation Calculator.* Accessed January 7, 2016. http://www.bls.gov/data/inflation_calculator.htm.

———. *Occupational Employment and Wages.* May 2014. Accessed July 6, 2015. http://www.bls.gov/ooh/management/medical-and-health-services-managers.htm.

Butler, Robert. "Geriatrics and Internal Medicine." *Annals of Internal Medicine* 91, no. 6 (1979): 903–8.

———. *Why Survive? Being Old in America.* New York: Harper and Row, 1975.

Bynum, Julie, Ellen Meara, Chiang-Hua Chang, and Jared Rhoads. "Our Parents, Ourselves: Health Care for an Aging Population: A Report of the Dartmouth Atlas Project." February 17, 2016. http://www.dartmouthatlas.org/downloads/reports/Our_Parents_Ourselves_021716.pdf.

Carreyrou, John. "Lab Reaches Tentative Deal with Government over Doctor Payment." *Wall Street Journal,* March 23, 2015.

Carreyrou, John, and Tom McGinty. "A Fast-Growing Medical Lab Tests Anti-Kickback Law." *Wall Street Journal,* September 8, 2014.

Carreyrou, John, and Maurice Tamm. "A Device to Kill Cancer, Lift Revenue." *Wall Street Journal.* December 7, 2010.

Carrier, Emily, Marisa Dowling, and Robert Berenson. "Hospitals' Geographic Expansion in Quest of Well-Insured Patients: Will the Outcome Be Better Care, More Cost, or Both?" *Health Affairs* 31, no. 4 (2012): 827–35.

Centers for Disease Control. "Lifetime Risk of Symptomatic Osteoarthritis, 2010–2012." Accessed July 19, 2016. http://www.cdc.gov/arthritis/data_statistics/arthritis-related-stats.htm.

———. "National Ambulatory Medical Care Survey: 2012 State and National Summary Tables." Accessed July 26, 2016. https://www.cdc.gov/nchs/data/ahcd/namcs_summary/2012_namcs_web_tables.pdf.

Centers for Medicare and Medicaid Services. "Accountable Care Organizations." Accessed March 15, 2016. https://www.cms.gov/Medicare/Medicare-Fee-for ServicePayment/ACO/index.html?redirect=/Aco/.

———. *Chronic Conditions among Medicare Beneficiaries. Chartbook, 2012 Edition.* Baltimore, 2012.

———. "Design for Nursing Home Compare Five-Star Quality Rating System. Technical Users Guide." Accessed August 25, 2016. http://www.medicare.gov /NursingHomeCompare/About/Ratings.html.

———. "Eliminating Serious, Preventable, and Costly Medical Errors—Never Events." May 18, 2006. Accessed December 10, 2015. https://www.cms.gov /Newsroom/MediaReleaseDatabase/Fact-Sheets/2006-Fact-Sheets-Items/2006 -05-18.html.

———. "Frequently Asked Questions about Billing the Physician Fee Schedule for Advance Care Planning Services." July 16, 2016. Accessed August 2, 2016. https://www .cms.gov/Medicare/Medicare-Fee-for-Service-Payment/PhysicianFeeSched/ Downloads/FAQ-Advance-Care-Planning.pdf.

———. *Hospital Compare*. Accessed December 24, 2014. https://www.medicare.gov /hospitalcompare/search.html.

———. "Hospital-Acquired Conditions." Accessed March 8, 2016. https://www .cms.gov/medicare/medicare-fee-for-service-payment/hospitalacqcond/hospital -acquired_conditions.html.

———. "Medicare Final CY 2015 Physician Fee Schedule." Accessed July 16, 2016. https://www.cms.gov/Medicare/Medicare-Fee-for-Service-Payment/ PhysicianFeeSched/PFS-Federal-Regulation-Notices-Items/CMS-1612-FC.html.

———. *Nursing Home Data Compendium*. 2013 ed. Accessed April 24, 2017. https://www .cms.gov/medicare/provider-enrollment-and-certification /certificationandcomplianc/downloads/nursinghomedatacompendium_508.pdf.

———. "New Hospitals and Health Care Providers Join Successful Cutting-Edge Federal Initiative that Cuts Costs and Puts Patients at the Center of their Care." CMS Press Release. Accessed April 29, 2016. https://www.hhs.gov.

Chaudhry, Basti, Jerome Wang, Shinyi Wu, et al. "Systematic Review: Impact of Health Information Technology on Quality, Efficiency, and Costs of Medical Care." *Annals of Internal Medicine* 144, no. 10 (2006): 742–52.

Chay, Kenneth, Daeho Kim, and Shailender Swaminathan. "Medicare Hospital Utilization and Mortality: Evidence from the Program's Origins." 2010. Accessed July 26, 2016. http://www8.gsb.columbia.edu/rtfiles/finance/Applied%20 Microeconomics/Fall%202009/Kenneth%20Chay.pdf.

Cherry, Donald, Christine Lucas, and Sandra Decker. "Population Aging and the Use of Office-Based Physician Services." NCHS Data Brief #41, August 2010. http://www .medicare.gov/hospitalcompare/About/Hospital-Info.html.

Clark, Cheryl. "If ACE Units Are So Great, Why Aren't They Everywhere?" *HealthLeaders Media*, April 25, 2013.

Clark, Eleanor, Suzanne Deutsche, Fred Frankel, et al. "Patient Care in Nursing Homes: A Look at Responsibility." *Journal of the American Medical Association* 200, no. 20 (1967): 144–47.

Clossey, Erin. "Coolidge House Nursing Home in Brookline to Close by End of Year." *Wicked Local Brookline*, October 14, 2014.

Cohen, Alan. "Biomedical Innovation and the Development of Medical Technology." In *Technology in American Health Care*, edited by Alan Cohen and Ruth Hanft, 45–78. Ann Arbor: University of Michigan Press, 2004.

———. "Critical Questions Regarding Medical Technology and its Effects." In *Technology in American Health Care*, edited by Alan Cohen and Ruth Hanft, 15–42. Ann Arbor: University of Michigan Press, 2004.

———. "Diffusion of New Medical Technology." In *Technology in American Health Care*, edited by Alan Cohen and Ruth Hanft, 79–104. Ann Arbor: University of Michigan Press, 2004.

Cohen, Deborah. "Concerns over Data in Key Dabigatran Trial." *BMJ*, no. 349 (2004): g4747.

Cohen, Harvey, John Feussman, Morris Weinberger, et al. "A Controlled Trial of Inpatient and Outpatient Geriatric Evaluation and Management." *New England Journal of Medicine* 346, no. 12 (2002): 905–12.

Cohen, Jonathan. "Argon Plasma Coagulation in the Management of Gastrointestinal Hemorrhage." *UpToDate*. Accessed June 29, 2016. http://www.uptodate.com.

Cohn, D'vera, Rich Morin, and Wendy Wang. "Who Moves? Who Stays Put? Where's Home?" Pew Research Center: A Social and Demographic Trends Report. December 17, 2008. http://www.pewsocialtrends.org/files/2010/10/Movers-and-Stayers.pdf.

Coleman, Eric, Carla Parry, Sandra Chalmers, and Sung-Joon Min. "The Care Transitions Intervention: Results of a Randomized Controlled Trial." *Archives of Internal Medicine* 166, no. 17 (2006): 1822–28.

Coleman, Matt. "Infection Rates Would Cut Hospitals' Bottom Lines." *Jacksonville Business Journal*, June 24, 2011.

Comondore, Vikram, P. J. Devereaux, Qi Zhou, et al. "Quality of Care in For-Profit and Not-for-Profit Nursing Homes. Systematic Review and Meta-Analysis." *BMJ*, no. 339 (2009): b2732.

Congressional Budget Office's April 2014 Medicare Baseline. April 2014. Accessed April 24, 2017. https://www.cbo.gov/sites/default/files/recurringdata/51302-2014-04-medicare.pdf.

Connolly, Stuart, Michael Ezekowitz, Salim Yusuf, et al. "Dabigatran versus Warfarin in Patients with Atrial Fibrillation." *New England Journal of Medicine* 361, no. 12 (2009): 1139–51.

Costa, Dora. "Causes of Improving Health and Longevity at Older Ages: A Review of the Explanations." *Genus* 61, no. 1 (2005): 21–38.

Counsell, Steven, Christopher Callahan, Daniel Clark, et al. "Geriatric Care Management for Low-Income Seniors: A Randomized Controlled Trial." *Journal of the American Medical Association* 298, no. 22 (2007): 2623–33.

Covinsky, Kenneth, Edgar Pierluissi, and C. Bree Johnston. "Hospitalization-Associated Disability." *Journal of the American Medical Association* 306, no. 16 (2011): 1782–93.

Cram, Peter, Xin Lu, Peter Kaboli, et al. "Clinical Characteristics and Outcomes of Medicare Patients Undergoing Total Hip Arthroplasty, 1991–2008." *Journal of the American Medical Association* 305, no. 15 (2011): 1560–67.

Cram, Peter, Xin Lu, Stephen L. Kates, et al. "Total Knee Arthroplasty by Volume, Utilization, and Outcomes among Medicare Beneficiaries, 1991–2010." *Journal of the American Medical Association* 308, no. 12 (2012): 1227–36.

Creditor, Morton. "Hazards of Hospitalization of the Elderly." *Annals of Internal Medicine* 118, no. 3 (1993): 219–23.

Creswell, Julie, and Reed Abelson. "A Giant Hospital Chain Is Blazing a Profit Trail." *New York Times*, August 14, 2012.

Cubanski, Juliette, and Tricia Neuman." The Facts on Medicare Spending and Financing." Kaiser Family Foundation, Issue Brief. July 2016.

Dafny, Leemore. "Hospital Industry Consolidation—Still More to Come." *New England Journal of Medicine* 370, no. 3 (2014): 198–99.

Dale, Stacy, Arkadipta Ghosh, Deborah Perlies, et al. "Two-Year Costs and Quality in the Comprehensive Primary Care Initiative." *New England Journal of Medicine* 376, no. 24 (2016): 2345–56.

Damadian, Raymond. "Tumor Detection by Nuclear Magnetic Resonance." *Science* 171, no. 3976 (1971): 1151–53.

The Dartmouth Atlas of Health Care. 2015. Accessed November 17, 2015. http://www .dartmouthatlas.org/data/table.aspx?ind=23&loct=2&tf=34&fmt=45&ch=1.

Davis, Feather. "Medicare Hospice Benefit: Early Program Experiences." *Health Care Financing Review* 9, no. 4 (1988): 98–111.

De Jonge, K. Eric, Namirah Jamshed, Daniel Gilden, Joanna Kubisiak, and Stephanie Bruce, Center for Workforce Studies. "Physician Specialty Data Book." November 2012.

De Jonge, K. Eric, Namirah Jamshed, Daniel Gilden, et al. "Effects of Home-Based Primary Care on Medicare Costs in High-Risk Elders." *Journal of the American Geriatrics Society* 62, no. 10 (2014): 1825–31.

DePuy Orthopaedics. 2013. Accessed January 2, 2013. http://www.depuy.com/about -depuy/depuy-divisions/depuy-orthopaedics/find surgeon/192.

DeVita, Vincent, and Edward Chu. "A History of Cancer Chemotherapy." *Cancer Research* 68, no. 21 (2008): 8643–53.

Devlin, John. "Einstein Hospital Opens in Bronx." *New York Times*, January 4, 1966.

The Diabetes Control and Complication Trial Research Group. "The Effect of Intensive Treatment of Diabetes on the Development of Long-Term Complications of Insulin-Dependent Diabetes Mellitus." *New England Journal of Medicine* 329, no. 14 (1993): 683–89.

Docteur, Elizabeth, and Robert A. Berenson. "How Does the Quality of US Health Care Compare Internationally?" Robert Wood Johnson Foundation and the Urban Institute, *Timely Analysis of Immediate Health Policy Issues*, August 2009. http://www .rwjf.org/content/dam/web-assets/2009/08/how-does-the-quality-of-u-s— health-care-compare-internationally.

Donnelly, Julie. "Genesis Health Care to Close 4th Massachusetts Nursing Home, Prompting Union Protest." *Boston Business Journal,* March 19, 2014.

———. "Steward Health Care: Layoffs Are Needed to Reduce Costs in Health Care Industry." *Boston Business Journal,* November 12, 2013.

Donohue, Julie. "A History of Drug Advertising: The Evolving Roles of Consumers and Consumer Protection." *Milbank Quarterly* 84, no. 4 (2006): 659–96.

Doyle, Cathal, Laura Lennox, and Derek Bell. "A Systematic Review of Evidence on the Links between Patient Experience and Clinical Safety and Effectiveness." *BMJ Open,* no. 3 (2013): e001570.

Duhigg, Charles. "At Many Homes, More Profit and Less Nursing." *New York Times,* September 23, 2007.

Dunn, Lindsey, and Scott Becker. "50 Things to Know about the Hospital Industry." *Becker's Hospital Review,* July 23, 2013.

Earle, Craig, Mary Beth Landrum, Jeffrey Souza, et al. "Aggressiveness of Cancer Care Near the End of Life: Is It a Quality-of-Care Issue?" *Journal of Clinical Oncology* 26, no. 23 (2008): 3860–66.

Eden, Joel, Donald Berwick, and Gail Wilensky, eds. *Graduate Medical Education That Meets the Nation's Health Needs.* Washington, DC: National Academies Press, 2014.

Edwards, Charles, and Raymond White. "About Nursing Homes." *Journal of the American Medical Association* 189, no. 2 (1964): 161–63.

Eggleston, Karen, Yu-Chu Shen, Joseph Lau, Chistopher Schmid, and Jia Chai. "Hospital Ownership and Quality of Care: What Explains the Different Results in the Literature?" *Health Economics* 17, no. 12 (2008): 1345–62.

Eisenberg, Floyd, Caterina Lasome, Annel Advani, et al. "A Study of the Impact of Meaningful Use Clinical Quality Measures." American Hospital Association, 2013. Accessed June 23, 2016. https://www.aha.org/content/13/13ehrchallenges-report-pdf.

Elyria Magazine and Community Guide, 2015. Accessed January 4, 2016. http://issuu .com/imagebuilders/docs/elyria15_low-res?e=10275665%2F9937130.

Ethgen, Olivier, Olivier Bruyère, Florent Richy, Charles Dardennes, and Jean-Yves Reginster. "Health Related Quality of Life in Total Hip and Total Knee Arthroplasty. A Qualitative and Systematic Review of the Literature." *Journal of Bone and Joint Surgery* 86-A, no. 5 (2004): 963–74.

The Evangelical Lutheran Good Samaritan Society. "Spiritual Well-Being." Accessed June 28, 2016. https://www.good-sam.com/about/ministry.

Evans, David, Jacquelin Wood, and Leonnie Lambert. "Patient Injury and Physical Restraint Devices: A Systematic Review." *Journal of Advanced Nursing* 41, no. 3 (2003): 274–82.

Evans, Melanie. "Juggling the Lineup." *Modern Healthcare,* January 14, 2012.

Federal Interagency Forum on Aging-Related Statistics. *Older Americans, 2012: Key Indicators of Well-Being.* Accessed June 29, 2016. http://www.agingstats.gov /agingstatsdotnet/Main_Site/Data/2012_Documents/Docs/EntireChartbook .pdf.

Ferrante, Lauren, Margaret Pisani, Terence Murphy, et al. "Functional Trajectories among Older Persons before and after Critical Illness." *JAMA Internal Medicine* 175, no. 4 (2015): 523–29.

Fisher, Elliott, David Wennberg, Therese Stukel, et al. "The Implications of Regional Variation in Medicare Spending. Part 2: Health Outcomes and Satisfaction with Care." *Annals of Internal Medicine* 138, no. 4 (2003): 288–98.

Fishman, Paul, Eric Johnson, Kathryn Coleman, et al. "Impact on Seniors of the Patient-Centered Medical Home: Evidence from a Pilot Study." *Gerontologist* 52, no. 5 (2012): 703–11.

Flory, James, Yinong Young-Xu, Ipek Gurol, et al. "Place of Death: US Trends since 1980." *Health Affairs* 23, no. 3 (2004): 194–200.

Forbes. "America's Largest Private Companies, 2015." Accessed June 26, 2016. http://www.forbes.com/largest-private-companies/list/2/#tab:rank.

Frack, Bill, and Nurry Hong. "Physician Practice Management: A New Chapter." *Becker's Hospital Review*, February 19, 2014.

Friedberg, Mark, Kristin Van Busun, Peggy Chen, et al. "Factors Affecting Physician Professional Satisfaction and Their Implications for Patient Care, Health Systems, and Health Policy." RAND. 2013. http://www.rand.org/pubs/research_reports/RR439.html.

Fry, Richard, and Jeffrey Passel. "The Growth in Multi-Generational Family Households." Pew Research Center: A Social and Demographic Trends Report. July 17, 2014. http://www.pewsocialtrends.org/2014/07/17/the-growth-in-multi-generational-family-households/.

Frydman, Carola, and Dirk Jenter. "CEO Compensation." *Annual Review of Financial Economics* 2, no. 1 (2010): 75–102.

Fuchs, Lior, Victor Novack, Stuart McLennan, et al. "Trends in Severity of Illness on ICU Admission and Mortality among the Elderly." *PLoS One*, no. 9 (2014): e93234.

Fye, W. Bruce. "The Origins and Evolution of the Mayo Clinic from 1864 to 1939: A Minnesota Family Practice Becomes an International 'Medical Mecca.'" *Bulletin of the History of Medicine* 84, no. 3 (2010): 323–57.

Gamble, Molly. "15 Things to Know about the Deal between Partners HealthCare, Massachusetts AG Martha Coakley." *Becker's Hospital Review*, July 18, 2014.

Gao, George. "American Ideal Family Size is Smaller than It Used to Be." Pew Research Center. May 8, 2015. http://www.pewresearch.org/fact-tank/2015/05/08/ideal-size-of-the-american-family/.

Gaynor, Martin, and Robert Town. "The Impact of Hospital Consolidation-Update." Robert Wood Johnson Foundation. *Synthesis Project.* June 2012. http://www.rwjf.org/content/dam/farm/reports/issue_briefs/2012/rwjf73261.

Gerteis, Margaret, Susan Edgman-Levitan, Jennifer Daley, and Thomas Delbanco. *Through the Patient's Eyes: Understanding and Promoting Patient-Centered Care.* San Francisco: Jossey-Bass, 1993.

Gillespie, Cathleen, and Kimberly Hurvitz. "Prevalence of Hypertension and Controlled Hypertension-United States, 2007–2010." *Morbidity and Mortality Weekly Report* 62, no. 3 (2013): 144–48.

Gillick, Muriel. "The Criteria of Choice in Medical Policy: Radiotherapy in Massachusetts." *Minerva* 15, no. 1 (1977): 15–31.

———. "How Medicare Shapes the Way We Die." *Journal of Health and Biomedical Law*, no. 7 (2012): 27–55.

———. "Long-Term Care Options for the Frail Elderly." *Journal of the American Geriatric Society* 37, no. 12 (1989): 1198–1203.

———. "Medicine as Ecoculture." *Annals of Internal Medicine* 151, no. 8 (2009): 577–80.

———. "Technological Innovations: Time for New Criteria?" *New England Journal of Medicine* 350, no. 21 (2004): 2199–2203.

Gillick, Muriel, Nancy Serrell, and Laurence Gillick. "Adverse Consequences of Hospitalization in the Elderly." *Social Science and Medicine* 16, no. 10 (1982): 1033–38.

Goffman, Erving. *Asylums: Essays on the Social Situation of Mental Patients and Other Inmates.* New York: Doubleday Anchor Books, 1961.

Gold, Jenny. "Proton Beam Therapy Heats Up Hospital Arms Race." *Kaiser Health News*, May 31, 2013.

Goldberg, Dan. "New York's Leading Health Systems Differ on Growth Strategy." *Politico*, February 9, 2015.

Goldstein/Eagan, Andrew. "Better than a Nursing Home?" *Time*, August 5, 2001.

Gomory, Ralph, and Richard Sylla. "The American Corporation." *Daedalus* 142, no. 2 (2013): 102–18.

Goodman, David, Amos Esty, Elliott Fisher, and Chiang-Hua Chang. "Trends and Variation in End-of-Life Care for Medicare Beneficiaries with Severe Chronic Illness: A Report of the Dartmouth Atlas Project." April 2011. Accessed March 27, 2017. http://www.dartmouthatlas.org/downloads/reports/EOL_Trend_Report _0411.pdf.

Goodman, David, Elliott Fisher, and Chiang-Hua Chang. Dartmouth Atlas Project. "After Hospitalization: A Dartmouth Atlas Report on Readmissions among Medicare Beneficiaries." Robert Wood Johnson. February 2013.

Goodman, David, Nancy Morden, Chiang-Hua Chang, Elliott Fisher, and John Wennberg. "Trends in Cancer Care near the End of Life: A Dartmouth Atlas of Health Care Brief." September 2013. Accessed March 27, 2017. http://www .dartmouthatlas.org/downloads/reports/Cancer_brief_090413.pdf.

Gorina, Yelena, Laura Pratt, Ellen Kramarow, and Nazik Elgaddal. "Hospitalization, Readmission, and Death Experience of Noninstitutionalized Medicare Fee-for-Service Beneficiaries Aged 65 and Older." National Health Statistics Reports 2015, #84.

Gorman, Anna. "Cedars-Sinai to Cut Most Psychiatric Services." *Los Angeles Times*, December 1, 2011.

Gornick, Marian, Joan Warner, Paul Eggers, et al. "Thirty Years of Medicare: Impact on the Covered Population." *Health Care Financing Review* 18, no. 2 (1996): 179–237.

Government Accounting Organization. "Group Purchasing Organizations: Funding Structure Has Potential Implications for Medicare Costs." GAO-15-3. October 24, 2014.

Gray, Bradford H., ed. *For-Profit Enterprise in Health Care*. Washington, DC: National Academy Press, 1986.

Grayson, Martha, Dale Newton, and Lori Thompson. "Payback Time: The Association of Debt and Income with Medical Student Career Choice." *Medical Education* 46, no. 10 (2012): 983–91.

Green, Alex. "Feds Drop Motion to Add Preston to Suit against Life Care Centers." *Chattanooga Times Free Press*, November 12, 2015.

———. "How Forrest Preston Built Life Care Centers into the Biggest Privately Held Company in the Industry." *Chattanooga Times Free Press*, April 27, 2015.

Greene, Jeremy. *Prescribing by the Numbers*. Baltimore: Johns Hopkins University Press, 2006.

Groves, Nancy. "Changing Demographics of Women in Medicine." *Ophthalmology Times*, February 2008.

Gu, Qiuping, Charles Dillon, and Vicki Burt. "Prescription Drug Use Continues to Increase. US Prescription Drug Data for 2007–2008." NCHS Data Brief #42, September 2010.

Gustke, Constance. "Small Residences for the Elderly Provide More Personal, Homelike Care." *New York Times*, November 20, 2015.

Guterman, Stuart, and Allen Dobson. "Impact of the Medicare Prospective Payment System for Hospitals." *Health Care Financing Review* 7, no. 3 (1986): 97–114.

Hajjar, Emily, Joseph Hanlon, Richard Sloane, et al. "Unnecessary Drug Use in Frail Older People at Hospital Discharge." *Journal of the American Geriatrics Society* 53, no. 9 (2005): 1518–23.

Hall, Margaret, Carol DeFrances, Sonja Williams, Aleksandr Golosinskiy, and Alexander Schwartzman. "National Hospital Discharge Survey, 2007." National Health Statistics Reports #29, October 2010.

Hall, Margaret, Shaleah Levant, and Carol DeFrances. "Hospitalization for Congestive Heart Failure: United States, 2000–2010." NCHS Data Brief #108, October 2012.

Halpern, Jake. "The Incredible, Perilous, Money-Making, People-Shrinking Machine." *Boston Magazine*, October 2005.

Hanover, Judy. "Business Strategy: The Current State of Ambulatory EHR Buyer Satisfaction." *IDC Health Insights: Healthcare Provider IT Strategies* #HI244027, November 2013. Accessed March 27, 2017. https://www.meddatagroup.com/wp-content/uploads/Final-IDC-Report-Ambulatory-EHR.pdf.

Hargrave, Elizabeth, Laura Summer, Jack Hoadley, Ayesha Mahmud, and Kate Quirk. "Retainer-Based Physicians: Characteristics, Impact, and Policy Considerations." MedPAC No. 10-9, October 2010. Accessed March 7, 2016. http://www.medpac.gov/documents/contractor-reports/Oct10_RetainerBasedPhysicians_CONTRACTOR_CB.pdf.

Harrington, Charlene, Brian Olney, Helen Carrillo, and Taewoon Kang. "Nurse Staffing and Deficiencies in the Largest For-Profit Nursing Home Chains and Chains Owned by Private Equity Companies." *Health Services Research* 47, no. 1 (2012): 106–28.

Hawes, Catherine, and Charles D. Phillips. "The Changing Structure of the Nursing Home Industry and the Impact of Ownership on Quality, Cost, and Access." In *For-Profit Enterprise in Health Care*, edited by Bradford H. Gray, 492–542. Washington, DC: National Academy Press, 1986.

Healthcare Cost and Utilization Project. "Bedsize of Hospitals." Accessed June 21, 2016. https://www.hcup-us.ahrq.gov/db/vars/h_bedsz/nisnote.jsp.

Hinami, Keiki, Chad Whelan, Robert Wolosin, Joseph Miller, and Tosha Wetterneck. "Worklife and Satisfaction of Hospitalists: Toward Flourishing Career." *Journal of General Internal Medicine* 27, no. 1 (2012): 28–36.

Hollmer, Mark. "The Pacemaker inside Me: What I Learned about the Industry as a Cardiac Patient." *FierceMedicalDevices*, February 4, 2014.

Horwitz, Jill R. "Making Profits and Providing Care: Comparing Nonprofit, For-Profit, and Government Hospitals." *Health Affairs* 24, no. 3 (2005): 790–801.

Hsiao, Chun-Ju, Donald Cherry, Paul Beatty, and Elizabeth Rechtsteiner. "National Ambulatory Medical Care Survey, 2007 Summary." *National Health Statistics Report*, no. 27 (2010): 1–32.

Husten, Larry. "Boehringer Ingelheim Settles US Pradaxa Litigation for $650 Million." *Forbes*, May 28, 2014.

IMS Institute for Healthcare Information. "Medicines Use and Spending Shifts: A Review of the Use of Medicines in the US in 2014." April 2015. https://www.imshealth.com/files/web/IMSH%20Institute/Reports/Medicines_Use_and_Spending_Shifts/Medicine-Spending-and-Growth_1995-2014.pdf.

Inouye, Sharon. "Delirium in Older Persons." *New England Journal of Medicine* 354, no. 11 (2006):1157–65.

Inouye, Sharon, Stephanie Studenski, Mary Tinetti, and George Kuchel. "Geriatric Syndromes: Clinical, Research and Policy Implications of a Core Geriatric Concept." *Journal of the American Geriatrics Society* 55, no. 5 (2007): 780–91.

Institute of Medicine. *Conflict of Interest in Medical Research, Education, and Practice.* Washington, DC: National Academies Press, 2009.

———. *Medical Devices and the Public's Health: the FDA 510(k) Clearance Process at 35.* Washington, DC: National Academies Press, 2011.

———. *Retooling for an Aging America: Building the Health Care Workforce.* Washington, DC: National Academies Press, 2008.

Integrated Health Care Association. "Orthopedics Data Compendium: Use, Cost, and Market Structure for Total Joint Replacement." August 2006. Accessed December 10, 2015. http://www.iha.org/pdfs_documents/medical_device/07_OrthopedicsDataCompendium.pdf.

Jackson, John. "Father of the Modern Hip Replacement: Professor Sir John Charnley (1911–1982). *Journal of Medical Biography* 19, no. 4 (2011): 151–56.

Jencks, Stephen, Mark Williams, and Eric Coleman. "Rehospitalizations among Patients in the Medicare Fee-for-Service Program." *New England Journal of Medicine* 360, no. 14 (2009): 1418–28.

Jha, Ashish, Jonathan Perlin, Kenneth Kizer, and R. Adams Dudley. "Effect of the Transformation of the Veterans Affairs Health Care System on the Quality of Care." *New England Journal of Medicine* 348, no. 22 (2003): 2218–27.

John Hartford Foundation. "A Brief History of Geriatrics." Accessed November 23, 2015. http://www.jhartfound.org/ar2005/2_a_brief_history.html.

Johnson, Shea. "Nursing Facility Sued for Wrongful Death." *The Daily Press (Victor Valley)*, August 4, 2015.

Johnson, Steven. "Kindred Seeks to Shake Up Post-Acute Care Continuum." *Modern Healthcare*, January 11, 2014.

Joynt, Karen, Sidney Le, E. John Orav, and Ashish Jha. "Compensation of Chief Executive Officers at Nonprofit US Hospitals." *JAMA Internal Medicine* 174, no. 1 (2014): 61–67.

Joynt, Karen, E. John Orav, and Ashish Jha. "Association between Hospital Conversion to For-Profit Status and Clinical and Economic Outcomes." *Journal of the American Medical Association* 312, no. 16 (2014): 1644–52.

Juo, Yen-Yi, Omar Hyder, Adil Haider, Melissa Camp, Anne Lidor, and Nita Ahuia. "Is Minimally Invasive Colon Resection Better than Traditional Approaches?" *JAMA Surgery* 149, no. 2 (2014): 177–84.

Kaiser Family Foundation. "Hospitals by Ownership Type." Accessed December 10, 2015. http://kff.org/other/state-indicator/hospitals-by-ownership/.

———. "Medicare Advantage." June 2015. http://kff.org/medicare/fact-sheet/medicare-advantage/.

———. "State Health Facts: Distribution of Medical School Graduates by Gender. June 2015. Accessed July 26, 2016. http://kff.org/other/state-indicator/medical-school-graduates-by-gender/.

———. "State Health Facts: Distribution of Medical School Graduates by Race/Ethnicity." Accessed April 13, 2016. http://kff.org/other/state-indicator/distribution-by-race-ethnicity/.

Kaiser Permanente. "Fast Facts about Kaiser Permanente." March 29, 2016. Accessed April 13, 2016. http://share.kaiserpermanente.org/article/fast-facts-about-kaiser-permanente/.

Kane, Carol. "Updated Data on Physician Practice Arrangements: Inching toward Hospital Ownership." American Medical Association, 2014.

Kane, Carol, and David Emmons. "New Data on Physician Practice Arrangements: Private Practice Remains Strong despite Shift toward Hospital Employment." American Medical Association, 2012.

Kane, Leslie, and Carol Peckham. *Medscape Physician Compensation Report, 2014.* April 15, 2014. http://www.medscape.com/features/slideshow/compensation/2014/public/overview.

Kassirer, Jerome. *On the Take: How Medicine's Complicity with Big Business Can Endanger Your Health*. New York: Oxford University Press, 2004.

Katz, Paul, and Jurgis Karuza. "Nursing Home Physician Specialists: A Response to the Workforce Crisis in Long-Term Care." *Journal of the American Medical Directors Association* 7, no. 6 (2006): 394–98.

Kaufman, Sharon. *Ordinary Medicine: Extraordinary Treatments, Longer Lives, and Where to Draw the Line*. Durham, NC: Duke University Press, 2015.

Kaye, Keith, Dror Marchaim, Ting-Yi Chen, et al. "Effect of Nosocomial Bloodstream Infections on Mortality, Length of Stay, and Hospital Costs in Older Adults." *Journal of the American Geriatrics Society* 62, no. 2 (2014): 306–11.

Kirchhoff, Suzanne. "Physician Practices: Background, Organization, and Market Consolidation." Congressional Research Service Report for Congress, January 2013.

Kitchener, Martin, Janis O'Meara, Ab Brody, Hyang Lee, and Charlene Harrington. "Shareholder Value and the Performance of a Large Nursing Home Chain." *Health Services Research* 43, no. 3 (2008): 1062–84.

Kizer, Kenneth, and R. Adams Dudley. "Extreme Makeover: Transformation of the Veterans Health Care System." *Annual Review of Public Health*, no. 30 (2009): 313–39.

Klevens, R. Monina, Jonathan Edwards, Chesley Richardson, et al. "Estimating Healthcare-Associated Infection in US Hospitals, 2002." *Public Health Reports* 122 (March–April 2007): 160–66.

Knatterud, Genell, Curtis Meinert, Christian Klimt, Robert Osborne, and Donald Martin. "Effects of Hypoglycemic Agents on Vascular Complications in Patients with Adult-Onset Diabetes." *Journal of the American Medical Association* 217, no. 6 (1971): 777–84.

Kohn, Linda, Janet Corrigan, and Molla Donaldson, eds. for Institute of Medicine. *To Err Is Human: Building a Safer Health System*. Washington, DC: National Academies Press, 1999.

Kolata, Gina. "Patients in Florida Lining Up for All that Medicare Covers." *New York Times*, September 13, 2003.

Kowalczyk, Liz. "Partners Hospitals, Doctors Top Health-Payment List." *Boston Globe*, August 14, 2013.

Kozak, Lola, Margaret Hall, and Maria Owings. "National Hospital Discharge Survey: 2000 Annual Survey with Detailed Diagnosis and Procedural Data." Vital and Health Statistics Series 13, No. 153. November 2002.

Krumholz, Harlan. "Post-Hospital Syndrome: An Acquired, Transient Condition of Generalized Risk." *New England Journal of Medicine* 368, no. 2 (2014): 100–102.

Kwok, Alvin, Marcus Semel, Stuart Lipsitz, et al. "The Intensity and Variation of Surgical Care at the End of Life: A Retrospective Cohort Study." *Lancet* 378, no. 9800 (2011): 1408–13.

Lam, Bourree. "Health-Care Mergers: Good for Health-Care Companies, Not So Good for Patients and Doctors." *Atlantic*, September 8, 2015.

Landefeld, C. Seth, Robert Palmer, Denise Kresevic, Richard Fortinsky, and Jerome Kowal. "A Trial of Care in a Hospital Medical Unit Especially Designed to Improve the Functional Outcomes of Acutely Ill Older Patients." *New England Journal of Medicine* 332, no. 20 (1995): 1338–44.

Lazar, Kay. "Complaints Follow Nursing Home Chain's Expansion." *Boston Globe,* May 5, 2015.

Leader, Shelah, and Marilyn Moon. "Medicare Trends in Ambulatory Surgery." *Health Affairs* 8, no. 1 (1989): 158–70.

Learmonth, Ian, Claire Young, and Cecil Rorabeck. "The Operation of the Century: Total Hip Replacement." *Lancet* 370, no. 9597 (2007): 1508–19.

Lee, Grace M., Ken Kleinman, Stephen B. Soumerai, Alison Tse, David Cole, Scott K. Fridkin, Teresa Horan, et al. "Effect of Nonpayment for Preventable Infections in U.S. Hospitals." *New England Journal of Medicine,* no. 367 (2012): 1428–37.

Lee, Thomas, Albert Bothe, and Glenn Steele. "How Geisinger Structures Its Physicians' Compensation to Support Improvements in Quality, Efficiency, and Volume." *Health Affairs* 31, no. 9 (2002): 2068–73.

Lenzer, Jeanne. "Majority of Panelists in Controversial New Cholesterol Guidelines Have Current or Recent Ties to Drug Manufacturers." *BMJ,* no. 347 (2013): f6989.

Levinson, Wendy, Pamela Hudab, and Andrea Tricco. "A Systematic Review of Surgeon-Patient Communication: Strengths and Opportunities for Improvement. *Patient Education and Counseling* 93, no. 1 (2013): 3–17.

Levinson, Wendy, and Philip Pizzo. "Physician Communications: It's about Time." *Journal of the American Medical Association* 305, no. 17 (2011): 1802–3.

Levy, Carl, Ron Fish, and Andrew Kramer. "Site of Death in the Hospital or Nursing Home of Medicare Skilled Nursing Facility Residents Admitted under Medicare Part A Benefit." *Journal of the American Geriatric Society* 52, no. 8 (2004): 1247–54.

Life Care Centers of America. "Mission and Values." Accessed January 4, 2015. https://lcca .com/mission/.

Lin, Grace, R. Adams Dudley, and Rita Redberg. "Cardiologists' Use of Percutaneous Intervention for Stable Coronary Artery Disease." *Archives of Internal Medicine* 167, no. 15 (2007): 1604–9.

LinkedIn. Profile for Walter Johnson. Accessed April 24, 2017. https://www.linkedin .com/in/walter-johnson-0566b015/.

Loftus, Peter. "For Doctors, Fewer Perks and Free Lunches." *Wall Street Journal,* April 12, 2013.

Loftus, Peter, and Joseph Walker. "Drug and Medical-Device Makers Paid $6.49 Billion to Doctors, Hospitals in 2014." *Wall Street Journal,* June 30, 2015.

Lopez, Ruth, Elaine Amelia, Neville Strumpf, Joan Teno, and Susan Mitchell. "The Influence of Nursing Home Culture on the Use of Feeding Tubes." *Archives of Internal Medicine* 170, no. 1 (2010): 83–88.

Lubitz, James, Linda Greenberg, Yelena Gorina, Lynne Wartzman, and David Gibson. "Three Decades of Health Care for the Elderly, 1965–1998." *Health Affairs* 20, no. 2 (2001): 19–32.

Ludmerer, Kenneth. *Let Me Heal: The Opportunity to Preserve Excellence in American Medicine.* New York: Oxford University Press, 2014.

———. *Time to Heal: American Medical Education from the Turn of the Century to the Era of Managed Care.* New York: Oxford University Press, 1989.

Lueck, Sarah. "In Nursing Homes, A Drug Middleman Finds Big Profits." *Wall Street Journal,* December 23, 2006.

Lundstrom, Marjie, and Phillip Reese. "California Falls Short in Disclosing Nursing-Home Ownership." *Sacramento Bee,* November 10, 2014.

———. "Unmasked: How California's Largest Nursing Home Chains Perform." *Sacramento Bee,* November 8, 2014.

———. "Unmasked: Who Owns California's Nursing Homes?" *Sacramento Bee,* November 9, 2014.

Lynn, Joanne. *MediCaring Communities: Getting What We Want and Need in Frail Old Age at an Affordable Cost."* Altarum Institute, 2016.

Maher, Robert, Joseph Hanlon, and Emily Hajjar. "Clinical Consequences of Polypharmacy in Elderly." *Expert Opinion on Drug Safety* 13, no. 1 (2014): 57–65.

Massachusetts Executive Office of Health and Human Services. "Regulations (2015)." Accessed December 11, 2015. http://www.mass.gov/eohhs/docs/dph/regs /105cms150.pdf.

Mattke, Soeren, Dan Han, Asa Wilks, and Elizabeth Sloss. "Medicare Home Visit Program Associated with Fewer Hospital and Nursing Home Admissions, Increased Office Visits." *Health Affairs* 34, no. 12 (2015): 2138–46.

May, Peter, Charles Norman, and R. Sean Morrison. "Economic Impact of Hospital Palliative Care Consultation: Review of Current Evidence and Directions for Future Research." *Journal of Palliative Medicine* 17, no. 90 (2014): 1054–63.

McCall, Nelda, Harriet Komisar, Andrew Peterson, and Stanley Moore. "Medicare Home Health Benefit Before and After the Balanced Budget Act." *Health Affairs* 20, no. 3 (2001): 189–98.

McCluskey, Priyanka. "Pay Continues to Rise for CEOs of Major Hospitals." *Boston Globe,* August 18, 2015.

McGee, Bill. "The Incredible Consolidating Travel Industry." *USA Today,* March 4, 2015.

McLaughlin, Jim. "Private Equity and Non-Profit Hospitals: Strange Bedfellows or Saving Grace?" *Becker's Hospital Review,* March 26, 2013.

McWilliams, J. Michael, Bruce Landon, Michael Chernew, and Alan Zaslavsky. "Change in Patients' Experience in Medicare Accountable Care Organizations." *New England Journal of Medicine* 371, no. 18 (2014): 1715–24.

MedPAC Report to the Congress. "Medical Education in the United States: Supporting Long-Term Delivery System Reforms." In *Improving Incentives in the Medicare Program,* chapter 1. Washington, DC, June 2009.

———. *Medicare Payment Policy.* Washington, DC, March 2013.

———. *Medicare Payment Policy.* Washington, DC, March 2015.

———. *Reforming the Delivery System.* Washington, DC, June 2008.

Meier, Barry. "Doctor Is Pressed Again on His Ties to Device Makers." *New York Times*, September 28, 2009.

Memorial Hospital. "Mission and Vision." Accessed June 21, 2016. http://memorial hospitaljax.com/about/mission-and-vision.dot.

Mendelson, Mary Adelaide. *Tender Loving Greed: How the Incredibly Lucrative Nursing Home "Industry" Is Exploiting America's Old People and Defrauding Us All.* New York: Knopf, 1974.

Meyer, Gregg, and Robert Gibbons. "Housecalls and the Elderly: A Vanishing Practice among Physicians." *New England Journal of Medicine* 337, no. 25 (1997): 1815–20.

Meyer, Harris. "Changing the Conversation in California about Care near the End of Life." *Health Affairs* 30, no. 3 (2011): 390–93.

———. "Group Health's Move to the Medical Home: For Doctors, It's Often a Hard Journey." *Health Affairs* 29, no. 5 (2010): 844–51.

Mezey, Mathy, Ethel Mitty, and Sarah Burger. "Rethinking Teaching Nursing Homes: Potential for Improving Long-Term Care." *Gerontologist* 48, no. 1 (2008): 8–15.

Miller, Gerald L., and Shari Miller Wagner. *Making the Rounds: Memoirs of a Small-Town Doctor.* Bradenton, FL: Booklocker.com, 2015.

Miller, Thomas. "Hospitalists in Community Hospitals." *American Society of Anesthesiologists* 78, no. 2 (2014): 10–13.

Millman, Jason. "Keeping Up with the Joneses, Hospital Edition." *Washington Post*, July 30, 2014.

Mitchell, Susan, Joan Buchanan, Steven Littlehale, and Mary Beth Hamel. "Tube-Feeding versus Hand-Feeding Nursing Home Residents with Advanced Dementia: A Cost Comparison." *Journal of the American Medical Directors Association* 4, no. 1 (2003): 27–33.

Mitchell, Susan, Dan Kiely, Lewis Lipsitz. "The Risk Factors and Impact on Survival of Feeding Tube Placement in Nursing Home Residents with Severe Cognitive Impairment." *Archives of Internal Medicine*, no. 157 (1997): 327–32.

Mitchell, Susan, Joan Teno, Dan Kiely, et al. "The Clinical Course of Advanced Dementia." *New England Journal of Medicine*, no. 361 (2009): 1529–38.

Mitchell, Susan, Joan Teno, Jason Roy, Glen Kabumoto, and Vincent Mor. "Clinical and Organizational Factors Associated with Feeding Tube Use among Nursing Home Residents with Advanced Cognitive Impairment." *Journal of the American Medical Association* 290, no. 1 (2003): 73–80.

Mizokami, Fumihiro, Yamiko Koide, Takeshi Noro, and Katsunori Furuta. "Polypharmacy with Common Diseases in Hospitalized Elderly Patients." *American Journal of Geriatric Pharmacotherapy* 10, no. 2 (2012): 123–28.

Monegain, Bernie. "Intermountain, Geisinger Share the Spotlight in Obama Talk." *HealthcareIT News*, June 12, 2009.

Mongan, Emily. "Kindred, RehabCare Settle False Claims Allegation for $125 Million." *McKnight's*, January 12, 2016.

Mor, Vincent, Orna Intrator, Zhanlian Feng, and David Grabowski. "The Revolving Door of Re-hospitalization for Skilled Nursing Facilities." *Health Affairs* 29, no. 1 (2010): 57–64.

Moriarty Leyendecker. "DePuy ASR Timeline." Accessed December 10, 2015. http://www
.moriarty.com/depuy_hip_recall/content/inline-images/depuy/depuy_asr
_timeline_110228.pdf.

Mother Jones. "How Banks Got Too Big to Fail." January/February 2010.

Nabel, Elizabeth, and Eugene Braunwald. "A Tale of Coronary Artery Disease and
Myocardial Infarction." *New England Journal of Medicine* 366, no. 1 (2012): 54–63.

Nascher, Ignatz. *Geriatrics: The Diseases of Old Age and Their Treatment.* Philadelphia:
P. B. Blakiston's Son and Co., 1916.

National Association of Long Term Care Administrator Boards. "Exam." Accessed
July 27, 2016. http://www.nabweb.org/nha-exam.

National Center for Health Statistics. *Health, United States, 2013: With Special Feature
on Prescription Drugs.* Hyattsville, MD, 2014.

———. *Health, United States, 2014: With Special Feature on Adults Aged 55–64.*
Hyattsville, MD, 2015.

———. "National Hospital Discharge Survey, 1965–1998." Advance Data No. 380,
July 12, 2007.

———. "National Hospital Discharge Survey: 2000 Annual Survey with Detailed
Diagnosis and Procedure Data." *Vital Health Statistics Series 13,* #153, 2002.

———. "Office Visits by Persons Age 65 and Over: National Ambulatory Medical
Care Survey, 1975." *AdvanceData* #22, 1978.

———. "Utilization of Short-Stay Hospitals: Summary of Non-Medical Statistics,
1967." *Vital and Health Statistics Series 13,* #9, 1972.

National Center for Quality Assurance. "The Future of Patient-Centered Medical
Homes." Accessed June 14, 2016. https://www.ncqa.org/Portals/0/Public%20
Policy/2014%20Comment%20Letters/The_Future_of_PCMH.pdf.

National Hospice and Palliative Care Organization. *NHPCO Facts and Figures.* 2015.

Neergaard, Lauran. "Doctor House Calls Can Save Money, Study Says." *Boston Globe,*
June 19, 2015.

Northeastern University, Bouvé College of Health Sciences. "Physician Assistant
Studies (MS) Overview." Accessed February 9, 2016. http://www.northeastern.edu
/bouve/physician-assistant/ms/.

Oberst, Jackie. "Dementia Care, Outpatient Therapy Popular Services. Top 50
Largest Nursing Facility Companies." *Provider,* June 2015, 45–49.

OECD. "OECD Health Statistics 2014: How Does the United States Compare?"
Accessed January 18, 2016. http://www.oecd.org/unitedstates/Briefing-Note
-UNITED-STATES-2014.pdf.

Office of the Inspector General. "Adverse Events in Skilled Nursing Facilities:
National Incidence among Medicare Beneficiaries." Department of Health and
Human Services: February 2014. https://oig.hhs.gov/oei/reports/oei-06-11
-00370.pdf.

Office of Inspector General. "The Medicare Payment System for Skilled Nursing
Facilities Needs to Be Reevaluated." Department of Health and Human Services:
September 2015. https://oig.hhs.gov/oei/reports/oei-02-13-00610.pdf.

Ornstein, Charles, Lena Groeger, Mike Tigas, and Ryann Jones. "Dollars for Docs: How Industry Dollars Reach Your Doctors." *Pro Publica*, March 17, 2016.

Osborn, Robin, Donald Moulds, David Squires, Michelle Doty, and Chloe Anderson. "International Survey Finds Shortcomings in Access, Coordination, and Patient-Centered Care." *Health Affairs* 33, no. 12 (2014): 2247–55.

Ouslander, Joseph, Gerri Lamb, Mary Perloe, et al. "Potentially Avoidable Hospitalizations of Nursing Home Residents: Frequency, Causes, and Costs." *Journal of the American Geriatrics Society* 58, no. 4 (2010): 627–35.

Ouslander, Joseph, and Robert Berenson. "Reducing Unnecessary Hospitalizations of Nursing Home Residents." *New England Journal of Medicine* 365, no. 13 (2011): 1165–67.

Ovbiagele, Bruce, Lee Schwamm, Eric Smith, et al. "Nationwide Trends in In-Hospital Mortality among Patients with Stroke." *Stroke* 4, no. 7 (2010): 1748–54.

Page, Leigh. "The Rise and Further Rise of Concierge Medicine." *BMJ*, no. 347 (October 28, 2013): f6465, doi: https://doi.org/10.1136/bmj.f6465.

Palo Alto Medical Foundation. "About Us: History." Accessed December 10, 2015. http://www.pamf.org/about/history/.

Papanikolaou, Panagiotis N., Georgia D. Christidi, and John P. A. Ioannidis. "Patient Outcomes with Teaching versus Nonteaching Healthcare: A Systematic Review." *PLoS Medicine*, September 12, 2006. http://dx.doi.org/10.1371/journal.pmed .0030341.

Paraprofessional Healthcare Institute (PHI). "Nurse Aide Training Requirements by State, 2016." Accessed July 6, 2015. http://phinational.org/policy/nurse_aide _training_requirements_state.

Park, Melissa, Donald Cherry, and Sandra Decker. "Nurse Practitioners, Certified Nurse Midwives, and Physician Assistants in Physician Offices." NCHS Data Brief #69, August 2011.

Patten, Eileen, and Richard Fry. "How Millennials Today Compare with Their Grandparents 50 Years Ago." Pew Research Center: A Social and Demographic Trends Report. March 19, 2015. http://www.pewresearch.org/fact-tank/2015/03/19 /how-millennials-compare-with-their-grandparents/.

Peckham, Carol. *Medscape Compensation Report, 2015*. Accessed July 13, 2016. http:/ /www.medscape.com/features/slideshow/compensation/2015/public /overview#page=1.

PerryUndem Research/Communication. "Survey of Adults 65 and Older." February 12, 2014. Accessed November 23, 2015. http://www.jhartfound.org /learning-center/wpcontent/uploads/2014/03/Topline_Results_Hartford_Med _Home_Poll.pdf.

Peterson, Lars, Steven Landers, and Andrew Bazemore. "Trends in Physician House Calls to Medicare Beneficiaries." *Journal of the American Board of Family Medicine* 25, no. 6 (2012): 862–68.

Pfuntner, Anne, Lauren Wier, and Carol Stocks. "Most Frequent Procedures Performed in US Hospitals, 2011." Healthcare Cost and Utilization Project

Statistical Brief #165, October 2013. https://www.hcup-us.ahrq.gov/reports /statbriefs/sb149.pdf.

The Physicians Foundation. *2014 Survey of America's Physicians: Practice Patterns and Perspectives*. Conducted by Merritt Hawkins, 2014. Accessed March 27, 2017. http://www.physiciansfoundation.org/uploads/default/2014_Physicians _Foundation_Biennial_Physician_Survey_Report.pdf.

Pioneer Network. Website. Accessed June 28, 2016. https://pioneernetwork.net/.

Plsek, Paul. "Complexity and the Adoption of Innovation in Health Care." Paper presented at Accelerating Quality Improvement in Health Care: Strategies to Speed the Diffusion of Evidence-Based Innovations, a conference, Washington, DC, January 2003.

Porter, Michael. "What Is Value in Health Care?" *New England Journal of Medicine* 363, no. 26 (2010): 2477–81.

Porter, Molly, and Meg Kellogg, "Kaiser Permanente: An Integrated Health Care Experience." *RISAI* 1, no. 1 (2008): 1–8.

Preston, Forrest. "Letter from the Chairman." *Life Care Leader, 2015 Edition*. http://lcca .com/images/publications/Leader-2015-Web.pdf. Page now defunct.

Provider Magazine. "Top 50 Largest Nursing Facility Companies." *Provider* 2014, 46–49.

Punke, Heather. "Hiring of Non-Physician Providers on the Rise." *Becker's Hospital Review*, November 2, 2012.

Rau, Jordan. "Medicare Fines 2,610 Hospitals in Third Round of Readmission Penalties." *Kaiser Health News*, October 2, 2014.

Redfoot, Donald L., and Sheel M. Pandya. *Before the Boom: Trends in Long-Term Supportive Services for Older Americans with Disabilities*. Washington, DC: AARP Public Policy Institute, 2002.

Reisman, Anna. "End of a Chapter." *Health Affairs* 29, no. 5 (2010): 1071–73.

Relman, Arnold. "The New Medical-Industrial Complex," *New England Journal of Medicine* 303, no. 17 (1980): 963–70.

Riley, Gerald, and James Lubitz. "Outcomes of Surgery among the Medicare Aged: Surgical Volume and Mortality." *Health Care Financing Review* 7, no. 1 (1985): 37–47.

Robinson, James. "Consolidation and the Transformation of Competition in Health Insurance." *Health Affairs* 23, no. 6 (2004): 11–24.

Rockoff, Jonathan. "As Doctors Lose Clout, Drug Firms Redirect the Sales Call." *Wall Street Journal*, September 10, 2014.

———. "Drug Reps Soften Their Sales Pitches." *Wall Street Journal*, January 10, 2012.

———. "Goodbye, Lipitor. Pfizer Bids a Farewell." *Wall Street Journal*, May 9, 2012.

———. "Helping Lipitor Live Longer." *Wall Street Journal*, November 22, 2011.

Rockoff, Jonathan, and Dionne Searcey. "Hip Joints Set Off New Rush to Court." *Wall Street Journal*, July 8, 2011.

Rodak, Sabina. "Structuring Hospital Service Line Management for Success." *Becker's Hospital Review*, June 14, 2012.

Rogers, Everett M. *Diffusion of Innovations*. 5th ed. New York: Free Press, 2003.

Rothberg, Michael B. "Coronary Artery Disease as Clogged Pipes: A Misconceptual Model." *Circulation: Cardiovascular Quality Outcomes* 6, no. 1 (2013): 129–32.

Rubenstein, Laurence, Karen Josephson, G. Darryl Wieland, et al. "Effectiveness of a Geriatric Evaluation Unit: A Randomized Clinical Trial." *New England Journal of Medicine* 311, no. 26 (1984): 1664–70.

Russo, C. Allison, and Anne Elixhauser. "Hospitalizations in the Elderly Population, 2003." Healthcare Cost and Utilization Project, Statistical Brief #6, May 2006.

Ryan, Andrew, Brahmajee Nallamothu, and Justin Dimick. "Medicare's Public Reports Initiative on Hospital Quality Had Modest or No Impact on Mortality in Three Conditions." *Health Affairs* 31, no. 3 (2012): 585–92.

Samuels, Alana. "Building Better Nursing Homes." *The Atlantic*, April 21, 2015.

Sandler, Michael. "CEO Pay Soars at Top Not-for-Profits." *Modern Healthcare*, August 8, 2015.

Schenker, Lisa. "Suit Alleges Abbott Supplier Omnicare Involved in Illegal Kickback Scheme." *Modern Healthcare*, December 22, 2014.

Schimmel, Elihu. "The Hazards of Hospitalization." *Annals of Internal Medicine* 60, no. 1 (1964): 100–110.

Schneider, Edward, Marcia Ory, and Maybelle Aung. "Teaching Nursing Homes Revisited." *Journal of the American Medical Association* 257, no. 20 (1987): 2725–55.

Schulte, Fred, and David Donald. "Cracking the Codes: How Doctors and Hospitals Have Collected Billions in Questionable Medicare Fees." Center for Public Integrity. September 15, 2012. Updated May 19, 2014. https://cloudfront-files-1 .publicintegrity.org/documents/pdfs/CPI%20Cracking%20the%20Codes.pdf.

Shaughnessy, Peter, Andrew Kramer, David Hittle, and John Steiner. "Quality of Care in Teaching Nursing Homes: Findings and Implications." *Health Care Financing Review* 16, no. 4 (1995): 55–83.

SHEP Cooperative Research Group. "Prevention of Stroke by Antihypertensive Drug Treatment in Older Persons with Isolated Systolic Hypertension. Final Results of the Systolic Hypertension in the Elderly Program (SHEP)." *Journal of the American Medical Association* 265, no. 24 (1991): 3255–64.

Shier, Victoria, Dmitry Khodyakov, Lauren Cohen, Sheryl Zimmerman, and Debra Saliba. "What Does the Evidence Really Say about Culture Change in Nursing Homes?" *Gerontologist* 54, no. S1 (2014): S6–S16.

Silverman, Ed. "Drug Makers Are Targeting Patients in Physician Offices More than Ever." *Wall Street Journal*, December 4, 2014.

Singer, Natasha. "Merck to Buy Schering-Plough for $41.1 Billion." *New York Times*, March 9, 2009.

Sinsky, Christine, and David Dugdale. "Medicare Payment for Cognitive vs Procedural Care: Minding the Gap." *JAMA Internal Medicine* 173, no. 18 (2013): 1733–37.

Sirovich, Brenda, Patricia Gallagher, David Wennberg, and Elliott Fisher. "Discretionary Decision Making by Primary Care Physicians and the Cost of U.S. Health Care." *Health Affairs* 27, no. 3 (2008): 813–23.

Smith-Bindman, Rebecca, Diana Miglioretti, and Eric Larson. "Rising Use of Diagnostic Medical Imaging in a Large Integrated Health System." *Health Affairs* 27, no. 6 (2008): 1491–1502.

Social Security Act, SEC. 1862. 42 U.S.C. 1395y.

Social Service Department of the Massachusetts General Hospital. "Patient Care in Nursing Homes." *Journal of the American Medical Association* 200, no. 2 (1967): 154–57.

Sorkin, Aaron. "Pfizer Said to Buy Large Drug Rival in $60 Billion Deal." *New York Times*, July 15, 2010.

Sorkin, Aaron, and Melody Peterson. "Glaxo and SmithKline Agree to Form Largest Drug Maker." *New York Times*, January 17, 2000.

Sorkin, Aaron, and Duff Wilson. "Pfizer Agrees to Pay $68 Billion for Rival Drug Maker Wyeth." *New York Times*, January 25, 2009.

South, Todd. "Judge Scolds Prosecutors in Whistle-Blower Medicare Fraud Investigation." *Chattanooga Times Free Press*, December 3, 2012.

Staats, Chere. "On the Case: Clues to Hospital Selling." *PharmExec.com*, July 1, 2003.

Staessen, Jan, Robert Fagard, Lugarde Thijs, et al. "Randomised Double-Blind Comparison of Placebo with Active Treatment for Older Patients with Isolated Systolic Hypertension: The Systolic Hypertension in Europe (Syst-Eur) Trial Investigators." *Lancet* 350, no. 9080 (1997): 757–64.

State Budget Crisis Task Force. "Report, July 31, 2012." Accessed July 6, 2015. https://www .minnpost.com/sites/default/files/attachments/Report-of-the-State-Budget -Crisis-Task-Force-Full.pdf.

Statista. "Density of Magnetic Resonance Imaging Units by Country." Accessed July 17, 2016. http://www.statista.com/statistics/282401/density-of-magnetic -resonance-imaging-units-by-country/.

Steiner, Claudia, Marguerite Barrett, Audrey Weiss, and Roxanne Andrews. "Trends and Projections in Hospital Stays for Adults with Multiple Chronic Conditions, 2003–2014." HCUP Statistical Brief #183, November 2014.

Stevenson, David, and David Grabowski. "Private Equity Investment and Nursing Home Care: Is It a Big Deal?" *Health Affairs* 27, no. 5 (2008): 1399–1408.

———. "Sizing Up the Market for Assisted Living." *Health Affairs* 29, no. 1 (2010): 35–43.

Stone, Robyn, Susan Reinhard, Barbara Bowers, et al. "Evaluation of the Wellspring Model for Improving Nursing Home Quality." New York: Commonwealth Fund, 2002.

SUPPORT Principal Investigators. "A Controlled Trial to Improve Care for Seriously Ill Hospitalized Patients: The Study to Understand Prognoses and Preferences for Outcomes and Risks of Treatments (SUPPORT)." *Journal of the American Medical Association* 274, no. 20 (1995): 1591–98.

Sutter Health, Palo Alto Medical Foundation. "Find the Doctor Who Is Right for You." Accessed January 18, 2016. http://www.pamf.org/providersearch/?sitecfg=41.

Temel, Jennifer S., Joseph A. Greer, Alona Muzikansky, et al. "Early Palliative Care for Patients with Metastatic Non–Small-Cell Lung Cancer." *New England Journal of Medicine* 363, no. 8 (2010): 733–42.

Teno, Joan, Pedro Gozalo, Julie Bynum, et al. "Change in End-of-Life Care for Medicare Beneficiaries: Site of Death, Place of Care, and Health Care Transitions in 2000." *Journal of the American Medical Association* 309, no. 5 (2013): 470–77.

Terry, Ken, Alison Ritchie, Donna Marbury, Lisa Smith, and Elaine Pofeldt. "Top 15 Challenges Facing Physicians in 2015." *Modern Medicine*, December 1, 2014.

Thomas, Katie. "Chain to Pay $38 Million over Claims of Poor Care." *New York Times*, October 10, 2014.

———. "In Race for Medicare Dollars, Nursing Home Care May Lag." *New York Times*, April 14, 2015.

———. "J&J to Pay $2.2 Billion in Risperdal Settlement." *New York Times*, November 4, 2013.

———. "$650 Million to Settle Blood Thinner Lawsuits." *New York Times*, May 28, 2014.

Tomes, Nancy. *Remaking the American Patient: How Madison Avenue and Modern Medicine Turned Patients into Consumers.* Chapel Hill: University of North Carolina Press, 2016.

Trust for America's Health. *The State of Obesity, 2014.* Robert Wood Johnson Foundation. Accessed December 24, 2015. http://www.rwjf.org/content/dam /farm/reports/reports/2014/rwjf414829.

Tschirhart, Evan, Qingling Du, and Amy Kelley. "Factors Influencing the Use of Intensive Procedures at the End of Life." *Journal of the American Geriatrics Society* 62, no. 11 (2014): 2088–94.

Tumlinson, Anne. "Physician Relationships Hold Key to SNF Success." *McKnight's*, January 22, 2014.

UK Prospective Diabetes Study Group. "Intensive Blood-Glucose Control with Sulphonylureas or Insulin Compared with Conventional Treatment and Risk of Complications in Patients with Type 2 Diabetes." *Lancet* 352, no. 9131 (1998): 837–53.

Unwin, Brian, and Paul Tatum. "House Calls." *American Family Physician* 83, no. 8 (2011): 925–38.

U.S. Department of Health, Education, and Welfare. "Arrangements for Physician Services to Residents of Nursing and Personal Care Homes. United States: May–June, 1964." National Center for Health Statistics Series 12, #13. February 1970.

———. "Characteristics of Residents in Institutions for the Aged and Chronically Ill. United States: April–June, 1963." National Center for Health Statistics Series 12, #2. September 1965.

———. "Chronic Illness among Residents of Nursing and Personal Care Homes. United States: May–June, 1964." PHS Publication No. 1000, Series 12, #7. March 1967.

———. "Institutions for the Aged and Chronically Ill. United States: April– June 1963." PHS Publication No. 1000, Series 12, #1. July 1965.

———. "Nursing and Personal Care Services Received by Residents of Personal Care Homes. United States: May–June, 1964." National Center for Health Statistics Series 12, #10. September 1968.

———. "Prevalence of Chronic Conditions and Impairments among Residents of Nursing Homes and Personal Care Homes. United States: May–June, 1964." National Center for Health Statistics Series 12, #8. July 1967.

———. "Volume of Physician Visits. United States—July 1966–June 1967, Data from the National Health Survey." Series 10, #49, November 1968.

U.S. Department of Health, Education, and Welfare, National Center for Health Statistics. "National Health Survey. Utilization of Short-Stay Hospitals, Summary of Nonmedical Statistics. United States—1967." Publication #72-1058, May 1972.

U.S. Department of Health and Human Services. "Characteristics of Office-Based Physicians and Their Practices." Vital and Health Statistics 2008, Series 13, #166.

———. "NIH Budget Overview (2016)." Accessed June 29, 2016. http://www.hhs .gov/about/budget/budget-in-brief/nih/index.html.

———. "Trends in Hospital Utilization: United States, 1965–86." Vital and Health Statistics, Series 13: Data from the National Health Survey, #101.

U.S. Department of Health and Human Services, Administration on Aging. "A Profile of Older Americans, 2014." https://aoa.acl.gov/aging_statistics/profile/2014/docs /2014-profile.pdf.

U.S. Department of Health and Human Services, CDC. *Health, United States, 2010. With Special Section on Death and Dying*. https://www.cdc.gov/nchs/data/hus /hus10.pdf.

U.S. Department of Health and Human Services, CDC, NCHS. *Health, United States, 2009. With Special Feature on Medical Technology*. https://www.cdc.gov/nchs/data /hus/hus09.pdf.

U.S. News and World Report. "Hospital Score Card (Memorial Hospital)." http://health .usnews.com/best-hospitals/area/fl/memorial-hospital-6390409.

Ventola, C. Lee. "Direct-to-Consumer Pharmaceutical Advertising: Therapeutic or Toxic?" *Pharmacy and Therapeutics* 36, no. 10 (2011): 669–74.

Wachter, Robert, and Lee Goldman. "The Emerging Role of 'Hospitalists' in the American Health Care System." *New England Journal of Medicine* 335, no. 7 (1996): 514–17.

———. "The Hospitalist Movement Five Years Later." *Journal of the American Medical Association* 287, no. 4 (2002): 483–94.

Walker, Joseph. "CVS to Buy Drug Providers for $10.4 Billion." *Wall Street Journal*, May 21, 2015.

Wall Street Journal Roundup. "Eli Lilly Agrees to Settle Zyprexa Marketing Cases." *Wall Street Journal*, January 15, 2009.

Weaver, Christopher, Anna Mathews, and Tom McGinty. "How Medicare Rewards Copious Nursing Home Therapy." *Wall Street Journal*, August 16, 2015.

Weiner, Joshua, Marc Freiman, and David Brown. "Nursing Home Quality: Twenty-Five Years after the Omnibus Budget Reconciliation Act of 1987." Kaiser Family Foundation, December 2007.

Weisman, Robert. "Steward Reshapes Mass. Health Care Business." *Boston Globe*, February 3, 2013.

Weiss, Audrey, and Anne Elixhauser, "Overview of Hospital Stays in the United States, 2012." HCUP Statistical Brief #180, October 2014.

Weiss, Rick. "A Tale of Politics: PET Scans' Change in Medicare Coverage." *Washington Post*, October 14, 2004.

Welch, W. Pete, Sally Stearns, Alison Cuellar, and Andrew Bindman. "Use of Hospitalists by Medicare Beneficiaries: A National Picture." *Medicare and Medicaid Research Review* 4, no. 2 (2014): E1–E8.

Wenger, Neil, David Solomon, Carol Roth, et al. "The Quality of Medical Care Provided to Vulnerable Community-Dwelling Older Patients." *Annals of Internal Medicine*, no. 139 (2003): 740–47.

Wennberg, John, Elliot Fisher, Therese Stukel, et al. "Use of Hospitals, Physician Visits, and Hospice Care during Last Six Months of Life among Cohorts Loyal to Highly Respected Hospitals in the United States." *BMJ* 328, no. 7440 (2004): 607.

Wennberg, John, and Alan Gittelsohn. "Small Area Variation in Health Care Delivery." *Science* 182, no. 4117 (1973): 1102–8.

West, Colin, and Denise Dupras. "General Medicine vs. Subspecialty Career Plans among Internal Medicine Residents." *Journal of the American Medical Association* 308, no. 21 (2012): 2241–47.

White, Heather, and Richard Glazier. "Do Hospitalist Physicians Improve the Quality of Inpatient Care Delivery? A Systematic Review of Process, Efficiency, and Outcome Measures." *BMC Medicine*, no. 9 (2011): 58.

Wier, Lauren, Anne Pfuntner, and Claudia Steiner. "Hospital Utilization among Older Adults." HCUP Statistical Brief #103, December 2010.

Witlox, Joost, Lisa Eurelings, Jos de Jonghe, et al. "Delirium in Elderly Patients and the Risk of Post-Discharge Mortality, Institutionalization, and Dementia: A Meta-Analysis." *Journal of the American Medical Association* 304, no. 4 (2010): 443–51.

Woolhandler, Steffie, and David U. Himmelstein. "Administrative Work Consumes One-Sixth of U.S. Physicians' Working Hours and Lowers Their Career Satisfaction." *International Journal of Health Services* 44, no. 4 (2014): 635–42.

Yahoo Finance. "Press Ganey Holdings: Profile." Accessed February 4, 2016. http://finance.yahoo.com/q/pr?s=PGND+Profile.

Yarbrough, Peter, Polina Kukhareva, Devin Horton, Karli Edholm, and Kensaku Kawamoto. "Multifaceted Intervention Including Education, Rounding Checklist Implementation, Cost Feedback, and Financial Incentives Reduces Inpatient Laboratory Costs." *Journal of Hospital Medicine* 11, no. 5 (2016). doi:10.1002/jhm.2552.

Young, Aaron, Humayun Chaudhry, Xiaomei Pei, et al. "A Census of Actively Licensed Physicians in the United States, 2014." *Journal of Medical Regulation* 101, no. 2 (2015): 8–23.

Yu, James, Pamela Soulos, Jeph Herrin, et al. "Proton versus Intensity-Modulated Radiotherapy for Prostate Cancer: Pattern of Care and Early Toxicity." *Journal of the National Cancer Institute* 105, no. 1 (2013): 25–32.

Zgierska, Aleksandra, David Rabago, and Michael Miller. "Impact of Patient Satisfaction Ratings on Physician and Clinical Care." *Patient Preference Adherence*, no. 8 (2014): 437–46.

Index

Studies in Social Medicine

Nancy M. P. King, Gail E. Henderson, and Jane Stein, eds., *Beyond Regulations: Ethics in Human Subjects Research* (1999).

Laurie Zoloth, *Health Care and the Ethics of Encounter: A Jewish Discussion of Social Justice* (1999).

Susan M. Reverby, ed., *Tuskegee's Truths: Rethinking the Tuskegee Syphilis Study* (2000).

Beatrix Hoffman, *The Wages of Sickness: The Politics of Health Insurance in Progressive America* (2000).

Margarete Sandelowski, *Devices and Desires: Gender, Technology, and American Nursing* (2000).

Keith Wailoo, *Dying in the City of the Blues: Sickle Cell Anemia and the Politics of Race and Health* (2001).

Judith Andre, *Bioethics as Practice* (2002).

Chris Feudtner, *Bittersweet: Diabetes, Insulin, and the Transformation of Illness* (2003).

Ann Folwell Stanford, *Bodies in a Broken World: Women Novelists of Color and the Politics of Medicine* (2003).

Lawrence O. Gostin, *The AIDS Pandemic: Complacency, Injustice, and Unfulfilled Expectations* (2004).

Arthur A. Daemmrich, *Pharmacopolitics: Drug Regulation in the United States and Germany* (2004).

Carl Elliott and Tod Chambers, eds., *Prozac as a Way of Life* (2004).

Steven M. Stowe, *Doctoring the South: Southern Physicians and Everyday Medicine in the Mid-Nineteenth Century* (2004).

Arleen Marcia Tuchman, *Science Has No Sex: The Life of Marie Zakrzewska, M.D.* (2006).

Michael H. Cohen, *Healing at the Borderland of Medicine and Religion* (2006).

Keith Wailoo, Julie Livingston, and Peter Guarnaccia, eds., *A Death Retold: Jesica Santillan, the Bungled Transplant, and Paradoxes of Medical Citizenship* (2006).

Michelle T. Moran, *Colonizing Leprosy: Imperialism and the Politics of Public Health in the United States* (2007).

Karey Harwood, *The Infertility Treadmill: Feminist Ethics, Personal Choice, and the Use of Reproductive Technologies* (2007).

Carla Bittel, *Mary Putnam Jacobi and the Politics of Medicine in Nineteenth-Century America* (2009).

Samuel Kelton Roberts Jr., *Infectious Fear: Politics, Disease, and the Health Effects of Segregation* (2009).

Lois Shepherd, *If That Ever Happens to Me: Making Life and Death Decisions after Terri Schiavo* (2009).

Mical Raz, *What's Wrong with the Poor? Psychiatry, Race, and the War on Poverty* (2013).

Johanna Schoen, *Abortion after Roe* (2015).

Nancy Tomes, *Remaking the American Patient: How Madison Avenue and Modern Medicine Turned Patients into Consumers* (2016).

Mara Buchbinder, Michele Rivkin-Fish, and Rebecca L. Walker, eds., *Understanding Health Inequalities and Justice: New Conversations across the Disciplines* (2016).

Muriel R. Gillick, *Old and Sick in America: The Journey through the Health Care System* (2017).